HYPERTENSION IN DIABETES

HYPERTENSION IN DIABETES

Edited by

Bryan Williams BSC MD FRCP
Professor of Medicine and Director
Cardiovascular Research Institute
University of Leicester
Leicester
UK

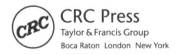

CRC Press
Taylor & Francis Group
Boca Raton London New York

CRC Press is an imprint of the
Taylor & Francis Group, an **informa** business

CRC Press
Taylor & Francis Group
6000 Broken Sound Parkway NW, Suite 300
Boca Raton, FL 33487-2742

© 2003 by Taylor & Francis Group, LLC
CRC Press is an imprint of Taylor & Francis Group, an Informa business

No claim to original U.S. Government works

Visit the Taylor & Francis Web site at
http://www.taylorandfrancis.com

and the CRC Press Web site at
http://www.crcpress.com

Contents

Contributors

George L Bakris MD
Rush Presbterian/St. Luke's Medical Center
1700 W. Van Buren, Suite 470
Chicago, IL 60612
USA

Suhkbinder Bassi
Clinical Research Fellow
Department of Medicine
University of Leicester School of Medicine
Leicester
UK

D John Betteridge BSc PhD MD FRCP FAHA
Professor of Endocrinology and Metabolism
Department of Medicine
Royal Free and University College Medical
School
University College London
London
UK

Mark E Cooper MB BS PhD FRACP
Professor of Medicine
Director of Division of Diabetic Complications
Baker Medical Research Institute
PO Box 6492
Melbourne, Vic 8008
Australia

Paul M Dodson MD FRCP FRCOphth
Department of Diabetes and Endocrinology
Birmingham Heartlands Hospital
Birmingham B9 5SS
UK

Richard E Gilbert MB PhD
Associate Professor
Department of Medicine
University of Melbourne
Austin and Repatriation Medical Centre
(Austin Campus)
Heidelberg, Vic 3084
Australia

Joanna C Girling MD
West Middlesex University Hospital
Isleworth
Middlesex TW7 6AF
UK

Aidan Halligan MD
Professor of Fetal Maternal Medicine
Department of Obstetrics and Gynecology
University of Leicester
Leicester LE2 7LX
UK

William B Kannel MD
Department of Preventive Medicine and
Epidemiology
Evans Department of Clinical Research
Boston University School of Medicine and
Framingham Heart Study
Framingham, MA 01701
USA

Eva Kohner
Professor, Division of Medicine
Department of Endocrinology
4th Floor, North Wing
St. Thomas' Hospital
Lambeth Palace Road
London SE1 7EH
UK

King Sun Leong
The University of Melbourne
Parkville, Victoria 3052
Australia

R Nithiyananthan MRCP
Undergraduate Centre
Birmingham Heartlands Hospital
Birmingham B9 5SS
UK

David O'Brien
Clinical Research Fellow
Department of Medicine
University of Leicester School of Medicine
Leicester
UK

Vinod Patel BSc MD MRCP MRCGP DRCOG
Consultant Physician
Diabetes & Endocrinology
George Eliot Hospital and
Honorary Senior Lecturer in Medicine
University of Warwick
UK

Gerald M Reaven MD
Professor of Medicine (Active Emeritus)
Stanford University School of Medicine and
Senior Vice President, Research
Shaman Pharmaceuticals
San Francisco, CA 94080-4812
USA

Andrew H Shennan MD
Consultant Obstetrician and Senior Lecturer
in Obstetric, Maternal and Foetal Medicine
St Thomas's Hospital
Lambeth Palace Road
London SE1 7EH
UK

Angela C Shore PhD BSc
Director of Biomedical and Clinical Science
Professor of Vascular Physiology
Institute of Biomedical and Clinical Science
Peninsula Medical School
Barrack Road
Exeter EX2 5AX
UK

Stephen M Thomas MCRP
Consultant Physician and Senior Lecturer
Diabetes Centre
King's College Hospital
Denmark Hill
London SE5 9RS
UK

Adam D Timmis MA MD FRCP
Department of Cardiology
Barts London NHS Trust
London
UK

John E Tooke MA MSc DM DSc (Oxon) FRCP FMedSci
Dean, Peninsula Medical School
ITTC Building
Tamar Science Park
Davy Road
Plymouth PL6 8BX
UK

Giancolo F Viberti MD FRCP
Professor of Diabetes and Metabolic Medicine
Department of Diabetes and Endocrinology
GKT School of Medicine, King's College
London
5th Floor Thomas Guy House
KCL Guy's Hospital
London SE1 9RT
UK

Philip Weston MD
Consultant Endocrinologist
The Royal Liverpool University Hospitals
Prescot Street
Liverpool L7 8XP
UK

Bryan Williams BSc MD FRCP
Professor of Medicine and Director
Cardiovascular Research Institute
Faculty of Medicine and Biological Sciences
University of Leicester
Leicester LE2 7LX
UK

Peter WF Wilson MD
Department of Preventive Medicine and
Epidemiology
Evans Department of Clinical Research
Boston University School of Medicine and
Framingham Heart Study
Framingham, MA 01701
USA

For
Sue, Tom and Amy

Preface

The interest in hypertension in diabetes cuts across many specialist disciplines beyond diabetology, including; cardiology, renal medicine, general medicine and therapeutics, among others. As such, much of the information about the epidemiology, pathophysiology, clinical consequences and impact of treatment of hypertension is scattered across many published works. The aim of this book was to bring this information together in a single authoritative and comprehensive compendium.

This has been a greater challenge than I originally envisaged, not least of all because there has recently been an explosion of interest in hypertension in diabetes, fuelled by the emergence of compelling data on the efficacy of antihypertensive therapy in people with diabetes. This challenge has been admirably met by the international panel of authors who agreed to contribute to this book. Their contributions are outstanding. Faced with a constant stream of new data as the manuscripts for the various chapters flowed in, I have had the formidable task of maintaining their high standards in updating their contributions, where necessary, to reflect the emergence of new data and to ensure that upon publication, this book is at the leading edge of current knowledge in this field. In so doing, I acknowledge that the wisdom is theirs and the

mistakes are mine! Needless to say, this book does not provide all of the answers to the clinical challenges faced by those treating hypertension in diabetes but I hope it does provide a solid foundation from which to move forward and tackle one of the most important risk factors for premature morbidity and mortality in people with diabetes. The very fact that there is a need for such a book at all reflects how far this area of medicine has moved in the past 10 years. There is much further to go.

I gratefully acknowledge the support of my fellow authors in producing this book, many of whom have remained friends throughout the process! I also acknowledge the patience of the publishers and in particular Alan Burgess, who commissioned the book, and Clive Lawson, whose editorial skills have helped make it happen. Finally, only those who have edited a multi-author medical textbook will recognize the enormity of the sacrifice of time required to complete a project such as this. That sacrifice has inevitably been borne by my wife, Sue, and children, Tom and Amy. Their support, understanding and forbearance are always an inspiration to me and a debt I can never repay. I dedicate this book to them.

Bryan Williams
Leicester, UK

Introduction: Diabetes is a cardiovascular disease

Bryan Williams

"It is often what we think we know already that prevents us from learning"
  Claude Bernard, 1878

Diabetes mellitus is traditionally defined as an endocrine disorder on the basis of impaired insulin production and/or action and is arbitrarily defined clinically as a consequence of the resulting glucose intolerance. This has led to the assumption that elevated circulating glucose concentrations *per se* are the prime cause of the excess morbidity and mortality associated with this common condition. There is much epidemiological data to support this hypothesis and recent studies have shown that glycosylated HbA1c is a powerful risk marker for cardiovascular disease, even when HbA1c levels are considered well into the conventional normal range.[1] However, epidemiology prompts hypotheses, it does not confirm a causal relationship. Nor does it confirm that therapeutic interventions designed to modify the risk marker will necessarily reduce the risk attributed to it. Nevertheless, until recently, it has been assumed that the prime driver of enhanced risk in people with diabetes is hyperglycaemia and consequently, for years, considerable clinical and financial resources have been directed towards the monitoring and correction of hyperglycaemia in type 1 and type 2 diabetic subjects. There is no doubt that this has been important with regard to microvascular protection, but alone it has been insufficient.

There are various ways of classifying a clinical disease process. One alternative, and perhaps more pragmatic approach to disease classification, is to consider its clinical impact both in terms of the pathological consequence of the disease and ultimately its effect on morbidity and mortality. From a pathological perspective, diabetes is readily classifiable as *a cardiovascular disease*. In diabetic patients, macrovascular disease (coronary heart disease, congestive cardiac failure, stroke and peripheral vascular disease) and microvascular disease (retinopathy, nephropathy and neuropathy), each by definition, have a primary or major vascular component and account for all of the well recognized complications of diabetes. Moreover, with regard to "clinical impact", diabetes is easy to classify as a cardiovascular disease. The major cause of premature morbidity and mortality in diabetic patients is cardiovascular disease.[2]

My third aspect of disease classification moves beyond the aforementioned epidemiological and pathophysiological associations and considers therapeutic manoeuvres that have been shown to prevent the morbidity and mortality associated with the disease process in prospective randomized controlled trials. With this criterion in mind, it is even more difficult to classify diabetes as anything other than a cardiovascular disease. Macrovascular complications are more than twice as common as microvascular disease in type 2 diabetes and are the major cause of mortality. In the United Kingdom Prospective Diabetes Study (UKPDS), more intensive glycaemic control had no significant impact on the mortality of type 2 diabetic patients, primarily because it had a disappointing impact on the development of macrovascular disease or its consequences.[3]

In stark contrast, the impact of more intensive treatment of hypertension has markedly and significantly reduced the rate of stroke, congestive cardiac failure, cardiovascular mortality and total mortality in a series of clinical trials.[4–16] This is important because it emphasizes that the treatment of an acknowledged cardiovascular disease risk factor, i.e. hypertension, improves the prognosis of people with diabetes, thereby supporting the classification of diabetes as a cardiovascular disease. Consistent with this view, therapeutic intervention directed at another major cardiovascular risk factor, notably LDL-cholesterol, notably with HMG-CoA inhibitors (statins), has also been shown to be remarkably effective at reducing heart disease and stroke and reducing mortality in people with diabetes.[17–20]

Mindful of these observations it is worth considering whether there is any clinical justification for considering diabetes as anything other than an accelerated cardiovascular disease, due to an aggregation of established cardiovascular risk factors. This key issue was addressed in another report from the UKPDS investigators who examined which cardiovascular risk factors predicted the development of clinically evident coronary artery disease in people with type 2 diabetes.[21] For those who have long-awaited the identification of a potent and unique "diabetes-specific factor", the results were disappointing. For those familiar with the management of a cardiovascular disease, there were no surprises. The UKPDS analysis revealed that a well recognized quintet of cardiovascular risk factors accounted for much of the excess risk of coronary heart disease in diabetic subjects, notably; high LDL-cholesterol and triglycerides, low HDL-cholesterol, hypertension, smoking and an increased HbA1c level.[21]

It would be too simplistic to conclude that people with diabetes are no different from any other population at high cardiovascular risk by virtue of a clustering of similar cardiovascular risk factors. Clearly, the risk factors themselves are more potent in diabetes as a consequence of their aggregation and modification by the diabetic milieu. For example, diabetic subjects are more vulnerable to hypertensive injury via a variety of mechanisms[22] and the lipid fractions are qualitatively and quantitatively disturbed in diabetes.[23] Both processes increase the potency of these important cardiovascular risk factors. Nevertheless, from a practical perspective, the principles guiding the monitoring and clinical management of these risk factors should be no different in diabetic subjects than those advocated for the general population. It is surely illogical that two patients with the same cardiovascular disease risk and the same likely cause of death, should be managed via two completely different care structures, with radically different priorities and resource allocation, by virtue of an arbitrary threshold defining glucose intolerance. The modern management of patients with diabetes must be re-focussed towards treatments that have been shown to prevent complications and save lives. These are primarily cardiovascular risk factor interventions.

In summary, diabetes is a cardiovascular disease by virtue of its predominant pathological complications, the aetiological factors contributing to the major causes of morbidity and mortality, and the major interventions proven to improve morbidity and mortality. Glycaemic control is, of course, important for microvascular protection but none more so than the other interventions, directed at traditional cardiovascular risk factors such as hypertension and LDL-cholesterol. Interventions, which if appropriately resourced and implemented, will also save lives. We learn and live.

References

1. Khaw KT, Wareham N, Luben R, et al. Glycated haemoglobin, diabetes, and mortality in men in Norfolk cohort of european prospective investigation of cancer and nutrition (EPIC-Norfolk). *BMJ* 2001; **322**: 15–18.
2. Garcia MJ, McNamara PM, Gordon T, Kannell WB. Morbidity and mortality in diabetics in the Framingham population. Sixteen year follow-up. *Diabetes* 1974; **23**: 105–11.
3. United Kingdom Prospective Diabetes Study group: Intensive blood glucose control with sulphonylureas or insulin compared with conventional treatment and risk of complications in patients with type 2 diabetes: UKPDS 33. *Lancet* 1998; **352**: 837–53.
4. Davis BR, Langford HG, Blaufox MD, et al. The association of postural changes in systolic blood pressure and mortality in persons with hypertension: The Hypertension Detection and Follow-up Programme (HDFP) experience. *Circulation* 1987; **75**: 340–46.
5. Curb JD, Pressel SL, Cutler JA, et al. Effect of diuretic based antihypertensive treatment on cardiovascular risk in people with diabetes. Systolic Hypertension in Elderly Program (SHEP) Cooperative research group. *JAMA* 1996; **276**: 1886–92.
6. United Kingdom Prospective Diabetes Study Group: Tight blood pressure control and risk of macrovascular and microvascular complications in type 2 diabetes: UKPDS 38. *BMJ* 1998; **317**: 703–13.
7. Hansson L, Zanchetti A, Carruthers SG, et al. Effects of intensive blood pressure lowering and low dose aspirin in patients with hypertension: principle results of the Hypertension Optimal Treatment (HOT) randomised trial. *Lancet* 1998; **351**: 1755–62.
8. Tuomilehto J, Rastenyte D, Birkenhager WH, et al. Effects of calcium channel blockade in older patients with diabetes and systolic hypertension. Systolic Hypertension in Europe Trial Investigators. *N Eng J Med* 1999; **340**: 677–84.
9. Estacio RO, Jeffers BW, Gifford N, Schrier RW. Effect of blood pressure control on diabetic microvascular complications in patients with hypertension and type 2 diabetes. *Diabetes Care* 2000; **23** (Suppl 2): B54–B64.
10. Schrier RW, Estacio RO, Esler A, Mehler P. The Heart Outcomes Prevention Evaluation Study Investigators. Effects of aggressive blood pressure control in normotensive type diabetic patients on albuminuria, retinopathy and strokes. *Kidney Int* 2002; **61**: 1086–97.
11. Effects of ramipril on cardiovascular and microvascular outcomes in people with diabetes mellitus: results of the HOPE study and MICRO-HOPE substudy. *Lancet* 2000; **355**: 253–59.
12. Lindholm L, Hansson L, Ekbom T, et al. Comparison of antihypertensive treatments in preventing cardiovascular event in elderly diabetic patients: results of the Swedish Trial in Old Patients with hypertension-2. *J Hypertension* 2000; **18**: 1671–5.
13. Niskanen L, Hedner T, Hansson L, Lanke J, Niklason A for the CAPPP study group. Reduced cardiovascular morbidity and mortality in hypertensive diabetic patients on first line therapy with an ACE inhibitor compared with a diuretic/β-blocker-based treatment regimen. *Diabetes Care* 2001; **24**: 2091–6.
14. Brown MJ, Palmer CR, Castaigne A, et al. Morbidity and mortslity in patients randomised to double-blind treament with long-acting calcium channel blocker or diuretic in the International Nifedpine GITS study: Intervention as a Goal in hypertension treatment (INSIGHT). *Lancet* 2000; **356**: 366–72.
15. Hansson L, Hedner T, Lund-Johansen P, et al. Randomised trial of effects of calcium antagonists compared to diuretics and β-blockers on cardiovascular morbidity and mortality in hypertension: the Nordic Diliazem (NORDIL) study. *Lancet* 2000; **356**: 359–65.
16. Lindholm LH, Ibsen H, Dahlof B, et al. Cardiovascular morbidity and mortality in patients with diabetes in the losartan intervention for endpoint reduction in hypertension study (LIFE): a randomised trial against atenolol. *Lancet* 2002; **359**: 1004–10.

17. Pyorala K, Pederson PR, Kjekshus J, et al. Cholesterol lowering with simvastatin improves prognosis of diabetic patients with coronary heart disease. *Diabetes Care* 1997; **20:** 614–20.

18. The Long-term Intervention with Pravastatin in Ischemic Diseae (LIPID) study group. Prevention of cardiovascular events and death with Pravastatin in patients with coronary heart disease and a broad range of initial cholesterol levels. *N Eng J Med* 1998; **339:** 1349–57.

19. Goldberg RB, Mellies MJ, Sacks FM, et al. for the CARE investigators. Cardiovascular events and their reduction with pravastatin in diabetic and glucose-intolerant myocardial infarction survivors with average cholesterol levels. Subgroup analysis in the cholesterol and recurrent events (CARE) trial. *Circulation* 1998; **98:** 2513–9.

20. Heart Protection Study Collaborative Group. MRC/BHF Heart Protection study of cholesterol lowering with simvastatin in 20,536 high risk individuals: a randomised placebo-controlled trial. *Lancet* 2002; **360:** 7–22.

21. UKPDS 23. Risk factors for coronary heart disease in non-insulin dependent diabetes mellitus: United Kingdom Prospective Diabetes Study. *BMJ* 1998; 823–8.

22. Williams B. Unique vulnerability of diabetic subjects to hypertensive injury. *J Hum Hypertension* 1999; **13:** 3–8.

23. Betteridge DJ. LDL heterogeneity: implications for atherogenicity in insulin resistance and NIDDM. *Diabetilogia* 1997; **40:** S149–S151.

I Epidemiology and Pathophysiology

1

Epidemiology and pathogenesis of hypertension in people with diabetes mellitus

Bryan Williams

Defining 'hypertension' in people with diabetes

Diabetes and hypertension are both common conditions in Western societies. They frequently co-exist, more often than can be accounted for by chance. It was recognized over 60 years ago that hypertension is more common in people with diabetes.[1] Subsequently it has often been stated that hypertension is at least twice as common in diabetic subjects when compared with the non-diabetic population, although the prevalence is clearly dependent on the definition of hypertension.[2] Hypertension can be defined as the level of blood pressure (BP) at which cardiovascular risk is measurably increased for the population and/or the level of blood pressure at which its treatment has been shown to significantly reduce cardiovascular morbidity and mortality in prospective randomized clinical trials. This definition is not without problems when endeavouring to define hypertension for people with diabetes mellitus. Firstly, at any level of blood pressure, people with diabetes are at higher cardiovascular risk than those without diabetes. Thus, if the definition of hypertension were to be based on an absolute level of cardiovascular risk, the blood pressure level demarcating 'hypertension' for the diabetic population would be substantially lower than that for the non-diabetic population. This is graphically illustrated by reference to the work

of Stamler and colleagues and their study of the MRFIT screenees.[3] At any level of BP adjusted for all other measured risk factors, coronary heart disease risk and cardiovascular death were consistently greater in diabetes when compared with the non-diabetic population. The risk of cardiovascular death for a man with known diabetes and systolic BP between 140 and 159 mmHg was *the same* as in men without diabetes with BP > 180 mmHg (Fig. 1.1). Thus on the basis of the epidemiology of the risk associated with hypertension, it could be argued that the threshold BP for the definition of hypertension should be substantially lower in diabetic people when compared with the non-diabetic population. Furthermore, in the United Kingdom Prospective Diabetes Study (UKPDS), a study of patients with type 2 diabetes, the risk associated with blood pressure was continuous, with no evidence of a safe threshold[4] (Fig. 1.2).

These observations highlight the second problem in defining hypertension in people with diabetes, notably, their apparent increased vulnerability to hypertensive injury, at much lower levels of blood pressure than for the non-diabetic population.[5] This impairment of self-defence against the injurious effects of hypertension supports the argument in favour of lower blood pressure thresholds for the definition of hypertension in diabetes. Nevertheless, it is important that the validity of such epidemiological associations and

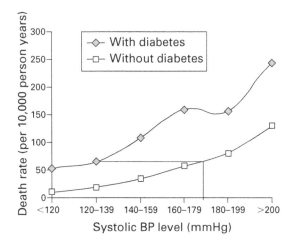

Figure 1.1

Impact of systolic blood pressure on age-adjusted cardiovascular disease death rates for men with and without diabetes at initial screening for MRFIT. (Redrawn from reference 3.)

pathophysiological predictions is tested in clinical trials of treatment of hypertension in people with diabetes. Such trials are essential to define whether the assumed risk can be reversed by the effective treatment of blood pressure, thereby defining the blood pressure threshold for treatment, i.e. hypertension, and the optimal target to which blood pressure should be lowered.

This brings us to the third problem in defining hypertension in people with diabetes, notably, the remarkable lack of prospective randomized clinical trial data documenting the benefits of antihypertensive therapy in people with diabetes. This deficit was crucial, because as stated above, an epidemiological association between a high level of cardiovascular risk and a specific BP level, and a compelling pathophysiological hypothesis for increased risk, does not necessarily mean that the introduction of antihypertensive therapy at that BP threshold would completely or even partially

reduce that risk. Data from prospective randomized clinical trials of antihypertensive therapy in diabetic patients were sorely needed.

In many of the early landmark antihypertensive therapy trials, diabetic subjects were excluded from the study. However, in two studies – HDFP and SHEP – diabetes was not an exclusion criterion and approximately 10% of the hypertensive participants were also diabetic.[6,7] Post-hoc examination of these cohorts suggested that the benefits of antihypertensive therapy in terms of reductions in cardiovascular disease (CVD) morbidity and mortality, were at least as great in diabetic as in non-diabetic subjects. Surprisingly, these reports gained little prominence and failed to prompt any obvious enthusiasm for antihypertensive therapy in diabetic subjects.

The evidence base for the substantial macrovascular and microvascular benefits of blood pressure reduction came in 1998 with the presentation of results from three significant trials: the diabetic cohort from the HOT study,[8] the diabetic cohort from the SystEur trial[9] and the blood pressure study embedded within the UKPDS.[10] Each yielded key and complementary messages and prompted revision of many previous guidelines for the management of hypertension. They also led to a widely accepted definition of hypertension in type 1 and 2 diabetes, i.e. a blood pressure ≥ 140 mmHg systolic and/or ≥ 90 mmHg diastolic.

Prevalence of hypertension in type 1 and type 2 diabetes

Defining the true prevalence of hypertension in diabetes is bedevilled by the fact that the many published surveys utilize various blood pressure thresholds for the definition of hyperten-

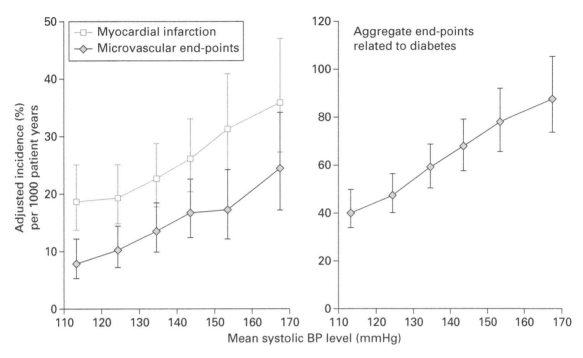

Figure 1.2
Incidence rates (95% confidence interval) of various end-points by category of updated mean systolic blood pressure adjusted for age, gender, ethnicity, smoking history, lipid levels and albuminuria, expressed for white men aged 50–54 at diagnosis of diabetes and a mean duration of diabetes of 10 years in UKPDS. (From reference 4.)

sion. Until recently, most published surveys used the old WHO definition of hypertension (blood pressure ≥160/95 mmHg) and reported hypertension prevalence rates of <25% for type 1 diabetes and approximately 50% for type 2 diabetes. From these reports it is not possible to deduce the prevalence of hypertension using the more recent definition of hypertension (≥140/90) but clearly it is much higher. The difficulty in defining the prevalence of hypertension in diabetes is compounded by the fact that it is also strongly influenced by the proportion of type 1 versus type 2 diabetic people included in the surveys and the prevalence of obesity, their gender and racial mix.

More recent surveys include the *Health*

Survey for England, a nationwide annual survey that documents the health and lifestyle characteristics of a large cohort of the English population.[11] Those included are representative of the national population in terms of geographic, ethnic and socio-demographic distribution. Between 1991 and 1994, 30,639 adults were included in the survey of whom 970 reported a history of diabetes. The respondents had blood pressure measured three times on a single occasion. Consistent with previous surveys, about half (51%) of those with diabetes had hypertension defined as a systolic blood pressure ≥160 mmHg or a diastolic pressure ≥95 mmHg diastolic or being on antihypertensive treatment. When a more stringent definition of hypertension (blood pressure $\geq 140/90$ mmHg) is applied, three-quarters of those with diabetes had a systolic BP ≥ 140 mmHg systolic or a diastolic BP ≥ 90 mmHg diastolic or were on antihypertensive treatment. Adjusted for age, those with diabetes were twice as likely to have hypertension as those without (odds ratio = 2.2, $p < 0.0001$). Moreover, the diagnosis of diabetes was still associated with a two-fold excess risk of hypertension after adjusting for obesity (body mass index) (Table 1.1). The corollary is also true, i.e. that hypertension per se, increases the risk of developing type 2 diabetes. Data were reported recently from a large prospective cohort study of 12,550 adults with hypertension who were followed for 6 years.[12] In the 1474 people with untreated hypertension, the risk of developing type 2 diabetes was increased 2.5 times when compared with their normotensive counterparts. Together, these observations confirm that hypertension is extremely common in people with diabetes, particularly type 2 diabetes. Indeed, we should regard a type 2 diabetic patient with a normal blood pressure ($<140/90$ mmHg) as a peculiar exception rather than the norm. Moreover, the diagnosis of primary hypertension more than doubles

the risk of that person developing type 2 diabetes. This is consistent with the hypothesis that primary hypertension is commonly an insulin-resistant state and supports the notion that common and/or other aetiological factors interact to predispose to both clinical states.

Influence of age on blood pressure in diabetes

In Western societies, ageing is associated with a progressive rise in systolic blood pressure and a smaller gradual decline in diastolic blood pressure beyond middle age.[13] This results in a progressive widening of pulse pressure and an earlier onset and increased prevalence of isolated systolic hypertension in older people with diabetes. These changes reflect age-dependent changes in conduit vessel structure and their impaired haemodynamic performance.[13–15] With ageing, the large conduit vessels become progressively stiffer due to a loss of elasticity, increased collagen cross-linking via advanced glycation and increased fibrosis of the vessel wall, thereby reducing vascular compliance.[13–15] Ageing has a marked effect on the prevalence of hypertension in both type 1 and type 2 diabetes (Fig. 1.3). The

Diabetes	Men (%)	Women (%)	All (%)
Type 1	34.5	29.5	32.3
Type 2	78.3	82.8	80.4
All diabetes	72.1	75.5	73.6

(From data in reference 11.)

Table 1.1
Percentage of patients with diabetes and hypertension ($\geq 140/90$ mmHg) and/or on antihypertensive therapy in the Health Survey for England 1991–1994

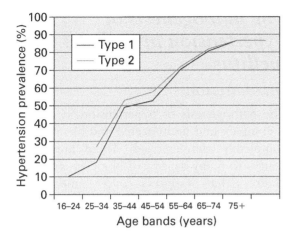

Figure 1.3
*Prevalence (%) of hypertension (>140/90 mmHg)
in people with diabetes. Data from the Health
Survey for England, 1991–1994 (drawn from data
derived from reference 11).*

effects of ageing on blood pressure are much
more pronounced in people with diabetes
when compared with the non-diabetic population. This latter observation appears to reflect
accelerated ageing, greater injury and/or
increased stiffening of conduit arteries in diabetic patients. This concept is supported by
the observation that age-adjusted pulse wave
velocity is markedly increased in patients with
diabetes.[16] Put simply, the blood vessels of
people with diabetes function as though they
are at least 10 years older than the patient.
This observation has enormous clinical significance because it suggests why isolated systolic
hypertension (systolic BP > 140 mmHg, diastolic BP < 90 mmHg) occurs more commonly
and earlier in people with diabetes when compared with the age-matched non-diabetic
population.

Influence of gender on blood pressure in diabetes

The role of gender in determining the prevalence of hypertension in diabetes is intriguing.
As shown in Fig. 1.4, hypertension is more
common in women with diabetes than in men.
The difference in the prevalence of hypertension between those with and without diabetes
was greater for women (OR = 2.8) than men
(OR = 2.0) ($p = 0.02$ for the diabetes/sex interaction adjusted for age). This greater risk of
diabetes-associated hypertension was mainly
accounted for by the greater body mass index
of diabetic women. Similarly, at baseline in the
UKPDS the prevalence of hypertension (blood
pressure ≥160/95 mmHg) in newly diagnosed
women (mean age 53) was 45% compared
with 32% in men (mean age 52).[17]

It is also interesting to note that the age-
related rise in blood pressure occurs earlier
and is steeper in diabetic women compared
with diabetic men. In the non-diabetic normotensive population, our own data have shown

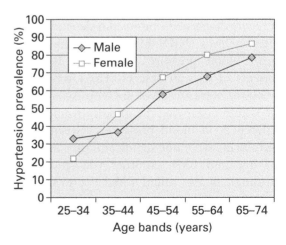

Figure 1.4
*Prevalence of hypertension (≥ 140/90 mmHg) in
type 2 diabetes, according to age and gender data
from the Health Survey for England, 1991–1994.[11]*

that the age-related rise in blood pressure during adulthood is also steeper in women, so that by their seventh decade, women have systolic blood pressure levels that equal or exceed those of men. In hypertensive non-diabetic women, this 'cross-over' occurs earlier with the prevalence of hypertension eventually reaching and then surpassing that of men at 45–55 years of age. However, it is clear from Fig. 1.3 that in people with diabetes this 'cross-over' occurs prematurely, so that the blood pressures of diabetic women exceed those of diabetic men at least a decade earlier than expected.

Influence of ethnicity on blood pressure in diabetes

In addition to age, BMI, the presence of renal disease and gender, another potentially important factor influencing blood pressure is ethnicity. In the USA multiple studies have concluded that hypertension is more prevalent, more severe and often associated with more target organ damage in both non-diabetic and diabetic black Americans. In the UKPDS study of newly diagnosed non-insulin-dependent diabetes mellitus (NIDDM) patients, the highest mean blood pressures were also found in patients of African descent. The lowest blood pressures were observed in Indo-Asians, with the whites occupying the middle ground.[17] The differences in blood pressure between whites and Asians were not significant after adjusting for age and BMI. Another UK study from Birmingham also found a higher prevalence of hypertension in diabetic patients of African descent (48.9%) when compared with whites (37.5%) and Indo-Asians (35.4%).[18]

The pathogenesis of hypertension in diabetes mellitus
Introduction

The pathogenesis of hypertension in diabetes is complex and multifaceted and has not been completely characterized. There are disturbances to many aspects of blood pressure regulation that progress over time. These disturbances are often subtle and lead to changes to 24 hour blood pressure load, long before they manifest as an increase in office blood pressure. The development of nephropathy magnifies these disturbances. The prevalence and time course of hypertension differ between type 1 and type 2 diabetic patients. In type 1 patients, clinic blood pressures are often normal at presentation and commonly remain normal during the first 10–15 years of diabetes. This reflects the younger age of this patient population. Thereafter, age-associated increases in blood pressure are evident (Figure 1.3). When hypertension is observed earlier in the course of type 1 diabetes, it is most often indicative of the development of nephropathy. In contrast, in type 2 diabetes, hypertension is frequently apparent at diagnosis and no doubt precedes the diagnosis of diabetes. If nephropathy develops in type 2 diabetes, it is associated with further increases in blood pressure but nephropathy is not the major factor driving the high prevalence of hypertension in type 2 diabetes.

The various components contributing to disturbed blood pressure regulation in diabetes are discussed individually below. It is worthy of emphasis, however, that these factors act in concert.

Disturbances to 24 hour blood pressure regulation

Office blood pressure measurements are an imperfect surrogate for 24 hour blood pressure load in people with diabetes. The emergence of 24 hour ambulatory blood pressure measurements (ABPM) has highlighted profound disturbances to blood pressure regulation in people with diabetes that occur before the detection of hypertension by conventional office blood pressure measurements.[19–27] This is important because it emphasizes that any level of office blood pressure corresponds to a higher 24 hour blood pressure load in people with diabetes when compared with those without diabetes. The characteristic disturbance in 24 hour blood pressure regulation in type 1 and type 2 diabetes is a reduction in the normal nocturnal dip in blood pressure, usually associated with a higher nocturnal heart rate, than in normotensive people without diabetes.[19–27] This has been demonstrated in otherwise seemingly healthy, 'normotensive' and normoalbuminuric diabetic patients. This results in a higher 24 hour blood pressure load despite normal office blood pressures and similar mean daytime BP readings to normotensive non-diabetic controls.

The normal circadian rhythm of blood pressure, characterized by the nocturnal dip, is strongly dependent on normal autonomic function.[28–30] The reduced nocturnal dip and the higher nocturnal heart rates point to subtle early disturbances to autonomic function that are not readily detectable by conventional bedside tests.[23,25,31] The mechanisms underpinning this early disturbance to autonomic function are unknown; however, it is inversely correlated with the quality of glycaemic control in early type 1 diabetes, suggesting that the hyperglycaemic state is important.[23] Whether these early disturbances in autonomic regula-tion of 24 hour blood pressure control can be reversed by improved glycaemic control has not been formally studied. Smoking may also be important in that day (+3.9 mmHg) and night (+3.5 mmHg) diastolic BP is significantly higher in type 1 diabetic normotensive, normoalbuminaemic smokers when compared with non-smokers.[32] This contrasts with the non-diabetic state in which smoking has been associated with a lower nocturnal BP.

Influence of microalbuminuria and proteinuria on 24 hour blood pressure regulation

Twenty-four hour ambulatory blood pressures are significantly increased in patients with type 1 or type 2 diabetes and microalbuminuria when compared with normoalbuminuric patients, despite comparable clinic blood pressures.[27,33–37] In cross-sectional studies of normo-albuminuric type 1 diabetic patients, patients with a 'high normal' urinary albumin excretion (UAE) rate had significantly higher 24 hour ambulatory BP than those with a 'low normal' UAE rate. The night:day BP ratio is particularly disturbed in patients with microalbuminuria (i.e. incipient nephropathy) and diabetes, although both day and night BP averages are increased when compared with normoalbumin-uric diabetics (Fig. 1.5). The transition from normoalbuminuria to microalbuminuria is also associated with a progressive year-on-year rise in office blood pressure (approximate rise in mean blood pressure of 3–4 mmHg/year), even though office BP may remain within the conventional normal range, i.e. <140/90 mmHg.[38] This progressive increase in blood pressure is paralleled by a progressive rise in urinary albumin excretion, so that after a few years, the patient is labelled hypertensive by conventional office blood pressure criteria and has developed proteinuria. Once type 1 or 2 diabetic patients develop overt proteinuria (i.e. nephropathy –

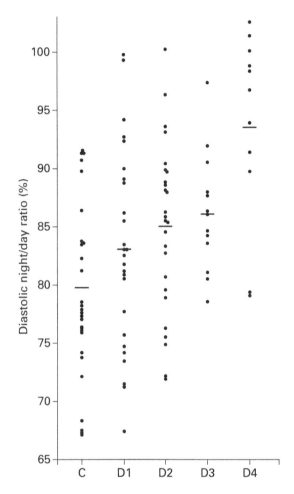

Figure 1.5
Night/day ratio for diastolic blood pressure in healthy people with type 1 diabetes. C, non-diabetic people with normoalbuminuria (n = 26); D1, diabetic, normoalbuminuria (n = 26); D2, diabetic, microalbuminuria; D3, diabetic, proteinuria, untreated hypertension; D4, diabetic, proteinuria, treated hypertension. (From reference 33.)

urinary albumin excretion >300 mg/24 hours), ambulatory BP and office BP increase further and the 24 hour BP profile is markedly disturbed. These disturbances are often accompanied by overt clinical evidence of autonomic dysfunction.

The aforementioned disturbances in BP regulation question the wisdom of labelling any diabetic patient with microalbuminuria or proteinuria as 'normotensive' on the basis of office BP readings. In my view, they are not normotensive in that the individual patient's BP regulation is profoundly disturbed and their BP load is markedly increased compared with the BP load before the onset of microalbuminuria. Moreover many diabetic patients – even with seemingly normal office blood pressures – already have evidence of target organ damage, notably an increased left ventricular mass, which is indicative of the increased blood pressure load. Table 1.2 summarizes a proposed classification of hypertension in diabetes, related to the level of albumin excretion, based on our improved understanding of the BP regulation and its disturbances in diabetes.

Volume homeostasis, extracellular sodium and the renin angiotensin aldosterone system

Exchangeable sodium is frequently elevated in patients with both type 1 and type 2 diabetes.[39–43] This is true whether or not the patient is normotensive or hypertensive. The fact that the total exchangeable sodium pool is expanded in diabetes has been recognized for many years and in the 1960s prompted Conn to suggest that diabetes is a form of hyper-aldosteronism. In both type 1 and type 2 diabetes, the exchangeable body sodium pool is expanded even in normotensive individuals by approximately 10%, independent of age, obesity, sex or the presence of complications.[39–43] Extracellular fluid volume is also expanded but this is not necessarily retained within the vascular space, indeed, blood volume is usually normal or contracted. This may be explained by increased microvascular permeability to albumin and fluids, particularly in

Blood pressure changes in diabetes mellitus

Early type I and type II 'normotensive'	• Subtle autonomic dysfunction
	• Decreased baroreceptor sensitivity
	• Increased blood pressure load +
	• TOD ±
Microalbuminuria 'normotensive' or hypertensive	• Disturbed autonomic function (±clinical)
	• Loss of nocturnal BP dip (±clinical)
	• Exaggerated BP responses
	• Increased blood pressure load ++
	• Progressive rise in blood pressure – TOD +
Proteinuria hypertensive	• Clinically evident autonomic dysfunction
	• Non-dipper – increased blood pressure load
	• Clinically hypertensive +++ TOD +++

Table 1.2
Association between normoalbuminuria, microalbuminuria and proteinuria and the development of progressively worsening disturbances to blood pressure regulation and target organ damage (TOD)

Parameter	No nephropathy		Incipient or overt nephropathy	
Exchangeable sodium	↑	↑	↑↑	↑↑
Extracellular volume	normal or ↑	normal or ↑	↑↑	↑↑
Intravascular volume	normal or ↓	normal or ↓	normal or ↓	normal or ↓
Plasma renin activity	normal or ↓	normal or ↓	↑	↑
Aldosterone	normal or ↓	normal or ↓	normal or ↓	normal or ↓
ANP	↑*	↑*	↑↑*	↑↑*
Sodium:renin product	normal	Normal	↑	↑

'Normal' refers to the normal range usually defined in people without diabetes or hypertension. *ANP (atrial natriuretic peptide) levels are increased but there is renal resistance to ANP. As the magnitude of proteinuria and renal impairment increases, the disturbances in the cited parameters get proportionately worse.

Table 1.3
Changes in various volume, electrolyte and hormonal parameters in people with diabetes and hypertension

those with established microvascular disease, which would lead to extravascular sequestration of fluids and albumin.

Once people with diabetes develop incipient or overt nephropathy, there is a marked increase in exchangeable sodium and fluid retention, often manifesting as oedema. This is positively related to the progressive rise in blood pressure and albumin excretion rate.[41,42] Despite marked sodium and volume retention, diabetic nephropathy is not usually associated with an expansion of intravascular volume. This is most likely due to the further enhancement of the trans-vascular escape of albumin as nephropathy progresses and blood pressure rises (Table 1.3).

Many factors contribute to the disturbed volume and sodium homeostasis in people with diabetes. The correlations between blood pressure, albumin excretion and exchangeable sodium suggest a primary renal defect underpinning the sodium retention associated with diabetes. Normotensive type 1 diabetic patients without any clinical evidence of nephropathy have an impaired ability to excrete a water load and diminished natriuresis in response to water immersion.[44] This occurs despite an enhanced glomerular filtration rate and an increase in filtered sodium, thereby implying enhanced tubular reabsorption of sodium. Furthermore, once nephropathy develops, plasma ANP concentrations are further elevated but the renal cyclic GMP responses to ANP are blunted suggesting renal resistance to ANP. These observations suggest that diabetes is a sodium-retaining state with the magnitude of sodium retention increasing with increasing severity of nephropathy.

Insulin may play a role in stimulating sodium retention by the kidney and this may be amplified by the presence of hyperglycaemia.[45] Plasma angiotensin II (Ang II) and aldosterone are generally normal or suppressed in type 1 and 2 patients in the absence of nephropathy. In contrast, plasma atrial natriuretic peptide (ANP) can be elevated in type 1 and 2 diabetics. Although the ANP response to saline infusion and water immersion appears normal in type 1 diabetes, the natriuretic response to a saline load is impaired during an ANP infusion, suggesting impaired renal tubular responses to ANP.

The role of the renin angiotensin system (RAS) in the pathogenesis of hypertension and sodium retention in diabetes has been the subject of enduring controversy.[45] In hypertensive type 1 diabetic patients, in the absence of overt nephropathy, plasma renin activity (PRA) appears to be suppressed or within the normal range. In patients with type 2 diabetes, in the absence of nephropathy, PRA is usually suppressed. This is the expected response of the RAS to the volume and sodium expanded state. Nevertheless, the relationship between sodium, volume and RAS activity is clearly more complex in diabetes.

PRA is a marker of circulating RAS activity but there may be differential activation of the RAS within tissues.[46] Many studies in experimental models of diabetes have shown that despite suppression of circulating RAS activity, key components of the RAS are expressed at normal or increased levels in diabetic renal tissues.[47–49] This supports the hypothesis that the renal tissue RAS is inappropriately activated in diabetes and that measurements of PRA are a poor surrogate for tissue RAS activity. In support of this hypothesis, studies in patients with type 2 diabetes have demonstrated increased functional renal RAS activity.[50–52] In type 2 diabetic patients receiving a high salt diet, PRA suppressed less well in diabetic subjects when compared with non-diabetic controls. Moreover, the renal vasodilator response to the ACE-inhibitor enalapril was substantially greater in salt-loaded type 2 diabetics when compared with salt-loaded non-diabetic controls, who exhibited a minimal response.[50–52] Together these observations support the hypothesis that the renal RAS is inappropriately active in patients with type 2 diabetes, even before the development of nephropathy.

Once diabetic patients develop nephropathy, the relationship between blood pressure, PRA and exchangeable sodium is more clear cut and similar to that seen in other forms of chronic renal disease. Notably, the raised blood pressure can be related to sodium retention and inappropriate activation of the RAS. Exchangeable sodium is elevated, PRA is inappropriately high and blood pressure is positively related to both exchangeable sodium and the sodium:renin product. It is also likely that nocturnal fluid retention/redistribution contributes to the frequently absent nocturnal dip in blood pressure in patients with nephropathy.

Disturbed endothelial function

The vascular endothelium plays an important role in regulating blood flow and blood pressure. Under normal conditions, the endothelium continuously liberates nitric oxide which acts as a potent vasodilator. Inhibition of this basal production of nitric oxide is associated with a rise in systemic blood pressure, suggesting that nitric oxide plays an important role in the regulation of basal vascular tone and blood pressure.[53] Endothelial-derived hyperpolarizing factor (EDHF) is another potent vasodilator liberated by the endothelium that plays a role in the maintenance of basal vascular tone. In addition to vasodilators, the endothelium also releases endothelins, extremely potent vasoconstrictors and various prostaglandins such as the vasoconstrictor PGH_2 or the vasodilator prostacyclin.

Many studies in man support the hypothesis that the normal balance of endothelial function is disturbed in type 1 and type 2 diabetes.[54–56] A variety of mechanisms appear to underpin the development of endothelial dysfunction in diabetes. These include: (1) decreased nitric oxide synthesis, (2) decreased nitric oxide bioavailability due to quenching by superoxide anions, (3) decreased production of EDHF, (4) increased vasoconstrictor prostaglandin synthesis. Many of these changes ante-date the development of overt diabetes and are demonstrable in people with insulin resistance.[57]

It is likely that hyperglycaemia per se plays an important role in the pathogenesis of endothelial dysfunction via mechanisms involving increased oxidative stress, which in part may be protein kinase C-dependent.[58] This leads to increased generation of superoxide anions, which can combine with NO, thereby quenching NO and increasing the production of the highly reactive radical peroxynitrite ($ONOO^-$). Abnormalities in glucose metabolism may also limit the production of NO. NADPH is a key co-factor required for NO production by endothelial nitric oxide synthase (eNOS). The availability of NADPH via the pentose phosphate pathway can be attenuated in the presence of hyperglycaemia, thereby leading to decreased NO synthesis. It has also been suggested that L-arginine (the substrate for NO synthesis) transport into the endothelium may be impaired in diabetes.[58] Dyslipidaemia, particularly oxidized LDL-cholesterol and increased circulating levels of free fatty acids, may also contribute to disturbed endothelial function and may also disturb NO production/consumption.

The disturbances to endothelial function in diabetes are of enormous significance with regard to blood pressure regulation and the haemodynamic performance of the vasculature. As NO normally counteracts vasoconstriction, the reduction in basal vasodilator tone will effectively increase vascular sensitivity to vasoconstrictors.[39,42,43] This phenomenon has been demonstrated previously in patients with diabetes and could contribute to the development of hypertension. In addition, NO is important in regulating arterial stiffness and wave reflection characteristics. Thus, impaired endothelial function would be expected to result in an aged vascular phenotype, with a widened pulse pressure and increased central arterial systolic blood pressure. This phenotype is characteristic of diabetes.

Abnormalities in vascular reactivity

Although plasma angiotensin II and catecholamine levels tend to be normal if not low in type 1 and type 2 diabetes, cardiovascular responsiveness to these agents is often exaggerated.[39,42,43] This increased vascular sensitivity, particularly to catecholamines, appears to occur independent of age, duration of diabetes or type of diabetic therapy. It is likely to arise via three possible mechanisms. (i) Sodium retention increases vascular responsiveness to pressor agents. The use of diuretics to reduce exchangeable sodium in diabetic patients has been shown to normalize the augmented vascular response of IDDM patients to catecholamines and promote a fall in blood pressure. (ii) Remodelling of the resistance vessels leading to an increase in the vascular wall:lumen ratio. These changes in vessel structure are accompanied by an increase in sensitivity to pressor agents. (iii) Impaired endothelial function resulting in a reduced basal vasodilator tone and increased sensitivity to vasoconstrictors.

Obesity and insulin resistance

There is a strong relationship between obesity, glucose tolerance and hypertension. This is a powerful and complex relationship. People who are hypertensive are more likely to develop obesity and people who are obese are more likely to become hypertensive. On average, mean blood pressure rises by approximately 1 mmHg for every 3 kg weight gain above ideal body weight. Moreover, women seem to be more sensitive than men to the pressor effects of weight gain.

Body fat distribution appears to be important in defining this relationship between blood pressure and body weight. Almost 50 years ago a French clinician, Jean Vague, reported that hypertension and the characteristic metabolic syndrome of obesity are more common in people with central adiposity.[59] Similar conclusions have been reached in sub-

sequent epidemiological surveys.[60] It is also well recognized that insulin resistance and the associated metabolic syndrome (impaired glucose tolerance, low HDL-cholesterol, high triglycerides and hyperuricaemia) also track with central adiposity, as does cardiovascular risk.[61] The fact that central adiposity is also powerfully predictive of type 2 diabetes provides a foundation for the association between hypertension and diabetes. However, even after correcting for body weight, there is still an excess of hypertension in type 1 and type 2 diabetes when compared with the non-diabetic population. Thus, weight gain and central adiposity account for some but not all of the excess prevalence of hypertension in people with diabetes.

Hypertension and glucose tolerance

Abnormalities in carbohydrate metabolism are common in people with hypertension and such people are 2.5 times more likely to develop type 2 diabetes.[12] Blood pressure is continuously associated with glucose tolerance and the converse is also true. Thus, there is likely to be a strong genetic basis for the interaction between risk of developing hypertension and type 2 diabetes which is powerfully influenced by environmental factors. Longitudinal surveys have confirmed the power of this relationship. In a long-term follow-up of middle-aged men in Finland who were normotensive when their blood pressure and glucose tolerance were assessed in 1968, those with the higher blood glucose values following a standard oral glucose load in 1968 had a higher prevalence of hypertension in 1986[62] (Table 1.4).

Similar findings were reported from the San Antonio Heart Study (SAHS). In an 8-year follow-up of 1254 normotensive, non-diabetic people, plasma glucose and blood pressure (systolic, diastolic and mean) were tracking

Blood glucose tertiles 1 hour after glucose load in 1968 (mmol/l)	Adjusted* odds ratio for developing hypertension by 1986
<5.15 (n = 198)	1.00
5.16–6.65 (n = 197)	1.36
≥6.66 (n = 185)	1.71

The odds ratios are adjusted* for age, body mass index, alcohol intake and initial systolic and diastolic blood pressure. No intervention was implemented during the period of follow-up. (Drawn from data in reference 62.)

Table 1.4
The odds ratio for development of hypertension after 18 years in 580 initially normotensive (BP< 160/95 mmHg) men according to tertiles of blood glucose values 1 hour after a standard oral glucose load.

variables that cross-predicted each other. For example, those with a plasma glucose at baseline which was at the higher end of the distribution were more likely to have a higher blood pressure after 8 years of follow-up. Likewise, those with a higher blood pressure at baseline were more likely to have a higher plasma glucose at follow-up.[63] This cross-predictivity is supported by the more recent finding from a 5-year follow-up study of 10,000 men from Israel in which systolic blood pressure was a significant predictor of diabetes regardless of age or obesity.[64]

Hypertension and insulin

In 1966 Welborn and colleagues noted that patients with hypertension had a heightened plasma insulin response to an oral glucose load, indicative of insulin resistance.[65] This has subsequently been confirmed by many other studies and the relationship is true even in lean individuals.[61,63,66] Thus, hypertension is commonly an insulin-resistant state. However, the strength of this relationship is variable and confounded by many factors, including age, gender, obesity and ethnicity. This is illustrated in Fig. 1.6, taken from the SAHS. Clearly, at similar insulin levels, the prevalence

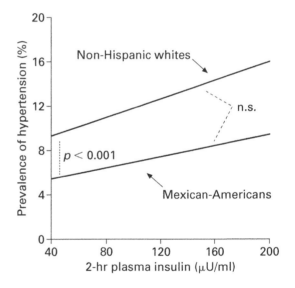

Figure 1.6
The association between plasma insulin and the prevalence of hypertension in Mexican-Americans and non-Hispanic whites in the San Antonio Heart Study. The gradient of the lines is similar (i.e. higher plasma insulin is associated with a higher prevalence of hypertension in both groups) but the intercepts are different (i.e. at any level of insulin, the prevalence of hypertension is higher in non-Hispanic whites). (From reference 67.)

of hypertension varies in different ethnic groups.[67] This may explain why certain ethnic groups with a very high prevalence of insulin resistance do not necessarily experience an excess prevalence of hypertension, e.g. the Southern Asian population in the UK.[18,68] It also explains how the ethnic mix of a population can strongly influence the strength of the relationship between insulin resistance and hypertension and why in some surveys this relationship has been weaker than in others. The characteristics of the insulin resistance associated with hypertension and the resultant metabolic syndrome are discussed elsewhere.

Obesity, insulin resistance and the pathogenesis of hypertension

The aforementioned studies suggest that the common association between hypertension and diabetes may be founded in the co-segregation of genes predisposing to both hypertension and diabetes and/or environmental factors (e.g. obesity and sedentary lifestyle) that increase the risk of developing hypertension and/or diabetes. How could abnormalities in glucose tolerance, insulin resistance and obesity lead to a higher blood pressure?

It has long been recognized that dietary intake, particularly fat and carbohydrate, influences the activity of the sympathetic nervous system (SNS).[69,70] Fasting suppresses, whereas feeding stimulates SNS activity. Activation of the SNS increases the metabolic rate in humans; thus, this mechanism is thought to provide a link between dietary intake and metabolic rate. For example, fasting decreases metabolic rate, whereas feeding increases it. This has been termed dietary thermogenesis and this process is regulated by insulin and the SNS.[71]

How do dietary intake and insulin influence SNS activity? One mechanism has been suggested to involve the metabolism of glucose in the ventromedial hypothalamus (VMH).[72,73] Decreased glucose metabolism by the VMH (i.e. during fasting when glucose and insulin levels are reduced) activates inhibitory pathways between the VMH and central sympathetic centres in the brain stem, thereby reducing central sympathetic outflow. Conversely, during feeding, insulin stimulates uptake and metabolism of glucose by cells within the VMH which results in suppression of the inhibitory pathway and increased central SNS activity (Fig. 1.7). According to this hypothesis, this would be designed to increase metabolism and thermogenesis and thereby maintain normal body weight.

In the obese, insulin levels are elevated as part of the insulin-resistant state that characterizes obesity. The resistance to the action of insulin is largely confined to insulin-mediated

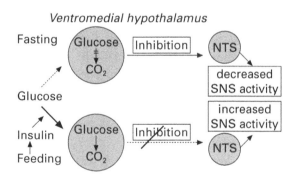

Figure 1.7

Relationship between glucose, insulin and central sympathetic outflow. In the fasting state, glucose metabolism in the neurones of the ventromedial hypothalamus (VMH) is suppressed thereby activating inhibitory pathways which suppress sympathetic nervous system (SNS) traffic from the nucleus tractus solitarus (NTS) in the brain stem. In the fed state, insulin promotes glucose uptake and metabolism by the VMH, thereby reducing the activity of the inhibitory pathway and allowing an increase in central SNS outflow. (Redrawn from reference 73.)

glucose uptake by skeletal muscle; the CNS responds normally to insulin. Thus obesity mimics the fed state and the neurones of the VMH respond to the increased insulin level by increasing their metabolism of glucose and suppressing the inhibition of central SNS outflow, thereby resulting in enhanced SNS activity associated with obesity. In support of this, it has been demonstrated that the obese are not resistant to the actions of insulin on the SNS[74] and that SNS activity is increased in the obese.[75]

Abnormalities in vascular stiffness – implications for systolic blood pressure and pulse pressure

As indicated above, there is evidence of a premature rise in systolic blood pressure in people with diabetes, associated with a premature widening of pulse pressure (Fig. 1.4). This mimics the recognized effects of ageing on blood pressure profiles in westernized societies; the major difference is that these occur earlier in people with diabetes.[13] This implies acceleration of the normal vascular ageing process which is characterized by progressive stiffening of the larger conduit arteries. This has been attributed to various mechanisms including: an age-related decline in endothelial dysfunction,[56] the progressive accumulation of vascular wall matrix proteins and the modification of vascular collagens by the development of cross-links via the formation of advanced glycation end-products (AGEs).[14,15] Ageing, mechanical strain, activation of the sympathetic nervous system and the renin-angiotensin-aldosterone system, along with elevated glucose concentrations may all play a role in promoting vascular matrix accumulation.[76–79] The matrix is then progressively modified by the formation of AGEs, the formation of which is accelerated by the diabetic state.[14,15]

Increased aortic stiffness has profound effects on blood pressure and increases the vascular load on the heart and the coupling efficiency between the heart and vasculature.[80] This premature stiffening of the aorta in diabetes explains the earlier development of systolic hypertension and a wider pulse pressure in diabetic subjects when compared with the non-diabetic population.[16,81] It also renders the systolic blood pressure more difficult to control with drug therapy.[82]

Secondary hypertension

Diabetics are also prone to develop hypertension due to causes other than those intrinsically related to their disease. Patients with diabetes are at increased risk of developing widespread vascular disease, which thereby increases their risk of developing atherosclerotic renovascular disease (see Chapter 00). There are also other clinical conditions in which diabetes and hypertension can co-exist, such as thyrotoxicosis, phaeochromocytoma, Cushing's syndrome, hyperaldosteronism and acromegaly. Other causes of secondary hypertension must also be considered such as coarctation, non-diabetic renal disease, etc. A classification of hypertension in diabetes mellitus is shown in Table 1.5.

Malignant or accelerated hypertension

There is little information regarding the prevalence of malignant or 'accelerated' hypertension in diabetic patients. Clinical experience and anecdotal reports suggest that malignant hypertension is no more common in diabetic patients than in the general population. Nevertheless, particular care must be taken to exclude renal artery stenosis or advanced

Parameter	Mechanisms
Type 1 diabetes	• Diabetic nephropathy (most common) • Primary hypertension of diabetes • Isolated systolic hypertension (with ageing)
Type 2 diabetes	• Primary hypertension of diabetes (most common) • Diabetic nephropathy • Isolated systolic hypertension (with ageing)
Endocrine causes for a combination of diabetes and hypertension	• Thyrotoxicosis • Cushing's syndrome • Phaeochromocytoma • Acromegaly • Some synthetic oestrogens/progestogens
Other causes of hypertension in diabetes	• Renovascular disease (usually atherosclerotic) • Hyperaldosteronism • Non-diabetic chronic renal disease • Aortic coarctation

Table 1.5
An outline classification of the various mechanisms potentially accounting for the development of hypertension in diabetic patients

nephropathy. Thereafter the evaluation of potential underlying causes and its subsequent clinical management are similar to those recommended for patients without diabetes.

Conclusions

This chapter has highlighted the common co-existence of hypertension and diabetes. This increased prevalence of hypertension in people with diabetes is dependent on a conspiracy of numerous mechanisms. The onset of nephropathy is an important cause of hypertension in people with type 1 diabetes but does not account for the very high prevalence of hypertension in type 2 diabetes. In type 2 diabetes, obesity appears to be an important contributor to the development of hypertension but is insufficient to account for it all. Subtle disturbances to blood pressure profiles are likely to result from abnormal blood pressure regulation, perhaps the earliest manifestation of diabetic autonomic dysfunction. Abnormal and/or inappropriate neurohumoral profiles are also likely to be important drivers of altered salt and water homeostasis and pathological disturbances of cardiovascular structures. Equally subtle and less well appreciated disturbances to endothelial and vascular wall function appear to be important for the premature development of systolic hypertension, a process of accelerated vascular ageing. The cross-predictivity of blood pressure and glucose homeostasis imply a genetic foundation for increased risk for developing diabetes and hypertension but there are clearly very powerful – indeed more powerful – environmental and lifestyle determinants. The various mechanisms are highlighted in Fig. 1.8, the complexity of which perhaps underscores our ignorance.

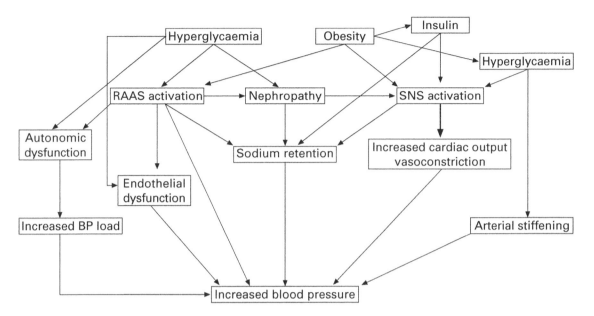

Figure 1.8
The many mechanisms contributing to an elevated blood pressure in people with diabetes.

References

1. Major SG. Blood pressure and diabetes – a statistical study. *Arch Intern Med* 1929; **44**: 797–812.
2. The National High Blood Pressure Education Programme Working Group report on hypertension in diabetes. *Hypertension* 1994; **23**: 145–58.
3. Stamler J, Vaccaro A, Neaton JD, Wentworth D. Diabetes and other risk factors and 12-year cardiovascular mortality for men screened in the Multiple Risk Factor Intervention Trial. *Diabetes Care* 1993; **263**: 2335–40.
4. Adler A, Stratton IM, Neil HAW, et al. Association of systolic blood pressure with macrovascular and microvascular complications of type two diabetes (UKPDS 36): prospective observational study. *BMJ* 2000; **321**: 412–19.
5. Williams B. The unique vulnerability of diabetic subjects to hypertensive injury. *J Hum Hyperten* 1999; **13**: 3–8.
6. Davis BR, Langford HG, Blaufox MD, et al. The association of postural changes in systolic blood pressure and mortality in persons with hypertension: The Hypertension Detection and Follow-up Program (HDFP) experience. *Circulation* 1987; **75**: 340–6.
7. Curb JD, Pressel SL, Cutler JA, et al. Effect of diuretic based antihypertensive treatment on cardiovascular risk in people with diabetes. Systolic Hypertension in Elderly Program (SHEP) Cooperative research group. *JAMA* 1996; **276**: 1886–92.
8. Hansson L, Zanchetti A, Carruthers SG, et al. Effects of intensive blood pressure lowering and low dose aspirin in patients with hypertension: principle results of the Hypertension Optimal Treatment (HOT) randomised trial. *Lancet* 1998; **351**: 1755–62.
9. Tuomilehto J, Rastenyte D, Birkenhager WH, et al. Effects of calcium channel blockade in older patients with diabetes and systolic hypertension. Systolic Hypertension in Europe Trial Investigators. *N Engl J Med* 1999; **340**: 677–84.
10. United Kingdom Prospective Diabetes Study Group. Tight blood pressure control and risk of macrovascular and microvascular complications in type 2 diabetes: UKPDS 38. *BMJ* 1998; **317**: 703–13.
11. Colhoun HM, Prescott-Clarke P. *Health Survey for England 1994.* HMSO: London, 1996.
12. Gress TW, Nieto J, Shahar E et al., for the Atherosclerosis Risk in Community (ARIC) Study. Hypertension and antihypertensive therapy as risk factors for type 2 diabetes mellitus. *N Engl J Med* 2000; **342**: 905–12.
13. Kelly RP, Hayward C, Aviolo A, O'Rourke M. Non-invasive determination of age-related changes in the human arterial pulse. *Circulation* 1989; **80**: 1652–9.
14. Bucala R, Cerami A. Advanced glycosylation: chemistry, biology and implications for diabetes and aging. *Adv Pharmacol* 1992; **23**: 1–24.
15. Valssara H, Fuh H, Makita Z, et al. Exogenous advanced glycation end-products induce complex vascular dysfunction in normal animals: a model for diabetic and aging complications. *Proc Natl Acad Sci USA* 1992; **89**: 12043–7.
16. Woolham Gl, Shner PL, Valbona BS, Hoff HE. The pulse wave velocity as an early indicator of atherosclerosis in diabetic subjects. *Circulation* 1962; **25**: 533–9.
17. The Hypertension in Diabetes Study Group. Hypertension in Diabetes Study: I. Prevalence of hypertension in newly presenting type 2 diabetic patients and the associated risk factors for cardiovascular and diabetic complications. *J Hypertens* 1993; **11**: 309–17.
18. Pacy PJ, Dodson PM, Beevers M, et al. Prevalence of hypertension in white, black and Asian diabetics in a district hospital diabetic clinic. *Diabetic Med* 1985; **2**: 125–30.
19. Rubler S, Abenavoli T, Greenblatt HA, et al. Ambulatory blood pressure monitoring in diabetic males: a method for detecting blood pressure elevations undisclosed by conventional

methods. *Clin Cardiol* 1982; **5**: 447–54.

20. White WB. Diurnal blood pressure and blood pressure variability in diabetic normotensive and hypertensive subjects. *J Hypertens* 1992; **10** (Suppl): S35–41.

21. Hansen KW, Poulsen PL, Ebbehoj E. Blood pressure elevation in diabetes: results from 24 hour ambulatory blood pressure recordings. In: *The Kidney and Hypertension in Diabetes Mellitus* (CE Mogensen, ed.). Kluwer Academic: Boston, 1998; 335–55.

22. Lurbe A, Redon J, Pascual JM, et al. Altered blood pressure during sleep in normotensive subjects with type 1 diabetes. *Hypertension* 1993; **21**: 227–35.

23. Weston PJ, James MA, Panerai RB, et al. Evidence of defective cardiovascular regulation in insulin dependent diabetic patients without clinical autonomic dysfunction. *Diabetes Res Clin Pract* 1998; **42**: 141–3.

24. Rubler S, Chu DA, Bruzzone CL. Blood pressure and heart rate responses during 24 hour ambulatory blood pressure monitoring and exercise in men with diabetes. *Am J Cardiol* 1985; **55**: 801–6.

25. Hornung RS, Mahler RF, Raftery EB. Ambulatory blood pressure and heart rate in diabetic patients: an assessment of autonomic function. *Diabetic Med* 1989; **6**: 579–85.

26. Fogari R, Zoppi A, Malamani GD, et al. Ambulatory blood pressure monitoring in normotensive and hypertensive type 2 diabetics; prevalence of impaired diurnal blood pressure patterns. *Am J Hypertens* 1993; **6**: 1–7.

27. Nielsen S, Schmitz A, Poulsen PL, et al. Albuminuria and 24-h ambulatory blood pressure in normoalbuminuric and microalbuminuric NIDDM patients. *Diabetes Care* 1995; **18**: 1434–41.

28. Mann S, Altman DG, Rafferty EB, Bannister R. Circadian variation of blood pressure in autonomic failure. *Circulation* 1988; **68**: 477–83.

29. Felici MG, Spallone V, Maiello MR, et al. Twenty-four hours blood pressure and heart rate profiles in diabetics with and without autonomic neuropathy. *Funct Neurol* 1991; **6**: 299–304.

30. Spallone V, Bernardi L, Ricordi L, et al. Relationship between the circadian rhythms of blood pressure and sympathovagal balance in diabetic autonomic neuropathy. *Diabetes* 1993; **42**: 1745–52.

31. Weston PJ, James MA, Panerai RB, et al. Abnormal baroreceptor-cardiac reflex sensitivity is not detected by conventional tests of autonomic function in patients with insulin dependent diabetes mellitus. *Clin Sci* 1996; **91**: 59–64.

32. Poulsen PL, Ebbehoj E, Hansen KW, Mogensen CE. Effects of smoking on 24-h ambulatory blood pressure and autonomic function in normoalbuminuric insulin dependent diabetic patients *Am J Hypertens* 1998; **11**: 1093–9.

33. Hansen KW, Mau Pedersen M, Marshall SM, et al. Circadian variation in blood pressure in patients with diabetic nephropathy. *Diabetologia* 1992; **35**: 1074–9.

34. Hansen KW, Christensen CK, Andersen PH, et al. Ambulatory blood pressure in microalbuminuria type 1 diabetic patients. *Kidney Int* 1992; **41**: 847–54.

35. Poulsen PL, Ebbehoj E, Hansen KW, Mogensen CE. 24-h blood pressure and autonomic function is related to albumin excretion within the normoalbuminuric range in IDDM. *Diabetic Med* 1994; **11**: 877–82.

36. Equiluz-Bruck S, Schnack C, Schemthaner G. Non-dipping of nocturnal blood pressure is related to urinary albumin excretion in patients with type 2 diabetes mellitus. *Am J Hypertens* 1996; **9**: 1139–43.

37. Hansen HP, Rossing P, Tarnow L, et al. Circadian rhythm of arterial blood pressure and albuminuria in diabetic nephropathy. *Kidney Int* 1996; **50**: 579–85.

38. Mathiesen ER, Ronn B, Jensen T, et al. Relationship between blood pressure and urinary albumin excretion in development of microalbuminuria. *Diabetes* 1990; **39**: 245–9.

39. Weidman P, Beretta-Picolli C, Trost BN. Pressor factors and responsiveness to hypertension accompanying diabetes mellitus. *Hypertension* 1985; **7** (Suppl 11): 33–42.

40. Brennan BL, Roginsky MS, Cohn S. Increased total body sodium as a mechanism for suppressed plasma renin activity in diabetes mellitus. *Clin Res* 1979; **27**: 51A.

41. O'Hare JA, Ferriss JB, Brady D, et al.

Exchangeable sodium and renin in hypertensive diabetic patients with and without nephropathy. *Hypertension* 1985; **7** (Suppl 11): 43–8.

42. Feldt-Rasmussen B, Mathiesen ER, Decjert T, et al. Central role for sodium in the pathogenesis of blood pressure changes independent of angiotensin, aldosterone and catecholamines in type 1 diabetes mellitus. *Diabetologia* 1987; **30**: 610–17.

43. Tuck ML, Corry D, Trujillo A. Salt sensitive blood pressure and exaggerated vascular reactivity in the hypertension of diabetes mellitus. *Am J Med* 1990; **88**: 210–16.

44. Firoretto P, Sambataro M, Cipollina MR, et al. Role of atrial natriuretic peptide in the pathogenesis of sodium retention in ID with and without nephropathy. *Diabetes* 1992; **41**: 936–45.

45. Weidmann P, Ferrari P, Shaw SG. Renin in diabetes mellitus. In: *The Renin Angiotensin System* (JIS Robertson and MG Nicholls, eds). Raven Press: New York, 1991; 75.1–75.26.

46. Campbell DJ. Circulating and tissue renin angiotensin systems. *J Clin Invest* 1987; **79**: 1–6.

47. Rosenberg ME, Smith LJ, Correa-Rotter, Hostetter TH. The paradox of the renin-angiotensin system in chronic renal disease. *Kidney Int* 1994; **45**: 403–10.

48. Kikkawa R, Kitamura E, Fujiwara Y, et al. Biphasic alteration of renin-angiotensin-aldosterone system in streptozotocin diabetic rats. *Renal Physiol* 1986; **9**: 187–92.

49. Anderson S, Jung FF, Ingelfinger JR. Renal renin-angiotensin system in diabetes: functional, immunohistochemical and molecular biological correlations. *Am J Physiol* 1993; **265**: F477–86.

50. Hollenberg NK. ACE inhibitors, AT1 receptor blockers and the kidney. *Nephrol Dial Transplant* 1997; **12**: 381–3.

51. Hollenberg NK, Fisher N. Renal circulation and blockade of the renin-angiotensin system. Is angiotensin converting enzyme inhibition the last word? *Hypertension* 1995; **26**: 602–9.

52. De'Oliveira JM, Proce DA, Fisher NDL, et al. Autonomy of the renin-angiotensin system in type 2 diabetes mellitus: dietary sodium and renal haemodynamic responses to ACE-inhibition. *Kidney Int* 1997; **52**: 771–7.

53. Vallance P. Nitric oxide in the human cardiovascular system. *Br J Clin Pharmacol* 1998; **45**: 433–9.

54. De Vriese AS, Verbeuren TJ, Van de Voorde J, et al. Endothelial dysfunction in diabetes. *Br J Pharmacol* 2000; **130**: 963–74.

55. Poston L, Taylor PD. Endothelium-mediated vascular function in insulin-dependent diabetes. *Clin Sci* 1995; **345**: 362–4.

56. Lekakis J, Papamichael C, Anastasiou H, et al. Endothelial dysfunction of conduit arteries in insulin-dependent diabetes without microalbuminuria. *Cardiovasc Res* 1997; **34**: 164–8.

57. Ueda S, Petrie JR, Cleeland SJ, et al. Insulin vasodilatation and the 'arginine paradox'. *Lancet* 1998; **351**: 959–60.

58. Tesfamariam B, Brown ML, Cohen RA. Elevated glucose impairs endothelium dependent relaxation by activating protein kinase C. *J Clin Invest* 1991; **87**: 1643–8.

59. Vague J. The degree of masculine differentiation of the obesities: a factor determining predisposition to diabetes, atherosclerosis, gout and uric calculous disease. *Am J Clin Nutr* 1956; **4**: 20.

60. Lapidus L, Bengtsson C, Larsson B, et al. Distribution of adipose tissue and risk of cardiovascular disease and death. *BMJ* 1984; **289**: 1257.

61. Williams B. Insulin resistance: the shape of things to come. *Lancet* 1994; **344**: 521–4.

62. Solomaa VV, Strandberg TE, Vanhanen H, et al. Glucose tolerance and blood pressure: long-term follow up of middle aged men. *BMJ* 1991; **302**: 493–6.

63. Ferrannini E. The phenomenon of insulin resistance: its possible relevance to hypertensive disease. In: *Hypertension Pathophysiology, Diagnosis and Treatment* (JH Laragh and BM Brenner, eds). Raven Press: New York, 1995; 2281–303.

64. Medalie JH, Papier CM, Goldbourt U, Herman JB. Major factors in the development of diabetes mellitus in 10,000 men. *Arch Intern Med* 1975; **135**: 811–17.

65. Welborn TA, Breckenridge A, Rubenstein AH, et al. Serum insulin in essential hypertension and in peripheral vascular disease. *Lancet* 1996; **1**: 1366–7.

66. Singer CB, Lucas P, Estigarribia JA, et al. Insulin and blood pressure in obesity. *Hypertension* 1985; **7**: 702–6.

67. Ferranini E, Haffner SM, Stern MP, et al. High blood pressure and insulin resistance: influence of genetic background. *Eur J Clin Invest* 1991; **21**: 280–6.

68. Williams B. Westernised Asians and cardiovascular disease: nature or nurture? *Lancet* 1995; **345**: 401–2.

69. Young JB, Landsberg L. Suppression of sympathetic nervous system during fasting. *Science* 1977; **196**: 1473.

70. Young JB, Landsberg L. Stimulation of the sympathetic nervous system during sucrose feeding. *Nature* 1977; **269**: 615.

71. Landsberg L. Diet, obesity and hypertension. A hypothesis involving insulin, the sympathetic nervous system and adaptive thermogenesis. *Q J Med* 1986; **236**: 1081.

72. Landsberg L, Young JB. Insulin-mediated glucose metabolism in the relationship between dietary intake and sympathetic nervous system activity. *Int J Obesity* 1985; **9** (Suppl 2): 63.

73. Landsberg L, Young JB. The role of sympathoadrenal system in modulating energy expenditure. *Clin Endocrinol Metab* 1984; **13**: 475.

74. O'Hare JA, Minaker KL, Meneilly GS, et al. Effect of insulin on plasma norepinephrine and 3,4 dihydroxyphenylalanine in obese men. *Metabolism* 1989; **38**: 322.

75. Grassi GH, Seravalle G, Cattaneo BM, et al. Sympathetic activation in obese normotensive subjects. *Hypertension* 1995; **25**: 560.

76. Williams B. Mechanical influences on vascular smooth muscle cell function. *J Hypertens* 1998; **16**: 1921–9.

77. Danne T, Spiro MJ, Spiro RG. Effect of high glucose on type IV collagen production by cultured glomerular epithelial, endothelial and mesangial cells. *Diabetes* 1993; **42**: 170–7.

78. O'Callaghan CO, Williams B. The regulation of human vascular smooth muscle extracellular matrix protein production by α- and β-adrenoceptor stimulation. *J Hypertens* 2002; **20**: 287–94.

79. Williams B. Mechanical influences on vascular smooth muscle cell function. *J Hypertens* 1998; **16**: 1921–9.

80. Lakatta E-G. Cardiovascular regulatory mechanisms in advanced age. *Physiol Rev* 1993; **73**: 413–67.

81. O'Rourke MF, Gallagher DE. Pulse wave analysis. *J Hypertens* 1996; **14** (Suppl 5): S147–57.

82. Brown MJ, Castaigne A, de-Leeuw PW, et al. Influences of diabetes and type of hypertension on response to antihypertensive treatment. *Hypertension* 2000; **35**: 1038–42.

2

Hypertension, macrovascular disease and diabetes mellitus: perspectives from the Framingham Study

William B Kannel and Peter WF Wilson

Introduction

Persistent inappropriate elevations of blood pressure and blood glucose are ominous harbingers of both small vessel and large vessel arteriosclerotic cardiovascular disease.[1-5] Because of their high prevalence in the general population, and their independent impact on the incidence of atherosclerotic cardiovascular disease, these conditions deserve a high priority for detection and treatment to prevent coronary disease, strokes, peripheral artery disease and cardiac failure. Hypertension and glucose intolerance appear to be metabolically linked and each plays a major and independent role in promoting accelerated atherogenesis. Adult onset type II diabetes is the most common variety of diabetes that affects the incidence of large vessel atherosclerotic disease. Interest in hyperglycaemia in adults has expanded to include lesser degrees of glucose intolerance, hyperinsulinaemia and insulin resistance and both are postulated to be components of an insulin resistance syndrome.[6] Atherosclerotic cardiovascular disease has replaced malignant hypertension and diabetic acidosis and coma as the feared outcomes of hypertension and diabetes. It may well be that insulin resistance is the common link between large vessel atherosclerosis, thrombogenesis, hypertension, obesity and diabetes.[7] As the population ages, the prevalence of these conditions will increase. Diabetic patients are prone to develop hypertension and hypertensive patients to develop diabetes. This chapter provides a contemporary perspective on the interaction of hypertension, insulin resistance and glucose intolerance as promoters of large vessel atherosclerotic disease and the implications for optimal preventive management of both hypertensive and diabetic patients.

Prevalence

The prevalence of type II diabetes in white Americans increases steeply with age from 0.5 per cent at age 20–44 years to 10 per cent at age 65–74 years (Fig. 2.1). Type I diabetes is much less prevalent, peaking at puberty with a lifetime prevalence of only 0.5 per cent.[8] Approximately half of type II diabetes goes undetected unless glucose tolerance testing is routinely done (Fig. 2.1).[9] The prevalence of lesser degrees of glucose intolerance is also largely undetected and increases steeply with age. The prevalence of this potentially dangerous impaired glucose tolerance often equals the prevalence of type II diabetes in middle-aged adults.[9] Approximately 10 per cent of young adults have some degree of glucose intolerance either manifested as overt diabetes or impaired glucose tolerance. This proportion rises to >40 per cent after age 65 years (Fig. 2.1). The prevalence of type II diabetes

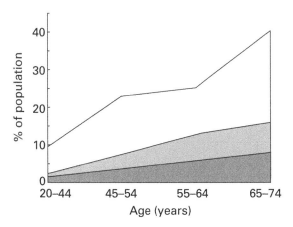

Figure 2.1
Prevalence of type II diabetes and impaired glucose tolerance (IGT) in the USA, 1976–1980.[9] (☐), IGT; (▨), undiagnosed type II diabetes; (▩), diagnosed type II diabetes.

also varies widely by region and ethnic origin. Its occurrence ranges from 10 to 15 per cent in the Americas and Europe, whereas it affects >50 per cent of Nauru Islanders in the South Pacific and Pima Indians in Arizona (Fig. 2.2). It does not necessarily follow, however, that the areas of increased diabetes prevalence have high rates of coronary disease.

The prevalence of diabetes in the USA has increased alarmingly and is now about three times as common as it was in 1958. This increase has been noted for all age groups greater than 45 years (Fig. 2.3). This increase has also been noted in the Framingham Study, even taking into account increased use of diuretic therapy in the population over the years.[7]

Diabetes is significantly more prevalent in persons with hypertension and its prevalence increases the more elevated the blood pressure (Table 2.1). In normotensive persons aged 35–64 years in the Framingham Study only 4.3 per cent of men and 2.1 per cent of women had diabetes. On the other hand, among hypertensive persons with pressures of ≥160/95 mmHg, the prevalence of diabetes in either sex was about 6.3 per cent. In persons over the age of 65 years the prevalence of diabetes in normotensive men and women respectively was 14 per cent and 10 per cent, whereas in those with this degree of hypertension (>160/95) the prevalence was 20 per cent and 15 per cent respectively.

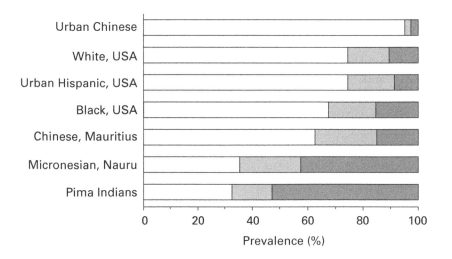

Figure 2.2
Prevalence of diabetes and impaired glucose tolerance (IGT) in adults (standardised to 30–64 years, both sexes combined). (☐), normal; (▨), IGT; (▩), diabetes mellitus. (From: King H, Rewers M. Global estimates for prevalence of diabetes mellitus and impaired glucose tolerance in adults. WHO Ad Hoc Diabetes Report Group. Diabetes Care 1993; 16: 157–77.)

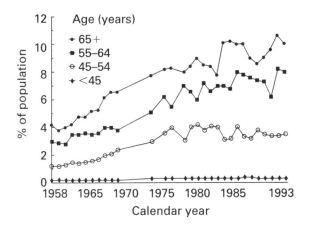

Figure 2.3
Time trends in the percentage of the population with diagnosed diabetes, by age: USA, 1958–1993. (From: Kenny SJ, Aubert RE, Geiss LS. Prevalence and incidence of non-insulin dependent diabetes. In: Harris MI, ed. Diabetes in America, 2nd edn. Bethesda, NIH, 1995: 47–68.)

Prevalence estimates from the National Health and Nutrition Examination Survey III indicate that there are 50 million adults in the USA, and one in every four adults who have hypertension defined at pressures of >140/95 mmHg.[10] The prevalence of hypertension increases with age from about 4 per cent

at age 18–24 years to 65 per cent at age 80 years or more (Fig. 2.4). Hypertension prevalence is lower in women than men until middle age, after which it is higher in women. With advancing age there is a disproportionate rise in systolic pressure resulting in a steeply rising prevalence of isolated systolic hypertension which characterises 60–65 per cent of the hypertension in the elderly. Hypertension is substantially more prevalent in diabetics than in non-diabetics. In the Framingham Study, about 50 per cent of diabetics had some degree of hypertension, a rate double that of non-diabetics of the same age (Table 2.1).[7]

Risk factor clustering

Both hypertension and diabetes show a distinct tendency to cluster with other metabolically linked risk factors. A tendency for hypertension to cluster with other risk factors has long been noted.[11,12] A metabolic basis for this clustering has been postulated[13–15] and many of the risk factors that tend to cluster with hypertension also predict its occurrence.[11,12] The extent of clustering of the hypertension with diabetes and other risk factors greatly influences its large vessel atherogenic potential. In individuals with elevated

| | Age 35–64 years | | | Age 65–94 years | | |
	Normal	*Mild*	*Moderate+*	*Normal*	*Mild*	*Moderate+*
Men	4.3%	4.7%	6.3%	14.0%	14.6%	20.1%
Women	2.1%	4.1%	6.4%	10.2%	12.2%	15.2%

Prevalence rates are age-adjusted. Trends significant at P<0.01. Mild HBP, ≥140/90 mmHg; moderate, ≥160/95 mmHg.

Table 2.1
Prevalence of diabetes by hypertensive status (1970–1982, Framingham Study).

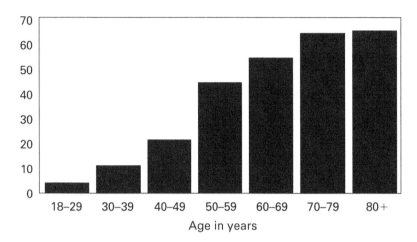

Figure 2.4
Hypertension prevalence by age (%): civilian non-institutionalised population, 1988–1991. Hypertension is defined as the average of three blood pressure measurements ≥140/90 mmHg on a single occasion or reported taking of antihypertensive medication. Source: Centers for Disease Control, National Center for Health Statistics, Third National Health and Nutrition Examination Survey, 1988–1991.

Diabetic status	Age-adjusted % prevalence	
	Men	Women
Non-diabetic	26.7	27.8
Diabetic	47.6*	51.8*
All subjects	28.9	29.6

HBP, ≥140/90 mmHg; *$P<0.001$.[6]

Table 2.2
Prevalence of hypertension by diabetic status (Framingham Study: subjects aged 55–64 years, exam 13).

blood pressure, clusters of three or more additional risk factors (including elevated blood glucose) occurred in 22 per cent of men and 27 per cent of women, a rate more than four times that expected by chance (Table 2.3).

Diabetes also tends to cluster with these other risk factors. Thus, diabetics tend to have higher blood pressures, be more obese, and have a variety of other abnormalities. The latter include higher triglycerides and VLDL-cholesterol, reduced HDL-cholesterol, adverse total/HDL cholesterol ratios, higher uric acid

and haematocrit values and twice as much left ventricular hypertrophy as persons of the same age without diabetes (Table 2.4).

Possible determinants of the observed risk factor clustering in diabetic and hypertensive persons include insulin resistance, abdominal obesity and autonomic imbalance.[13-15] Obesity and weight gain have been identified as important determinants of both hypertension and diabetes.[16] Abdominal obesity, promoting insulin resistance and abnormal sympatho-adrenal activity, has been implicated as a

Number of additional risk factors	Prevalence (%)	
	Men	Women
None	22	18
One	29	28
Two or more	49	54
Three or more	22	27

Prevalence is age-adjusted; HBP, ≥138 mmHg (men); ≥130 mmHg (women). Other risk factors are top quintile of total cholesterol, BMI, triglycerides, glucose and bottom quintile of HDL-cholesterol.

Table 2.3
Clustering of other risk factors with elevated blood pressure (Framingham Offspring Study, subjects aged 30–65 years).

Risk factors	Men Diabetes		Women Diabetes	
	Present	Absent	Present	Absent
Glucose (mg/dl)	147‡	87	134‡	86
Systolic BP	145‡	137	149‡	140
BMI (kg/m^2)	27.4‡	26.0	28.0‡	25.4
HTC (%)	46.6‡	45.2	43.9	41.9
Uric acid (mg/dl)	5.3‡	4.9	4.4‡	3.9
LVH (%)	14.5†	7.1	12.4‡	5.8
Cigarettes (%)	35.6*	43.0	32.3	33.6
Total cholesterol (mg/dl)	223	223	248	243
HDL-cholesterol (mg/dl)	42.1‡	46.1	53.0‡	57.6
LDL-cholesterol (mg/dl)	138	143	156	156
VLDL-cholesterol (mg/dl)	37.3‡	30.1	33.1‡	27.9
Total/HDL ratio	5.3†	4.8	4.7†	4.2

BMI, body mass index; HTC, hematocrit; LVH, left ventricular hypertrophy.
*$P<0.05$; †$P<0.01$; ‡$P<0.001$.

Table 2.4
Comparison of cardiovascular risk factors in diabetics versus non-diabetics, Framingham Study (age-adjusted means).

major instigator of accelerated atherogenesis in diabetes and hypertension.[17,18] It has been estimated that about 50 per cent of hyperten-sive persons have some degree of insulin resis-tance.[19,20] Abnormalities of lipoprotein metab-olism, insulin resistance and glucose tolerance

Men BMI (kg/m²)	Average number of risk factors	Women BMI (kg/m²)	Average number of risk factors
<23.7	1.65 (±0.91)	<20.8	1.80 (±0.87)
23.7–25.5	1.85 (±0.95)	20.8–22.3	2.00 (±1.02)
25.6–27.2	2.06 (±1.05)	22.4–23.9	2.22 (±1.06)
27.3–29.5	2.28 (±1.09)	24.0–26.8	2.20 (±0.99)
>29.5	2.35 (±1.08)	>26.8	2.66 (±1.09)

Other risk factors include: top quintiles of total cholesterol, BMI, triglycerides, glucose and bottom quintile of HDL-cholesterol.

Table 2.5
Risk factor clustering according to body mass index (Framingham Offspring Study, subjects aged 18–74 years with elevated blood pressure).

are common in persons with essential hypertension, even in their normotensive first-degree relatives.[14] Weight gain worsens all the elements of the insulin resistance syndrome, including glucose intolerance and hypertension, and weight loss improves them (Table 2.5).[21]

Whatever the cause of risk factor clustering in persons with either hypertension or diabetes, it is evident that these conditions seldom occur in isolation and that when confronted with patients with either condition, it is prudent to screen for the presence of the other metaboli-

cally linked atherogenic traits which are likely to be present 75–80 per cent of the time.

Atherosclerotic hazards

Hypertension and diabetes each independently predispose to the development of large vessel atherosclerotic cardiovascular disease. Risk of such cardiovascular events increases in a continuous graded fashion with the blood pressure, even within the range of blood pressures usually considered normotensive (Fig. 2.5). It

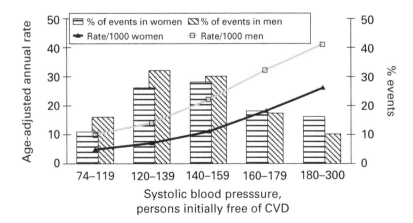

Figure 2.5
Risk of cardiovascular events by level of systolic blood pressure, 38-year follow-up: Framingham Study, subjects aged 35–64 years. (From: Kannel WB. Cardiovascular risk assessment in hypertension. In: Braunwald E, Hollenberg N, eds. Atlas of heart diseases. Hypertension: mechanisms and therapy, vol II. Philadelphia, Current Medicine, 1998; 5.1–5.16)

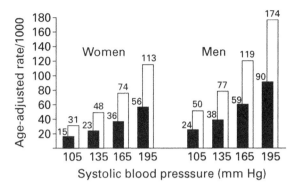

Figure 2.6
Risk of cardiovascular events according to systolic blood pressure and diabetic status. Framingham Study, 26-year follow-up, cholesterol 185 mg/dl, no left ventricular hypertrophy, non-smokers: (■), non-diabetic subjects; (□), diabetic subjects.

is important to recognise that a substantial proportion of the cardiovascular events promoted by hypertension occur at blood pressures in the high normal and mild blood pressure elevations. This is particularly important when there is coexistent diabetes, because at any level of blood pressure the risk of a cardiovascular event is doubled when glucose intolerance is present (Fig. 2.6). In general, persons with blood pressures of $\geqslant 140/90$ mmHg have a 2–4-fold increased risk of developing atherosclerotic cardiovascular events such as coronary disease, strokes, peripheral artery disease or cardiac failure (Table 2.6). The incidence of coronary disease in hypertensive persons equals that of all the other diseases combined, making it the chief and most lethal hazard to be prevented. Although the absolute risk imposed by hypertension in women is only half that of men, the relative risk, comparing hypertensives with

Cardiovascular events	Age-adjusted biennial rate/1000		Age-adjusted risk ratio		Excess risk/1000	
	Men	Women	Men	Women	Men	Women
Coronary heart disease	45	21	2.0*	2.2*	23	12
Stroke	12	6	3.8*	2.6*	9	4
Peripheral arterial disease	10	7	2.0*	3.7*	5	5
Cardiac failure	14	6	4.0*	3.0*	10	4
Cardiovascular events	65	35	2.2*	2.5*	36	21

*$P < 0.0001$.

Table 2.6
Risk of cardiovascular events in subjects with hypertension: 36-year follow-up (Framingham study, persons aged 35–64 years).

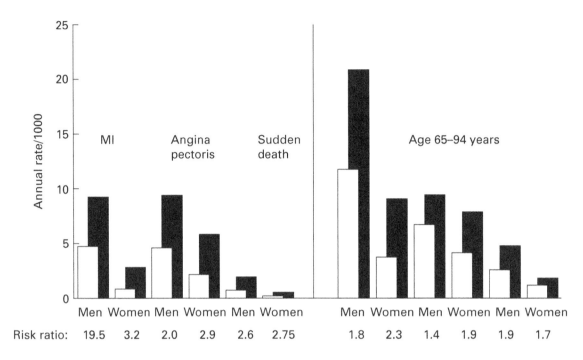

Figure 2.7
Risk of clinical manifestations of coronary disease by hypertensive status (≥140/90 mmHg). Framingham Study, 40-year follow-up. (□), non-high blood pressure; (■), high blood pressure (≥140/90 mmHg). MI, myocardial infarction.

normotensives within each sex, is similar in men and women. Hypertensive persons with diabetes are a particularly high risk segment of the population because of the doubling of cardiovascular disease imposed by glucose intolerance.

Hypertension predisposes to all of the clinical manifestations of coronary disease, including angina pectoris, myocardial infarction and sudden death (Fig. 2.7). Although the absolute risk is lower in women, the risk ratios for all varieties are larger in women. As currently defined, the impact of hypertension on the development of cardiovascular disease (2.2–2.5 risk ratios for men and women) is somewhat lower than that for diabetes

(2.2–3.7 risk ratios for men and women). The attributable risk for coronary disease is substantially greater for hypertension than for diabetes. Because of the much higher prevalence of hypertension in the population, 38–55 per cent of cardiovascular events are attributable to hypertension, whereas only 4–5 per cent are attributable to overt diabetes.

In addition to coronary and cerebrovascular diseases, diabetes also predisposes to peripheral artery disease and heart failure (Table 2.7). The absolute risk is greatest for coronary disease, but the relative risk is greatest with heart failure. The relative risk, comparing diabetic with non-diabetic individuals within each sex, is substantially greater in women than

Cardiovascular events	Age-adjusted biennial rate/1000		Age-adjusted risk ratio		Excess risk/1000	
	Men	Women	Men	Women	Men	Women
Coronary heart disease	39	21	1.5*	2.2**	12	12
Stroke	15	6	2.9**	2.6**	10	4
Peripheral arterial disease	18	18	3.4**	6.4**	13	15
Cardiac failure	23	21	4.4**	7.8**	18	18
Cardiovascular events	76	65	2.2**	3.7**	42	47

*P<0.001, **P<0.0001.

Table 2.7
Risk of cardiovascular events in diabetics: 36-year follow-up (Framingham study, persons aged 35–64 years).

men for all the cardiovascular disease outcomes except stroke. Diabetes tends to eliminate the female advantage women have over men as candidates for all cardiovascular disease (Table 2.7).

Diabetes, as well as hypertension, is associated with an increased risk of all clinical manifestations of coronary disease including angina, myocardial infarction and sudden death.[22] The risk ratios are larger for myocardial infarction than angina in women, but not in men (Fig. 2.8). Risk ratios imposed by diabetes are greater in women than men for specific clinical manifestations of coronary disease, including coronary mortality, myocardial infarction and angina pectoris.[23]

Despite the fact that myocardial infarction size is usually no greater in diabetics than non-diabetics, early mortality, cardiogenic shock, myocardial rupture and rhythm disturbances appear to occur more often in diabetics.[24–27] Heart failure, postinfarction angina, infarct extension and death have been found to be more common in diabetics than non-diabetics during hospitalisation for myocardial infarction.[27]

More extensive coronary artery disease and myocardial lesions have been reported in diabetics than non-diabetics and diabetic hearts have low capillary densities.[28,29] Diabetics are also reported to have higher rates of restenosis after angioplasty than non-diabetics and those with more severe diabetes and poor glycaemic control have worse long-term outcome after coronary artery bypass grafting (CABG).[30,31]

Population studies consistently report an increased prevalence of unrecognised or silent myocardial infarctions in diabetics.[32] Myocardial ischaemia provoked by exercise testing may be more likely to be painless in diabetics than non-diabetics,[33,34] although all studies do not concur.[35,36] An increased propensity to unrecognised myocardial infarctions has also been observed in diabetic participants from

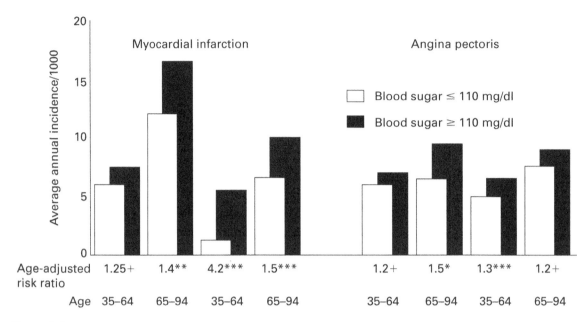

Figure 2.8
*Risk of myocardial infarction and angina pectoris according to hyperglycaemia status. Framingham Study, 30-year follow-up. (□), blood sugar ⩽ 110 mg/dl; (■), blood sugar ⩾ 110 mg/dl. +, not significant; *P<0.05; **P<0.01; ***P<0.001.*

the Framingham Study, but only in men (Table 2.8). The proportion of infarctions that went unrecognised in women was actually substantially lower in diabetics than non-diabetics.

Less well appreciated is the fact that hypertensive persons of either sex are also predisposed to silent or unrecognised myocardial infarctions. In the Framingham Study, half of all infarctions in hypertensive women went unrecognised. In men, about 38 per cent of infarctions went unrecognised, a proportion twice that of non-hypertensives. Thus the diabetic propensity to myocardial infarction may be confined to men, whereas hypertensive patients of both sexes are at greater risk of silent or unrecognised infarctions.[7] Hypertensive men aged 35–64 years who also have dia-

betes further increase their risk of silent infarction two-fold (Fig. 2.9).[7] The increased risk of unrecognised infarction in hypertensive persons was found to hold even when those who were on treatment, had left ventricular hypertrophy or were diabetic were excluded.[37] Because both hypertensive and diabetic patients are each particularly prone to silent or unrecognised myocardial infarctions, a high degree of vigilance with routine periodic electrocardiogram (ECG) examinations is mandatory in patients who have both these conditions.

Heart failure is a common end-stage of hypertension and diabetes. Hypertension and coronary disease are the dominant causes, but 24 per cent of men and 28 per cent of women who had hypertensive heart failure in the

Glucose intolerance	Men		Women	
	All MI	Unrecognised	All MI	Unrecognised
Absent	13.1	3.2	3.8	1.4
Present	24.8	9.7	13.8	2.4
Risk ratio	1.8*	3.0***	3.6***	1.7+
Percentage unrecognised				
Without glucose intolerance		18	37	
With glucose intolerance		39	17	

Table 2.8
Unrecognised myocardial infarction according to glucose intolerance (Framingham Study, subjects aged 35–44 years, 26-year follow-up). +, not significant; *p<0.05; ***p<0.001.

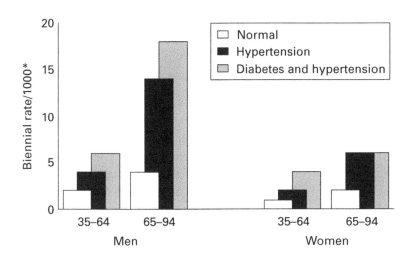

Figure 2.9
Risk of unrecognised myocardial infarction by hypertensive and diabetic status. Framingham Study, 30-year follow-up. *Age- and risk factor-adjusted.

Framingham Study had diabetes on the examination prior to their developing failure.[38] In persons with hypertension, diabetes increases the risk of their developing heart failure 1.8-fold in men and 3.6-fold in women (Table 2.9). Despite its similar age and risk factor adjusted risk ratio, diabetes is relatively uncommon among those who experience a myocardial infarction.[39] Heart failure in diabetics may be due to epicardial coronary disease resulting in association with a myocardial infarction, long-standing hypertension or

Risk factor	Sex	Age- and risk factor-adjusted hazard ratio† (95% CI)
Myocardial infarction	M	5.54 (3.96–7.77)
	F	5.99 (4.33–8.27)
Angina pectoris	M	1.35 (0.95–1.92)
	F	1.71 (1.25–2.34)
Diabetes	M	1.78 (1.23–2.59)
	F	3.57 (2.59–4.94)
Left ventricular hypertrophy	M	1.97 (1.31–2.96)
	F	2.80 (1.93–4.05)
Valvular heart disease	M	2.40 (1.62–3.56)
	F	1.96 (1.41–2.73)

*Based on 165 congestive heart failure events in 1707 men and 192 events in 2118 women with hypertension prior to congestive heart failure. Based on dynamic model with reclassification of hypertension and risk factors at each follow-up examination. CI, confidence interval.
†Adjusted for angina pectoris, myocardial infarction, diabetes, left ventricular hypertrophy and valvular heart disease.

Table 2.9
*Risk factors for congestive heart failure among hypertensive subjects**

microvascular disease.[40] Diabetics dying of heart failure have been reported to have myocardial arteriolar thickening, microaneurysms and basement membrane thickening lesions that are typical of diabetic angiopathy.[29] Diastolic dysfunction characterised by increased left ventricular end diastolic pressure, reduced end diastolic volume and normal ejection fraction, is more common in diabetics and may precede progressive impairment of systolic function that is characteristic of the later stage.[41]

Failure in the hypertensive diabetic may be due to a cardiomyopathy induced by insulin resistance.[40] Echocardiographic evidence of increased left ventricular wall thickness and mass has been reported in the Framingham Study diabetics.[42] Insulin resistance has been reported to be a determinant of left ventricular mass even in non-diabetics.[43] Diabetics have also been found to have a depressed ejection fraction and a subnormal increase in this indicator of left ventricular function in response to exercise.[41] It is difficult to know how much of the impaired cardiac function and heart failure in the diabetic is due to more severe coronary disease and hypertension, and how much is attributable to a primary diabetic cardiomyopathy.

Preventive implications

Four decades of epidemiological research indicate that both hypertension and diabetes are powerful and independent predisposing factors for large vessel atherosclerotic disease in all vascular territories. Evidence now indicates that levels of impaired glucose tolerance and blood pressure formerly considered innocuous are important contributors to accelerated atherogenesis. It is now apparent that hypertension is a common problem in the diabetic patient and that many hypertensive persons have impaired glucose tolerance and insulin resistance. Both hypertension and diabetes are often accompanied by a cluster of atherogenic risk factors promoted by abdominal obesity and weight gain, now characterised as an insulin resistance syndrome. The presence of either hypertension or diabetes should trigger a search for the other metabolically linked risk factors, one or more of which is present most of the time. The risk of clinical large vessel atherosclerosis in hypertensive individuals is worsened when concomitant diabetes is present. Such risk escalates even further when the other risk factors that tend to cluster with either of these conditions are also present. The

risk of developing macrovascular cardiovascular sequelae of either of these conditions (e.g. coronary disease) varies widely depending on the accompanying risk factors (Figs 2.10 and 2.11). This is an important consideration in assessing the treatment requirements for diabetic or hypertensive patients encountered in clinical practice. Patients with hypertension and diabetes are especially vulnerable to large vessel atherosclerotic sequelae, making the control of the blood pressure elevation and the often accompanying dyslipidaemia particularly important. The best opportunity for preventing the macrovascular disease of diabetes lies in the management of the associated risk factors. For hypertensive patients with diabetes or glucose intolerance, the blood pressure should be reduced to ≤130/85 mmHg. Obesity is common in middle-aged Americans and especially so in those who develop hypertension and diabetes. All the atherogenic accompaniments of hypertension and diabetes, as well as these conditions themselves, can be

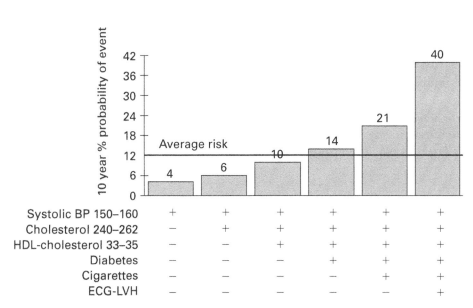

Figure 2.10
Probability of CHD event in mild hypertension by intensity of associated risk factors. Framingham Study, men aged 45 years. (From: Kannel WB. Epidemiology of essential hypertension. Proc R Coll Phys Edin 1991; 21: 273–87.)

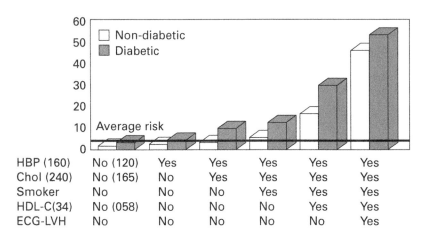

HBP (160)	No (120)	Yes	Yes	Yes	Yes	Yes
Chol (240)	No (165)	No	Yes	Yes	Yes	Yes
Smoker	No	No	No	Yes	Yes	Yes
HDL-C(34)	No (058)	No	No	No	Yes	Yes
ECG-LVH	No	No	No	No	No	Yes

Figure 2.11
Risk of CHD by diabetic status according to level of other factors. Framingham Study, 50-year-old women. HBP, high blood pressure; Chol, cholesterol; Smoker, cigarette smoker; HDL-C, HDL-cholesterol; ECG-LVH, left ventricular hypertrophy on ECG.

improved by weight reduction (Table 2.5). Of particular relevance to the atherosclerosis-prone hypertensive or diabetic patient, obesity promotes rises in low-density lipoprotein (LDL)-cholesterol, triglyceride, blood glucose, blood pressure, uric acid, left ventricular mass and reductions in HDL-cholesterol and insulin sensitivity. Weight control and exercise are major features of a preventive programme for hypertensive and diabetic candidates for atherosclerotic cardiovascular disease.

No antihypertensive agent is specifically prohibited for use in diabetic hypertensive patients, but ACE inhibitors and alpha-blockers appear to have certain advantages, including a tendency to decrease insulin resistance or benefit proteinuria in patients with diabetic renal disease and retard deleterious ventricular remodelling. Diuretic-induced hypokalaemia may further impair glucose tolerance, and beta-blockers may also worsen glucose intolerance and mask hypoglycaemic symptoms. Alpha-blockers may aggravate postural hypotension and ACE-inhibitors can induce hyperkalaemia.

It is essential to treat hypertension urgently in those who have any hint of impaired glucose tolerance. The often associated dyslipidaemia, characterised by an elevated triglyceride and reduced HDL-cholesterol, should be sought out and corrected with a statin or fibrate drug. Multivariate assessment before and after treatment, using cardiovascular risk profiles, provides the best clinical indication of success in improving the underlying insulin resistance.[44,45]

References

1. Kannel WB, McGee DL. Diabetes and cardio-vascular risk factors: the Framingham Study. *Circulation* 1979; **59**: 8–13.
2. Ruderman NB, Haudenshild C. Diabetes as an atherogenic factor. *Prog Cardiovasc Dis* 1984; **26**: 373–400.
3. Fuller JH, Shipley MJ, Rose G, Jarrett RJ, Keen H. Coronary heart disease risk and impaired glucose tolerance: the Whitehall Study. *Lancet* 1980; **1**: 1373–6.
4. Kannel WB. Risk factors in hypertension. *J Cardiovasc Pharmacol* 1989; **13** (Suppl 1): 4–10.
5. Adler A, Stratton IM, Neil HAW, et al. Association of systolic blood pressure with macrovascular and microvascular complications of type two diabetes (UKPDS 36): Prospective observational study. *BMJ* 2000; **321**: 412–19.
6. Reaven GM. Role of insulin resistance in human disease (syndrome X): an expanded definition. *Annu Rev Med* 1993; **44**: 121–31.
7. Kannel WB, Wilson PWF, Zhang T-J. The epidemiology of impaired glucose tolerance and hypertension. *Am Heart J* 1991; **121**: 1268–73.
8. Atkinson MA, Maclaren NK. The pathogenesis of insulin-dependent diabetes mellitus. *N Engl J Med* 1994; **331**: 1428–36.
9. Harris MI, Hadden WC, Knowler WC, Bennett PH. Prevalence of diabetes and impaired glucose tolerance and plasma glucose levels in US population aged 20–74 yrs. *Diabetes* 1987; **36**: 523–34.
10. The fifth report of the Joint National Committee on detection, evaluation and treatment of high blood pressure. National High Blood Pressure Education Program. National Institutes of Health. National Heart Lung and Blood Institute, 1993: NIH Publication No. 93-1088.
11. Kannel WB. Potency of vascular risk factors as the basis for antihypertensive therapy. *Eur Heart J* 1992; **13** (Suppl G): 34–42.
12. Kannel WB. Implications of Framingham Study data for treatment of hypertension: impact of other risk factors. In: Laragh JH, Buhler FR, Seldin DW, eds. *Frontiers in hypertension research*. New York, Springer-Verlag, 1981: 17–21.
13. Weber MA, Smith DH, Neutel JM, Graettinger WF. Cardiovascular and metabolic characteristics of hypertension. *Am J Med* 1991; **91**: 4S–10S.
14. Reaven GM, Chen YD. Insulin resistance, its consequences and coronary disease. Must we choose one culprit? [editorial comment]. *Circulation* 1996; **93**: 1780–3.
15. Julius S, Gudbrandsson T, Jamerson K, Andersson O. The interconnection between sympathetics, microcirculation and insulin resistance in hypertension. *Blood Press* 1992; **1**: 9–19.
16. Garrison RJ, Kannel WB, Stokes J, Castelli WP. Incidence and precursors of hypertension in young adults: the Framingham Offspring Study. *Prev Med* 1987; **16**: 234–51.
17. Despres JP. Abdominal obesity as important component of insulin-resistance syndrome. *Nutrition* 1993; **9**: 452–9.
18. Gray RJ, Matloff JM, Canklin CM, et al. Perioperative myocardial infarction: late clinical course after coronary artery bypass surgery. *Circulation* 1982; **66**: 1185–9.
19. Reaven GM. Insulin resistance, hyperinsulinemia, and hypertriglyceridemia in the etiology and clinical course of hypertension. *Am J Med* 1991; **90**: 7S–12S.
20. Pollare T, Lithel H, Berne C. A comparison of the effects of hydrochlorothiazide and captopril on glucose and lipid metabolism in patients with hypertension. *N Engl J Med* 1989; **321**: 868–73.
21. Stamler R, Stamler J, Grimm R, et al. Nutritional therapy for high blood pressure. Final report of a four year randomized controlled trial: the Hypertension Control Program. *JAMA* 1987; **257**: 1484–91.
22. Cupples LA, D'Agostino RB. Some risk factors related to the annual incidence of cardiovascu-

lar disease and death using pooled repeated biennial measurements: The Framingham Study, 30 year follow-up. In: Kannel WB, Wolf PA, Garrison RJ, eds. The Framingham Study: an epidemiological investigation of cardiovascular disease. Bethesda, MD, National Heart, Lung and Blood Institute, 1987: (NIH) Publication No. 87-2703.

23. Barrett-Conner EL, Cohen BA, Wingard DL, Edelstein SL. Why is diabetes mellitus a stronger risk factor in women than in men? *JAMA* 1991; **265**: 627–32.

24. Stone PH, Muller JE, Hartwell T, et al. The effect of diabetes mellitus on prognosis of serial left ventricular function after acute myocardial infarction: contribution of both coronary disease and diastolic left ventricular dysfunction to the adverse prognosis. The MILIS Study Group. *J Am Coll Cardiol* 1989; **14**: 49–57.

25. Woods KL, Samanta A, Burden AC. Diabetes mellitus as a risk factor for acute myocardial infarction in Asians and Europeans. *Br Heart J* 1989; **62**: 118–22.

26. Herlitz J, Malmberg K, Karlson BW, Ryden L, Hjalmarson A. Mortality and morbidity during a five-year follow-up of diabetics with myocardial infarction. *Acta Med Scand* 1988; **224**: 31–8.

27. Hands ME, Rutherford JD, Muller JE, et al. The in-hospital development of cardiogenic shock after myocardial infarction: incidence, predictors of occurrence, outcome and prognostic factors. The MILIS Study Group. *J Am Coll Cardiol* 1989; **14**: 40–6, 47–8.

28. Burchiel CM, Reed DM, Marcus EB, Strong JP, Hayashi T. Association of diabetes mellitus with coronary atherosclerosis and myocardial lesions. An autopsy study from the Honolulu Heart Program. *Am J Epidemiol* 1993; **137**: 1328–40.

29. Yarom R, Zirkin H, Stammler G, Rose AG. Human coronary microvessels in diabetes and ischemia. Morphometric study of autopsy material. *J Pathol* 1992; **166**: 265–70.

30. Stein B, Weintraub WS, Gebhart SB, et al. Influence of diabetes mellitus on early and late outcome after percutaneous transluminal coronary angioplasty. *Circulation* 1995; **91**: 979–89.

31. Lawrie GM, Morris GC Jr, Glaeser DH. Influence of diabetes mellitus on the results of coronary bypass surgery. Follow-up of 212 diabetic patients 10 to 15 years after surgery. *JAMA* 1986; **256**: 2967–71.

32. Wingard DL, Barrett-Conner EL. Heart disease and diabetes. In: Harris MI, ed. *Diabetes in America*. Bethesda, National Institutes of Health, 1995: 429–48.

33. Murray DP, O'Brien T, Mulrooney R, et al. Autonomic dysfunction and silent myocardial ischemia on exercise testing in diabetes mellitus. *Diabetic Med* 1990; **7**: 580–4.

34. Nesto RW, Phillips RT, Kett KG, et al. Angina and exertional myocardial ischemia in diabetic and non-diabetic patients: assessment by exercise thallium scintigraphy. *Ann Int Med* 1988; **108**: 170–5.

35. Callaham PR, Frolicher VF, Klein J, et al. Exercise-induced silent ischemia: age, diabetes mellitus, previous myocardial infarction and prognosis. *J Am Coll Cardiol* 1989; **14**: 1175–80.

36. Chipkin SR, Frid D, Alpert JS, et al. Frequency of painless myocardial ischemia during exercise tolerance testing in patients with and without diabetes mellitus. *Am J Cardiol* 1987; **59**: 61–5.

37. Kannel WB, Dannenberg AL, Abbott RD. Unrecognized myocardial infarction and hypertension: the Framingham Study. *Am Heart J* 1985; **109**: 581–5.

38. Levy D, Larson MG, Vasan RS, Kannel WB, Ho KL. The progression from hypertension to congestive heart failure. *JAMA* 1996; **275**: 1557–62.

39. Abbott RD, Donahue RP, Kannel WB, Wilson PWF. The impact of diabetes on survival following myocardial infarction in men versus women. The Framingham Study. *JAMA* 1988; **260**: 3456–60.

40. Schaffer SW. Cardiomyopathy associated with noninsulin-dependent diabetes. *Mol Cell Biochem* 1991; **107**: 1–20.

41. Mustonen JN, Uusitupa MI, Laakso M, et al. Left ventricular systolic function in middle aged patients with diabetes mellitus. *Am J Cardiol* 1994; **73**: 1202–8.

42. Galderisi M, Anderson KM, Wilson PWF, Levy D. Echocardiographic evidence for the existence of a distinct diabetic cardiomyopathy (The Framingham Study). *Am J Cardiol* 1991; **68**: 85–9.

43. Sasson Z, Rasooly Y, Bhesania T, Rasooly I. Insulin resistance is an important determinant of left ventricular mass in the obese. *Circulation* 1993; **88**: 1431–6.

44. Anderson KM, Wilson PWF, Odell PM, et al. An updated coronary risk profile: a statement for health professionals. *Circulation* 1991; **83**: 357–63.

45. Wolf PA, D'Agostino RB, Belanger AJ, et al. Probability of a stroke: a risk profile from the Framingham Study. *Stroke* 1991; **22**: 312–18.

3

Does insulin resistance play a role in the pathogenesis and clinical course of patients with hypertension?

Gerald M Reaven

Introduction

Essential hypertension is a multifactorial disease, and it is unlikely that any given abnormality will prove to be the 'cause' of this syndrome. Rather, a number of abnormalities are likely to predispose individuals to develop high blood pressure. In this context, recent evidence has raised the likelihood that resistance to insulin-mediated glucose uptake and/or compensatory hyperinsulinaemia may play such a role. It seems even more likely that abnormalities of glucose, insulin and lipoprotein metabolism have a profound effect on the clinical course of patients with high blood pressure. In this chapter an attempt will be made to review both these issues by addressing the following four questions. Do insulin resistance and its associated metabolic abnormalities exist in patients with essential hypertension? Do insulin resistance and/or compensatory hyperinsulinaemia play a role in the regulation of blood pressure? What are the pathophysiological mechanisms that might serve as the link between insulin resistance and essential hypertension? And finally, is there a relationship between insulin resistance and/or its consequences and the clinical course of individuals with high blood pressure?

Do insulin resistance and its associated metabolic abnormalities exist in patients with essential hypertension?

In 1966, Welborn et al.[1] studied 19 individuals diagnosed as having essential hypertension and demonstrated that patients with high blood pressure had significantly higher plasma insulin concentrations than a control population. Hyperinsulinaemia was noted before and at every time point measured after an oral glucose load, and was present in both treated and untreated patients with high blood pressure.

Until relatively recently, little attention was directed toward the relationship between high blood pressure and hyperinsulinaemia. However, approximately 20 years later, several research groups[2-6] confirmed the original observation of Welborn et al.[1] There is also evidence that hypertension may be associated with glucose intolerance,[5,6] an observation that had been made previously.[7] The combination of glucose intolerance and hyperinsulinaemia strongly suggested that a defect in insulin-stimulated glucose uptake was likely to exist in some patients with hypertension, and there is now considerable evidence indicating that this is the case.[4-6,8] These observations served as a catalyst to stimulate an extraordinary amount of research activity in the last 20 years

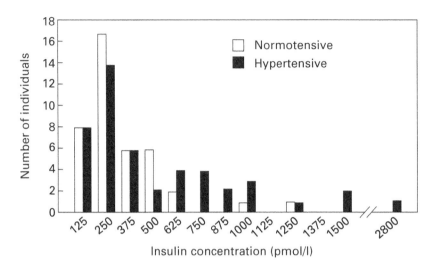

Figure 3.1
Frequency distribution of the plasma insulin response 2 h after a 75-g oral glucose challenge in normotensive (□) and hypertensive (■) volunteers. (Reprinted from J Intern Med 1992; 231: 235, with kind permission of the authors and the journal.)

focusing on the potential role that insulin resistance and/or compensatory hyperinsulinaemia might play in the regulation of blood pressure. As a result of this activity, there appears to be widespread agreement that insulin resistance and compensatory hyperinsulinaemia are characteristic of patients with essential hypertension. On the other hand, not all patients with essential hypertension are insulin resistant and hyperinsulinaemic. Obtaining a precise estimate of the frequency of abnormalities of insulin metabolism in patients with essential hypertension is not as simple as it may seem. Resistance to insulin-mediated glucose uptake and compensatory hyperinsulinaemia are continuous variables, not dichotomous ones, as demonstrated in Fig. 3.1 which shows the distribution of plasma insulin concentrations 2 h after the ingestion of 75 g of glucose in 41 patients with hypertension and 41 normotensive subjects.[9] These hypertensive patients were identified as part of a routine health survey and the normotensive subjects were participants in the same survey, selected to match the patients with

respect to variables such as sex, degree of obesity, ethnic background, type of employment and level of physical activity. Only 10 per cent of the normotensive subjects had 2 h plasma insulin concentrations >80 μU/ml, as compared with 45 per cent of the patients with hypertension. On the basis of these and other findings,[8] approximately 50 per cent of patients with hypertension can be considered to have insulin resistance and hyperinsulinaemia.

Normotensive individuals who are insulin-resistant and hyperinsulinaemic are at risk of developing a cluster of other abnormalities;[10] in addition to glucose intolerance, they tend to have a high plasma triglyceride (TG) and a low high density lipoprotein (HDL)-cholesterol concentration. Therefore, it should not be surprising that similar metabolic abnormalities are commonly present in patients with essential hypertension.[11–14]

Based upon the above considerations, it seems reasonable to conclude that a substantial proportion of patients with essential hypertension are resistant to insulin-mediated glucose disposal and are hyperinsulinaemic. In addition, they will tend to be somewhat glucose intolerant, with elevated plasma TG and low HDL-cholesterol concentrations.

Do insulin resistance and/or compensatory hyperinsulinaemia play a role in the regulation of blood pressure?

Perhaps the simplest answer to this question is that insulin resistance and compensatory hyperinsulinaemia are neither necessary nor sufficient for essential hypertension to develop. The results shown in Fig. 3.1 made it abundantly clear that a significant proportion of patients with essential hypertension were insulin sensitive. Furthermore, blood pressure does not increase in all subjects who are insulin-resistant and hyperinsulinaemic. On the other hand, I believe that insulin-resistant subjects are more likely to develop hypertension than are insulin-sensitive individuals. In this regard, the situation closely resembles the role of insulin resistance in the development of type II diabetes.[10,15] Hyperglycaemia only develops in insulin-resistant individuals when they no longer are able to secrete the large amount of insulin necessary to overcome the insulin resistance. In a similar fashion, it seems likely that hypertension only develops when some unknown compensatory response(s) is no longer able to overcome the metabolic changes associated with insulin resistance and compensatory hyperinsulinaemia that favour an increase in blood pressure. Evidence, both for and against the notion that insulin resistance and hyperinsulinaemia play a role in the regulation of blood pressure, will be reviewed in the remainder of this section.

What comes first: hypertension or insulin resistance?

Once it became apparent that insulin resistance and hyperinsulinaemia existed in a substantial proportion of patients with essential hypertension, it was necessary to consider the possibility that these variables were related in a causal manner. Although it may not have been apparent at the outset which was cause and which was effect, it now seems quite clear from several lines of evidence that high blood pressure does not cause insulin resistance. For example, neither insulin resistance nor hyperinsulinaemia develop in either human beings or rodents with secondary forms of hypertension.[16-20] Additional evidence that insulin resistance and compensatory hyperinsulinaemia may lead to hypertension, but not *vice versa*, can be derived from evidence that insulin resistance exists in normotensive, first degree relatives of patients with high blood pressure.[21-25] An example of this can be seen in Fig. 3.2, which displays the results of insulin resistance measurements in normotensive individuals, with or without a family history of hypertension.[23] The two groups were essentially identical in terms of age, gender distribution, body mass index and blood pressure. However, the steady-state plasma glucose (SSPG) concentration was higher in those with a family history of hypertension at the end of a 3-h infusion of somatostatin, insulin and glucose. As the steady-state plasma insulin concentrations were similar in the two groups, the subjects with a positive family history of hypertension were relatively resistant to the ability of insulin to dispose of the glucose load. In addition to being insulin-resistant, the group with a family history of hypertension was also relatively dyslipidaemic as shown in Table 3.1.[23]

The results in Fig. 3.2 and Table 3.1 demonstrate that first-degree relatives of

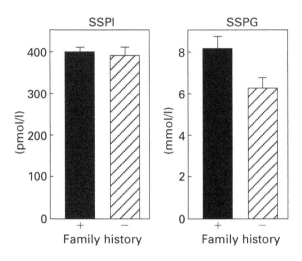

Figure 3.2
Steady-state plasma insulin (SSPI) and glucose (SSPG) concentrations during the insulin suppression test in volunteers with (+, ■) and without (−,▨) a family history of hypertension. (Reprinted from Am J Hypertens 1992; 5: 694, with kind permission of the authors and the journal.)

Variable (mmol/l)	Positive family history	Negative family history	P
Cholesterol	4.80 ± 0.15	4.44 ± 0.12	<0.07
VLDL-CHOL	0.50 ± 0.06	0.23 ± 0.03	<0.001
IDL-CHOL	0.34 ± 0.07	0.21 ± 0.02	<0.08
LDL-CHOL	2.65 ± 0.12	2.54 ± 0.10	NS
HDL-CHOL	1.34 ± 0.06	1.47 ± 0.05	<0.10
VLDL + IDL + LDL-CHOL	3.47 ± 0.14	3.00 ± 0.11	<0.003
Ratio of CHOL/HDL-CHOL	3.84 ± 0.18	3.09 ± 0.11	<0.001
Triglyceride	1.15 ± 0.07	0.76 ± 0.05	<0.001
VLDL-TG	0.71 ± 0.07	0.40 ± 0.04	<0.001
IDL-TG	0.14 ± 0.02	0.10 ± 0.01	NS
LDL-TG	0.19 ± 0.01	0.16 ± 0.01	<0.05
HDL-TG	0.11 ± 0.01	0.09 ± 0.01	<0.06

CHOL, cholesterol; TG, triglyceride; NS, not significant.

Table 3.1
Plasma lipid and lipoprotein concentrations.

patients with hypertension display the same metabolic defects as do patients with essential hypertension. These data not only show that the metabolic changes associated with essential hypertension can exist in the absence of any increase in blood pressure, they are also consistent with the view that these changes may predispose an individual to develop high blood pressure.

Population studies

Cross-sectional studies

The earliest concerns as to the existence of a causal relationship between insulin resistance and compensatory hyperinsulinaemia evolved from cross-sectional population studies.[26–29] On the other hand, there are a large number of published cross-sectional studies indicating that blood pressure and insulin resistance and/or compensatory hyperinsulinaemia are significantly correlated.[2,3,8,30–32] In an effort to resolve these discordant results, the European Group for the Study of Insulin Resistance examined the relationship between a specific measure of insulin resistance and blood pressure in 333 normotensive individuals, studied in 20 different clinical research centres.[33] The results indicated that blood pressure was directly related to both insulin resistance and insulin concentration. Furthermore, these relationships were independent of differences in age, gender and degree of obesity.

The enormous size of the European study provides strong evidence for a link between insulin resistance, hyperinsulinaemia and blood pressure. There are at least two possible reasons for the fact that this relationship was not seen in all studies. First, as discussed earlier, not all patients with hypertension are insulin-resistant and hyperinsulinaemic, nor do all insulin-resistant subjects have increases in blood pressure. Based on these considerations, and given all the factors known to modulate blood pressure, not finding a correlation between plasma insulin concentration and blood pressure in an epidemiological study does not rule out the possibility that it may still play a role in blood pressure regulation.

Second, it has been postulated that the relationship between insulin resistance, hyperinsulinaemia and blood pressure varies as a function of race. For example, in one study of 42 healthy African Americans,[29] it was argued that the lack of a relationship between either insulin resistance or hyperinsulinaemia and blood pressure in black people suggests that insulin resistance does not predispose this ethnic group to develop hypertension. On the other hand, there is published evidence that black hypertensive patients are insulin-resistant and hyperinsulinaemic when compared with black subjects with normal blood pressure, whether living in the USA[34] or in Tanzania.[35] Furthermore, in a much larger epidemiological study involving >14,000 participants,[36] evidence was published indicating that hypertension clustered with other manifestations of insulin resistance in both white and African American subjects.

Based upon the considerations discussed above, there seems to be no reason to reject the hypothesis that insulin resistance and/or compensatory hyperinsulinaemia predispose an individual to develop hypertension. Indeed, it seems that the available cross-sectional data are reasonably supportive of this notion.

Longitudinal studies

Unfortunately, we are unaware of any prospective studies in which it is possible to assess the effect of specific measures of insulin resistance on the development of hypertension. The most relevant extensive study seems to have been performed by Skarfors et al.,[37] who evaluated risk factors for the development of hypertension in 2130 men observed over a

10-year period. Not surprisingly, they found that baseline blood pressure was the strongest predictor of the development of hypertension. In addition, baseline characteristics of normotensive men who became hypertensive were compared with individuals who remained normotensive. The analysis showed that individuals who subsequently developed hypertension were more obese, had higher insulin (fasting and after intravenous glucose) and TG concentrations. When baseline blood pressure was excluded from multivariate analysis, independent predictors of the progression to hypertension were obesity (as estimated by body mass index), fasting and post-glucose insulin concentrations, and a family history of hypertension.

A somewhat similar prospective study was performed by Lissner et al.,[38] who evaluated risk factors for the development of hypertension in 278 women followed over a 12-year period. In addition, they examined the relationship between blood pressure and risk factors in 219 women not receiving antihypertensive medication. Hypertension developed in approximately one-third of the population in the 12-year period. In multiple logistic regression analysis, fasting insulin concentration was found to be a predictor of the transition from normal to high blood pressure, independent of adjustment for initial body mass index, waist/hip ratio and weight gain. The power of hyperinsulinaemia was further emphasised by finding that the women in the upper quartile in terms of fasting insulin concentration were more than three-fold more likely to develop hypertension than those in the lowest quartile. Essentially similar conclusions were observed when changes in blood pressure over the 12-year period were considered as a continuous variable in the 219 women not taking antihypertensive medication. However, in this instance, increases in

body weight over the period of observation were also found to be related to increases in blood pressure.

The ability of insulin to predict changes in blood pressure over time has also been shown in Finnish children and adolescents.[39] The ages of the study population ranged from 3 to 18 years at baseline, and they were followed for 16 years. The results of this study indicated that fasting insulin concentrations 'seem to regulate actual blood pressure within the normal range and to predict future blood pressure'. It was also pointed out that these conclusions applied to boys and girls, and were independent of differences in age and weight.

Essentially similar conclusions were reached from a somewhat more complicated study of 1865 children and adolescents, followed over a 6-year period.[40] In general, the results of this study demonstrated that the higher the fasting insulin concentration at baseline, the greater the increase in blood pressure over the 6-year period of observation. Perhaps of greater interest was the finding that 'high insulin levels seem to precede the development of a potentially atherogenic risk factor profile including low HDL-cholesterol, high triglyceride, and high systolic blood pressure'.

Based on the above summary, there appears to be substantial evidence that the presence of hyperinsulinaemia, as a surrogate measure of insulin resistance, is a risk factor for the development of hypertension. This was true both in adults and children, and the relationship appeared to be independent of differences in gender and both overall and regional obesity. Furthermore, hyperinsulinaemia also predicted the development of the dyslipidaemia characteristic of insulin-resistant individuals.[10,15] These data provide substantial support for the view that insulin resistance and/or compensatory hyperinsulinaemia may play a role in the pathogenesis of hypertension in at least some individuals.

Intervention studies

Perhaps the evidence that is most often advanced to argue against a role for insulin resistance and compensatory hyperinsulinaemia is that the acute administration of insulin to normal volunteers causes vasodilation and does not increase blood pressure.[41] On the other hand, there is no *a priori* reason to believe that the chronic effects of compensatory hyperinsulinaemia on blood pressure regulation in insulin-resistant subjects should be the same as the acute effects of a primary increase in insulin concentration. Furthermore, in studies addressing the more chronic effects of insulin resistance and compensatory hyperinsulinaemia on blood pressure, a more complicated situation exists. For example, weight loss – which enhances insulin sensitivity and lowers plasma insulin concentrations in non-diabetic individuals[42] – can also decrease blood pressure in patients with essential hypertension,[43] and this change seems to be correlated with the improvement in insulin resistance.[44] Similarly, there is evidence that blood pressure can be lowered in obese individuals by physical training without any change in weight, but only in those individuals who were hyperinsulinaemic and/or hypertriglyceridaemic before the training programme was initiated.[45] Because there is also evidence that insulin sensitivity is directly related to level of habitual physical activity,[46] it is reasonable to conclude that the decrease in blood pressure was associated with an improvement in insulin-stimulated glucose uptake. Finally, it has been shown that blood pressure falls when insulin dose is reduced in obese patients with type II diabetes and hypertension,[47] and that insulin treatment increases blood pressure in patients with type II dia-

betes.[48] Both these reports lend support to the view that ambient insulin concentration modulates blood pressure.

Based upon the above data from interventional studies, the evidence that the acute administration of insulin does not increase blood pressure appears to be, at the least, counter-balanced by evidence that more chronic changes in insulin level and/or insulin action are closely associated with changes in blood pressure. Therefore, it does not seem prudent to discard the view that insulin resistance and compensatory hyperinsulinaemia increase the risk of developing hypertension on the basis of acute studies in normal volunteers.

Animal studies

Although discretion is advisable when attempting to assess the relevance of animal studies to human pathophysiology, it is difficult not to be overly enthusiastic regarding the evidence from studies of rodent hypertension as to the relationship between insulin resistance, hyperinsulinaemia and hypertension. To begin with, it was shown some time ago that substituting fructose for the carbohydrate conventionally present in rat chow led to insulin resistance and hyperinsulinaemia in Sprague-Dawley rats.[49] These changes could be seen within 1 week and were not associated with obesity. It is now clear that this dietary manipulation also leads to a consistent increase in blood pressure of ~20 mmHg.[50–52] The increase in blood pressure develops within 10 days, lasts for as long as 3 months, and disappears once the fructose-enriched diet is removed. Furthermore, prevention of fructose-induced insulin resistance and/or hyperinsulinaemia by exercise training[51] or the infusion of somatostatin[52] markedly attenuated the degree of fructose-induced hypertension.

Insulin resistance, hyperinsulinaemia and dyslipidaemia are not unique to fructose-induced

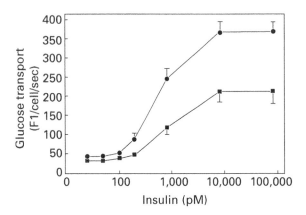

Figure 3.3
Glucose transport in the absence or presence of varying amounts of insulin by adipocytes isolated from WKY (●) or SHR (■) rats. Results are means ± SE of eight experiments. (Reprinted from Diabetes 1989; 38: 1155, with kind permission of the authors and the journal.)

hypertension in rats, and similar changes have been described in three genetic forms of rodent hypertension – rats with spontaneous hypertension (SHR), Dahl salt-sensitive rats and Milano hypertensive rats.[53–58] In the case of SHR, the data in Fig. 3.3 demonstrate that insulin-mediated glucose disposal is decreased in their isolated adipocytes.[54] Furthermore, blood pressure – as well as plasma insulin and triglyceride concentrations – is correlated with the degree of adipocyte insulin resistance in SHR and WKY rats.[56]

Another approach to evaluating the possibility that insulin resistance and/or hyperinsulinaemia play a causal role in rodent hypertension has been to test the effect of insulin-sensitising agents in various rodent models. This topic has been the focus of an excellent recent review[59] and a thorough discussion of this issue would not be appropriate within the context of this chapter. Although the studies evaluating the putative relationship provide substantial evidence for the link between a treatment-induced improvement in insulin sensitivity and a decrease in blood pressure in various hypertensive models, there is also evidence that the relationship may not necessarily be causal. On the one hand, there is evidence that thiazolidenedione compounds – known to enhance insulin sensitivity[60] – decrease blood pressure in Dahl salt-sensitive rats, SHR and fructose-fed Sprague-Dawley rats.[61–63] Furthermore, administration of vanadium compounds reduces both insulin resistance and blood pressure in SHR.[64,65] On the other hand, pioglitazone, a thiazolidenedione compound, also lowers blood pressure in rats with renal hypertension, an example of hypertension in rats that is not associated with either insulin resistance or hyperinsulinaemia.[66] Furthermore, evidence has also been presented that administration of troglitazone, another thiazolidenedione, to SHR, improved insulin sensitivity without affecting blood pressure.[67]

The confounding effects of species differences in experimental results add further confusion to the evidence from animal studies concerning the relationship between insulin resistance, hyperinsulinaemia and hypertension. For example, as the infusion of insulin to normal dogs for several days does not increase blood pressure, it has been concluded that insulin does not regulate blood pressure.[68] However, the same research group has shown that insulin infused in a similar manner to rats increases blood pressure.[69] The most reasonable explanation for these discordant data is derived from the previously emphasised point that insulin resistance and compensatory hyperinsulinaemia increase the risk of developing hypertension, but that neither abnormality, by itself, will necessarily lead to an increase in blood pressure. This general principle is further supported by the observation that although feeding fructose-enriched diets will induce insulin resistance and hyperinsulinaemia in several species of rats, an associated increase in blood pressure is species-specific.[70,71]

In conclusion, the results of studies in animal models of hypertension closely resemble the results of observations in human beings. More specifically, there is abundant evidence of associations between insulin resistance, hyperinsulinaemia and hypertension. However, not all animals that are insulin resistant or hyperinsulinaemic become hypertensive.

How can insulin resistance and/or compensatory hyperinsulinaemia cause hypertension?

The simplest answer to this question is that it is highly unlikely that either insulin resistance or hyperinsulinaemia cause hypertension by themselves. It is obvious that not all patients with high blood pressure are insulin resistant and hyperinsulinaemic (see Fig. 3.1), nor are all insulin-resistant subjects hypertensive. As stated earlier, insulin resistance and compensatory hyperinsulinaemia appear to increase the risk of development of hypertension. Thus, the question posed above can be broken down into two related questions: 1) how does insulin resistance and/or compensatory hyperinsulinaemia predispose an individual to develop high blood pressure and 2) what compensatory mechanisms fail in this situation and permit the increase in blood pressure?

Before addressing the two additional questions posed above, it is necessary to devote some attention to what is meant by the phrase insulin resistance. In particular, it is important

to establish the fact that differences in tissue sensitivity to insulin exist. Specifically, a defect in the ability of insulin to stimulate glucose disposal by muscle can be present in an individual, without evidence of any abnormality in the ability of insulin to either stimulate renal sodium retention[72] or enhance sympathetic nervous system (SNS) activity.[73] Indeed, in the remainder of this section arguments will be made that the retention of a normal tissue response to insulin in the kidney and SNS in individuals whose muscles and adipose tissue are insulin-resistant helps to explain why such individuals are at increased risk of developing hypertension.

Why are insulin-resistant and hyperinsulinaemic individuals at risk of developing hypertension?

Perhaps the simplest link between muscle insulin resistance, compensatory hyperinsulinaemia and hypertension is related to the effect of insulin on renal sodium metabolism. It has been known for some time that the infusion of insulin into normal individuals increases sodium retention.[74] More recently, evidence has been presented that this is also true of patients with hypertension.[75] If the link between insulin resistance and hypertension is attributable to enhanced sodium retention, as a consequence of compensatory hyperinsulinaemia, it might be predicted that such patients would also be salt sensitive. Although this issue has not been definitely settled, there is evidence in both normotensive and hypertensive individuals that the blood pressure is sensitive to salt in insulin-resistant individuals.[76,77]

Although still involving the kidney to some extent, insulin activation of the SNS provides a somewhat broader approach to understanding why insulin-resistant and hyperinsulinaemic individuals are at increased risk of developing hypertension. An increase in heart rate is recognised not only as a manifestation of enhanced SNS activity, but as a significant predictor of the development of hypertension.[78,79] The fact that heart rate is also related to both insulin resistance and hyperinsulinaemia[73] is consistent with the view that these abnormalities of insulin metabolism predispose individuals to develop hypertension via stimulation of the SNS. This formulation has been reviewed recently in great detail, and evidence describing the relationship between insulin resistance, hyperinsulinaemia and SNS in the modulation of blood pressure has been summarised.[80] As initially proposed by Landsberg,[81] hyperinsulinaemia, secondary to insulin resistance, stimulates the SNS, leading to increases in heart rate, cardiac output, vascular resistance and sodium retention. Given this panoply of changes, it should not be too surprising that insulin-resistant and hyperinsulinaemic individuals are at risk of developing hypertension.

The discussion up to this point has focused on two somewhat related mechanisms to help explain why insulin-resistant and hyperinsulinaemic individuals are at risk of developing hypertension. Obviously, these are not the only possibilities. On the other hand, they seem to be the explanations for which there is the most evidence at this time. At the least, they provide a hypothesis as to the nature of these relationships that can be evaluated.

What compensatory mechanisms must fail for hypertension to develop in insulin-resistant individuals?

As emphasised earlier, not all insulin-resistant and hyperinsulinaemic individuals develop high blood pressure. Therefore, although enhanced sodium retention may increase the likelihood that insulin-resistant and hyperinsulinaemic individuals will become hypertensive, this defect is not sufficient, by itself, to increase blood pressure. In many ways, this situation is analogous to the difference in the effect of dietary salt on blood pressure in Dahl salt-sensitive (Dahl S) and Dahl salt-resistant (Dahl R) rats, and evocative of the link between insulin resistance and salt sensitivity addressed above. Evidence has been published that insulin-stimulated glucose disposal is decreased by isolated adipocytes from both Dahl S and R rats.[82] This defect does not change in response to a high salt diet, an intervention that only increases blood pressure in Dahl S rats. Thus, it could be hypothesised that there is a compensatory response to insulin-induced sodium retention in Dahl R rats that permits them to overcome this physiological response and remain normotensive. In contrast, it could be argued that Dahl S rats lack some factor that compromises their ability to compensate for the insulin-induced increase in sodium retention, permitting their blood pressure to increase in response to the high salt diet. Obviously, the existence of such a factor – regardless of whether it plays a role in blood pressure regulation in Dahl rats and its relevance, if any, to the human situation – is totally speculative. However, the observations in Dahl rats offer an experimental paradigm to explain why only some insulin-resistant patients develop hypertension. One possible contender for the putative factor that prevents a sodium-induced increase in blood pressure may be atrial natriuretic peptide (ANP). For example, ANP levels have been shown to be inappropriately low in the offspring of hypertensive families,[83] and evidence has also been published showing a direct relationship between ANP and insulin levels.[84] Could a defective ANP response to enhanced sodium retention explain why salt-sensitive hypertension is common in insulin-resistant individuals? This seems to be a possibility worth exploring in future experiments. On the other hand, it is probably unlikely that failure of only one defence mechanism will permit blood pressure to increase in all insulin-resistant and hyperinsulinaemic individuals. It seems more likely that different defects will exist in different individuals, and the unravelling of all these issues will require more thoughtful and complete phenotypic characterisation of insulin-resistant individuals in the future.

Insulin resistance, its consequences and the clinical course of patients with hypertension

The advent of more effective antihypertensive drugs has greatly decreased morbidity and mortality in patients with high blood pressure. However, the clinical benefit of lowering blood pressure has been much more dramatic in decreasing the risk of stroke as compared with heart attack.[85] As heart attack is the major cause of morbidity and mortality in patients with hypertension, this apparent paradox has received a great deal of attention. Not surprisingly, many different explanations have been proposed to account for this unwelcome finding. For example, it has been argued that stroke is more directly related to blood pressure than is heart attack, and that the apparent difference in outcome is a function of the relatively short duration of the intervention trials. Another suggestion has been that the problem lies with the fact that thiazide diuretics and/or beta-receptor antagonists, the drugs used in the controlled clinical trials, have an untoward effect on carbohydrate and lipid metabolism that tended to mitigate their bene-

ficial effects on blood pressure. Although this may be true to some extent, there is a much simpler explanation for the apparent paradox between lowering blood pressure and coronary heart disease (CHD). Specifically, as a group patients with high blood pressure tend to be insulin resistant, glucose intolerant, hyperinsulinaemic and dyslipidaemic – changes recognised as increasing the risk of CHD in normotensive individuals.[10,14,15] More direct evidence that the metabolic changes associated with hypertension may be the link between high blood pressure and CHD can be derived from the results of a recent study showing that untreated hypertensive patients, without clinical evidence of CHD, who have ischaemic heart disease by the Minnesota Code criteria, are insulin-resistant, glucose intolerant and hyperinsulinaemic as compared with a matched group of equally hypertensive individuals with normal electrocardiograms (ECGs).[86] The glucose tolerance test results from this study are shown in Fig. 3.4. These results indicate that the hypertensive patients with ECG evidence of ischaemic heart disease were somewhat glucose intolerant and very hyperinsulinaemic as compared with healthy volunteers and patients with high blood pressure and normal ECGs. Patients with high blood pressure and an abnormal ECG were significantly more insulin-resistant, and the data in Table 3.2 indicate that they were also dyslipidaemic as compared with normotensive individuals or hypertensive patients with normal ECGs. The existence of these CHD risk factors in the hypertensive patients with abnormal ECGs was seen in the absence of pharmacological treatment of their high blood pressure.

Furthermore, the magnitude of the abnormalities in insulin, glucose and lipid metabolism when present in patients with high blood pressure is much greater than the untoward

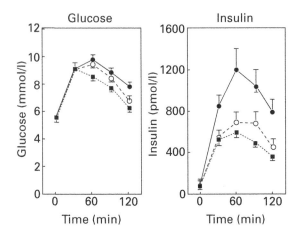

Figure 3.4
Plasma glucose and insulin responses to an oral glucose challenge in control (■--■) and hypertensive patients with either a normal (○--○) or an abnormal (●--●) ECG as defined by the Minnesota Code criteria. (Reprinted from Am J Hypertens 1992; 5: 444, with kind permission of the authors and the journal.)

the evidence that these metabolic changes increase the risk of CHD in normotensive individuals, it seems reasonable to suggest that their impact would be at least as great in patients with high blood pressure. As these metabolic abnormalities were not addressed in the clinical trials that have been conducted, it is not too surprising that CHD did not decrease when the therapeutic focus was solely on lowering blood pressure. The obvious clinical corollary to this explanation for the relative ineffectiveness of antihypertensive drug treatment in decreasing CHD is that therapeutic attention must be directed toward alleviating all CHD risk factors, not just blood pressure.

Conclusion

There is considerable evidence that patients with high blood pressure, as a group, are insulin-resistant, glucose intolerant, hyperinsulinaemic and dyslipidaemic. Studies in both man and rodent models of hypertension suggest that insulin resistance and/or compensatory hyperinsulinaemia have a role in blood pressure regulation and may predispose individuals to develop

effect of any antihypertensive treatment.[87] Finally, lowering blood pressure with antihypertensive treatment does not return these metabolic abnormalities to normal.[5,6] Given all

Group	Cholesterol (mmol/l)	LDL-cholesterol (mmol/l)	HDL-cholesterol (mmol/l)	Cholesterol/HDL-cholesterol (ratio)	Triglyceride (mmol/l)
Control (n = 25)	5.05 ± 0.24	3.11 ± 0.22	1.36 ± 0.08	3.95 ± 0.31	1.16 ± 0.12
Normal ECG (n = 24)	4.79 ± 0.19	3.03 ± 0.18	1.28 ± 0.07	4.00 ± 0.25	1.21 ± 0.14
Abnormal ECG (n = 29)	5.36 ± 0.18	3.39 ± 0.17	1.10 ± 0.06*	5.04 ± 0.23**	1.81 ± 0.13**

*Different from control ($P < 0.01$);
**different from control and normal ECG ($P < 0.02$).

Table 3.2
Lipid and lipoprotein concentrations (mean ± SEM).

high blood pressure. Of greater immediate clinical import is the fact that the abnormalities of glucose, insulin and lipid metabolism that exist in substantial numbers of patients with high blood pressure increase their risk of CHD. Given this information, it seems prudent to enlarge the scope of our therapeutic approach to patients with hypertension, and initiate efforts to both lower blood pressure and improve all risk factors for CHD.

References

1. Welborn TA, Breckenridge A, Rubinstein AH, Dollery CT, Fraser TR. Serum-insulin in essential hypertension and in peripheral vascular disease. *Lancet* 1966; **1**: 1136-7.
2. Lucas CP, Estigarribia JA, Darga LL, Reaven GM, Insulin and blood pressure in obesity. *Hypertension* 1985; **7**: 702-6.
3. Modan M, Halkin H, Almog S, et al. Hyperinsulinemia: a link between hypertension, obesity and glucose intolerance. *J Clin Invest* 1985; **75**: 809-17.
4. Ferrannini E, Buzzigoli G, Bonadona R. Insulin resistance in essential hypertension. *N Engl J Med* 1987; **317**: 350-7.
5. Shen D-C, Shieh S-M, Fuh M, Wu D-A, Chen Y-DI, Reaven GM. Resistance to insulin-stimulated glucose uptake in patients with hypertension. *J Clin Endocrinol Metab* 1988; **66**: 580-3.
6. Swislocki ALM, Hoffman BB, Reaven GM. Insulin resistance, glucose intolerance and hyperinsulinemia in patients with hypertension. *Am J Hypertens* 1989; **2**: 419-23.
7. Jarret RJ, Keen H, McCartney M, et al. Glucose tolerance and blood pressure in two population samples: their relation to diabetes mellitus and hypertension. *Int J Epidemiol* 1978; **7**: 15-24.
8. Pollare T, Lithell H, Berne C. Insulin resistance is a characteristic feature of primary hypertension independent of obesity. *Metabolism* 1990; **39**: 167-74.
9. Zavaroni I, Mazza S, Dall'Aglio E, Gasparini P, Passeri M, Reaven GM. Prevalence of hyperinsulinaemia in patients with high blood pressure. *J Intern Med* 1992; **231**: 235-40.
10. Reaven GM. Role of insulin resistance in human disease. *Diabetes* 1988; **37**: 1595-607.
11. MacMahon SW, Macdonald GJ, Blacket RB. Plasma lipoprotein levels in treated and untreated hypertensive men and women. *Arteriosclerosis* 1985; **5**: 391-6.
12. Shieh S-M, Shen M, Fuh MM-T, Chen Y-DI, Reaven GM. Plasma lipid and lipoprotein concentrations in Chinese males with coronary artery disease, with and without hypertension. *Atherosclerosis* 1987; **67**: 49-55.
13. Fuh M-T, Shieh SM, Wu D-A, et al. Abnormalities of carbohydrate and lipid metabolism in patients with hypertension. *Arch Intern Med* 1987; **147**: 1035-8.
14. Reaven GM. Relationship between insulin resistance and hypertension. *Diabetes Care* 1991; **14**: 33-8.
15. Reaven GM. Pathophysiology of insulin resistance in human disease. *Physiol Rev* 1995; **75**: 473-86.
16. Marigliano A, Tedde R, Sechi LA, Para A, Pisanu G, Pacifico A. Insulinemia and blood pressure: relationships in patients with primary and secondary hypertension, and with or without glucose metabolism impairment. *Am J Hypertens* 1990; **3**: 521-6.
17. Shamiss A, Carroll J, Rosenthall T. Insulin resistance in secondary hypertension. *Am J Hypertens* 1992; **5**: 26-8.
18. Buchanan TA, Sipos GF, Gadalah S, et al. Glucose tolerance and insulin action in rats with renovascular hypertension. *Hypertension* 1991; **18**: 341-7.
19. Reaven GM, Ho H. Renal vascular hypertension does not lead to hyperinsulinemia in Sprague-Dawley rats. *Am J Hypertens* 1992; **5**: 314-17.
20. Dall'Aglio E, Tosini P, Ferrari P, Zavaroni I, Passeri M, Reaven GM. Abnormalities of insulin and lipid metabolism in Milan hypertensive rats. *Am J Hypertens* 1991; **4**: 773-5.
21. Ferrari P, Weidmann P, Shaw S, et al. Altered insulin sensitivity, hyperinsulinemia and dyslipidemia in individuals with a hypertensive parent. *Am J Med* 1991; **91**: 589-96.
22. Allemann Y, Horber FF, Colombo M, et al. Insulin sensitivity and body fat distribution in normotensive offspring of hypertensive parents. *Lancet* 1993; **341**: 327-31.
23. Facchini F, Chen Y-DI, Clinkingbeard C, Jeppesen J, Reaven GM. Insulin resistance,

hyperinsulinemia, and dyslipidemia in nonobese individuals with a family history of hypertension. *Am J Hypertens* 1992; **5**: 694–9.

24. Ohno Y, Suzuki H, Yamakawa H, Nakamura M, Otsuka K, Saruta T. Impaired insulin sensitivity in young, lean normotensive offspring of essential hypertensives: possible role of disturbed calcium metabolism. *J Hypertens* 1993; **11**: 421–6.

25. Beatty OL, Harper R, Sheridan B, Atkinson AB, Bell PM. Insulin resistance in offspring of hypertensive parents. *BMJ* 1993; **307**: 92–6.

26. Mbanya J-C, Wilkinson R, Thomas T, Alberti K, Taylor R. Hypertension and hyperinsulinemia: a relation in diabetes but not in essential hypertension. *Lancet* 1988; **I**: 733–4.

27. Donhaue RP, Skyler JS, Sneiderman N, Prineas RJ. Hyperinsulinemia and elevated blood pressure: cause, confounder, or coincidence? *Am J Epidemiol* 1990; **132**: 827–36.

28. Collins VR, Dowse GK, Finch CF, Zimmet PZ. An inconsistent relationship between insulin and blood pressure in three Pacific Island populations. *J Clin Epidemiol* 1990; **43**: 1369–78.

29. Saad MF, Lillioja S, Nyomba BL, et al. Racial differences in the relation between blood pressure and insulin resistance. *N Engl J Med* 1991; **324**: 733–9.

30. Manicardi V, Camellini L, Bellodi G, Caselli C, Ferrannini E. Evidence for an association of high blood pressure and hyperinsulinemia in obese man. *J Clin Endocrinol Metab* 1986; **62**: 1302–4.

31. Fournier AM, Gadia MT, Kubrusly DB, Skylar JS, Sosenko JM. Blood pressure, insulin, and glycemia in nondiabetic subjects. *Am J Med* 1986; **80**: 861–4.

32. Denker PS, Pollok VE. Fasting serum insulin levels in essential hypertension. A meta analysis. *Arch Intern Med* 1992; **152**: 1649–51.

33. Ferrannini E, Natali A, Capaldo B, Lehtovirta M, Jacob S, Yki-Järvinen H, for the European Group for the Study of Insulin Resistance (EGIR). Insulin resistance, hyperinsulinemia, and blood pressure. Role of age and obesity. *Hypertension* 1992; **30**: 1144–9.

34. Falkner B, Hulman S, Kushner H. Insulin-stimulated glucose utilization and borderline hypertension in young adult blacks. *Hypertension* 1993; **22**: 18–25.

35. Mgonda YM, Ramaiya KL, Swai ABM, McLarty DG, Alberti KGMM. Insulin resistance and hypertension in non-obese Africans in Tanzania. *Hypertension* 1998; **31**: 114–18.

36 Schmidt MI, Brancati FL, Duncan BB, Heiss GH, Watson RL, Sharrett AR. A metabolic syndrome in whites and African-Americans: the atherosclerosis risk in communities baseline study. *Diabetes Care* 1996; **19**: 414–19.

37. Skarfors ET, Lithell HO, Selinus I. Risk factors for the development of hypertension: a 10-year longitudinal study in middle-aged men. *J Hypertension* 1991; **9**: 217–23.

38. Lissner L, Bengtsson C, Lapidus L, Kristjansson K, Wedel H. Fasting insulin in relation to subsequent blood pressure changes and hypertension in women. *Hypertension* 1992; **20**: 797–801.

39. Taittonen L, Uhari M, Nuutinen M, Turtinen J, Pokka T, Akerblom HK. Insulin and blood pressure among healthy children. *Am J Hypertens* 1996; **9**: 193–9.

40. Raitakari OT, Porkka KVK, Rönnemaa T, et al. The role of insulin in clustering of serum lipids and blood pressure in children and adolescents. *Diabetologia* 1995; **38**: 1042–50.

41. Anderson AE, Mark AL. The vasodilator action of insulin: implications for the insulin hypothesis of hypertension. *Hypertension* 1993; **21**: 136–41.

42. Olefsky JM, Reaven GM, Farquhar JW. Effects of weight reduction on obesity: studies on carbohydrate and lipid metabolism. *J Clin Invest* 1974; **53**: 64–76.

43. Reisin E, Abel R, Modan M, Silverberg DS, Eliahou HF, Modan B. Effect of weight loss without salt restriction on the reduction of blood pressure in overweight hypertensive patients. *N Engl J Med* 1978; **298**: 1–6.

44. Su H-Y, Sheu WH-H, Chin H-ML, Jeng C-Y, Chen Y-DI, Reaven GM. Effect of weight loss on blood pressure and insulin resistance in normotensive and hypertensive obese individuals. *Am J Hypertens* 1995; **8**: 1016–71.

45. Krotkiewski M, Mandroukas K, Sjostrom L, et al. Effects of long-term physical training on body fat, metabolism and blood pressure in obesity. *Metabolism* 1979; **28**: 650–8.

46. Rosenthal M, Haskell WL, Solomon R,

Widstrom A, Reaven GM. Demonstration of a relationship between level of physical training and insulin-stimulated glucose utilization in normal humans. *Diabetes* 1983; **32**: 408–11.

47. Tedde R, Sechi LA, Marigliano A, Pala A, Scano L. Antihypertensive effect of insulin reduction in diabetic-hypertensive patients. *Am J Hypertens* 1989; **2**: 163–70.

48. Randeree HA, Omar MAK, Motala AA, Seedat MA. Effect of insulin therapy on blood pressure in NIDDM patients with secondary failure. *Diabetes Care* 1992; **15**: 1258–63.

49. Zavaroni I, Sander S, Scott S, Reaven GM. Effect of fructose feeding on insulin secretion and insulin action in the rat. *Metabolism* 1980; **29**: 970–3.

50. Hwang I-S, Ho H, Hoffman BB, Reaven GM. Fructose-induced insulin and hypertension in rats. *Hypertension* 1987; **10**: 512–16.

51. Reaven GM, Ho H, Hoffman BB. Attenuation of fructose-induced hypertension in rats by exercise training. *Hypertension* 1988; **12**: 129–32.

52. Reaven GM, Ho H, Hoffman BB. Somatostatin inhibition of fructose-induced hypertension. *Hypertension* 1989; **14**: 117–20.

53. Mondon CE, Reaven GM. Evidence of abnormalities of insulin metabolism in rats with spontaneous hypertension. *Metabolism* 1988; **37**: 303–5.

54. Reaven GM, Chang H, Hoffman BB, Azhar S. Resistance to insulin-stimulated glucose uptake in adipocytes isolated from spontaneously hypertensive rats. *Diabetes* 1989; **38**: 1155–60.

55. Reaven GM, Ho H, Chang H. Hypertriglyceridemia in Dahl rats: effect of sodium intake and gender. *Horm Metab Res* 1991; **23**: 44–5.

56. Reaven GM, Chang H. Relationship between blood pressure, plasma insulin and triglyceride concentration, and insulin action in spontaneous hypertensive and Wistar-Kyoto Rats. *Am J Hypertens* 1991; **4**: 34–8.

57. Dall'Aglio E, Tosini P, Ferrari P, Zavaroni I, Passeri M, Reaven GM. Abnormalities of insulin and lipid metabolism in Milan hypertensive rats. *Am J Hypertens* 1991; **4**: 773–5.

58. Reaven GM, Twersky J, Chang H. Abnormalities of carbohydrate and lipid metabolism in Dahl rats. *Hypertension* 1991; **18**: 630–5.

59. Kotchen TA. Attenuation of hypertension by insulin-sensitizing agents. *Hypertension* 1996; **28**: 219–23.

60. Hofmann CA, Colca JR. New oral thiazolidinedione antidiabetic agents act as insulin sensitizers. *Diabetes Care* 1992; **12**: 1075–8.

61. Dubey RK, Zhang HY, Reddy SR, Boegehold MA, Kotchen TA. Pioglitazone attenuates hypertension and inhibits growth of renal arteriolar smooth muscle in rats. *Am J Physiol* 1993; **265**: R726–R732.

62. Pershadsingh HA, Szollosi J, Benson S, Hyun WC, Feuerstein BG, Kurtz TW. Effect of ciglitazone on blood pressure and intracellular calcium metabolism. *Hypertension* 1993; **21**: 1020–3.

63. Kotchen TA, Reddy S, Zhang HY. Increasing insulin sensitivity lowers blood pressure in the fructose-fed rat. *Am J Hypertens* 1997; **10**: 1020–6.

64. Bhanot S, McNeill JH. Vanadyl sulfate lowers plasma insulin and blood pressure in spontaneously hypertensive rats. *Hypertension* 1994; **24**: 625–32.

65. Bhanot S, Bryer-Ash M, Cheung A, McNeill JH. Bis(maltolato)-oxovanadium(IV), attenuates hyperinsulinemia and hypertension in spontaneously hypertensive rats. *Diabetes* 1994; **43**: 857–61.

66. Zhang HY, Reddy SR, Kotchen TA. Antihypertensive effect of pioglitazone is not invariably associated with increased insulin sensitivity. *Hypertension* 1994; **24**: 106–10.

67. Katayama S, Abe M, Kashiwabara H, Kosegaza T, Ishii J. Evidence against a role of insulin in hypertension in spontaneously hypertensive rats: CS-045 does not lower blood pressure despite improvement of insulin resistance. *Hypertension* 1994; **23**: 1071–4.

68. Hall JE, Brands MW, Kivlighn SD, Mizelle HL, Hildebrandt A, Gaillard CA. Chronic hyperinsulinemia and blood pressure. *Hypertension* 1990; **15**: 519–27.

69. Brands MW, Hildebrandt DA, Mizelle HL, Hall JE. Sustained hyperinsulinemia increases arterial pressure in conscious rats. *Am J Physiol* 1991; **260**: R764–R768.

70. Reed MJ, Ho H, Donnelly R, Reaven GM. Salt-sensitive and carbohydrate-sensitive rodent hypertension: evidence of strain differences. *Blood Pressure* 1994; **3**: 197–201.

71. Donnelly R, Ho H, Reaven GM. Effects of low sodium diet and unilateral nephrectomy on the development of carbohydrate-induced hypertension. *Blood Pressure* 1995; **4**: 164–9.

72. Skott P, Vaag A, Bruum NE, et al. Effect of insulin on renal sodium handling in hyperinsulinemic type 2 (non-insulin-dependent) diabetic patients with peripheral insulin resistance. *Diabetologia* 1991; **34**: 275–81.

73. Facchini FS, Riccardo A, Stoohs A, Reaven GM. Enhanced sympathetic nervous system activity – the linchpin between insulin resistance, hyperinsulinemia, and heart rate. *Am J Hypertens* 1996; **9**: 1013–17.

74. DeFronzo RA, Cooke C, Andres R, Faloona GR, David PJ. The effect of insulin in renal handling of sodium, potassium, calcium and phosphate in man. *J Clin Invest* 1975; **55**: 845–55.

75. Muscelli E, Natali A, Bianchi S, et al. Effect of insulin on renal sodium and uric acid handling in essential hypertension. *Am J Hypertens* 1996; **9**: 746–52.

76. Sharma AM, Schorr U, Distler A. Insulin resistance in young salt-sensitive normotensive subjects. *Hypertension* 1993; **21**: 273–9.

77. Zavaroni I, Coruzzi P, Bonini L, et al. Association between salt sensitivity and insulin concentrations in patients with hypertension. *Am J Hypertens* 1995; **8**: 855–8.

78. Paffenbarger RS, Thorne MC, Wing AL. Chronic disease in former college students: VIII. Characteristics in youth predisposing to hypertension in later years. *Am J Epidemiol* 1968; **88**: 25–32.

79. Selby JV, Friedman GD, Quesenberry CP. Precursors of essential hypertension: pulmonary function, heart rate, uric acid, serum cholesterol and other serum chemistries. *Am J Epidemiol* 1990; **131**: 1017–27.

80. Reaven GM, Lithell H, Landsberg L. Hypertension and associated metabolic abnormalities – the role of insulin resistance and the sympathoadrenal system. *N Engl J Med* 1996; **334**: 374–81.

81. Landsberg L. Diet, obesity and hypertension: a hypothesis involving insulin, the sympathetic nervous system, and adaptive thermogenesis. *Q J Med* 1986; **61**: 1081–90.

82. Reaven GM, Twersky J, Chang H. Abnormalities of carbohydrate and lipid metabolism in Dahl rats. *Hypertension* 1991; **18**: 630–5.

83. Rune MO, Myking OL, Lund-Johansen P, Omvik P. The Bergen blood pressure study: inappropriately low levels of circulating atrial natriuretic peptide in offspring of hypertensive families. *Blood Pressure* 1994; **3**: 223–30.

84. Ferri C, Piccoli A, Laurenti O, et al. Atrial natriuretic factor in hypertensive and normotensive diabetic patients. *Diabetes Care* 1994; **17**: 195–200.

85. Collins R, Peto R, MacMahon S, et al. Blood pressure, stroke and coronary heart disease. Pt. 2. Short-term reductions in blood pressure: overview of randomised drug trials in their epidemiological context. *Lancet* 1990; **335**: 827–38.

86. Sheu WH-H, Jeng C-Y, Shieh S-M, et al. Insulin resistance and abnormal electrocardiograms in patients with high blood pressure. *Am J Hypertens* 1992; **5**: 444–8.

87. Reaven GM. Treatment of hypertension: focus on prevention of coronary heart disease. *J Clin Endocrinol Metab* 1993; **76**: 537–40.

4

Dyslipidaemia: implications for cardiovascular risk in hypertensive diabetic subjects

D John Betteridge

Introduction

Patients with diabetes mellitus and particularly those with concurrent hypertension are at high risk of premature and extensive atherosclerotic disease. Dyslipidaemia is an important additional risk factor which is open to therapeutic manipulation. Subgroup analyses of the coronary heart disease (CHD) secondary prevention trials with statin drugs indicate that diabetics do well in terms of risk reduction. In this short review the burden of atherosclerosis-related disease in diabetes will be discussed together with the impact of dyslipidaemia and hypertension. The pathophysiology of dyslipidaemia will be described and an approach to management outlined. In addition, the impact of diabetic nephropathy and the potential impact of various antihypertensive drugs on dyslipidaemia will be discussed.

Atherosclerosis-related disease

Although the possibility of a specific diabetic large vessel disease has been raised in the past, it is likely that the major underlying cause of cardiovascular disease in diabetic populations is atherosclerosis.[1] Several pathological studies have indicated the more extensive and premature nature of atherosclerosis in patients with diabetes. The degree of atherosclerosis in diabetics varies from country to country, as

demonstrated by the International Atherosclerosis Project;[2] however, the additional impact of diabetes is evident for each country. It would appear from this and other studies[3] that diabetes accelerates the progression of atherosclerosis in all populations studied.

Coronary heart disease

CHD accounts for 75 per cent of the cardiovascular deaths seen in diabetic patients. In fact, 80 per cent of all deaths are attributable to cardiovascular disease and >75 per cent of all hospitalisations are attributable to cardiovascular disease.[1,4–6] In specific pathological studies of the coronary vessels, diabetics have been found to have a more diffuse distribution of lesions together with a larger number of vessels involved and also more severe narrowing of the left main coronary artery.[7,8]

In angiography analyses carried out as part of thrombolytic and PTCA studies, a higher frequency of multi-vessel disease in diabetic patients has been observed compared with non-diabetic individuals.[9–11]

Both the risk of developing acute myocardial infarction and mortality – particularly in hospital mortality associated with acute infarction – are increased 2–3-fold in diabetic patients compared with non-diabetic individuals.[1,5,9,12] This appears to be related to increased left ventricular failure, cardiogenic shock and conduction disturbances.[6] Furthermore, the long-term prognosis after myocardial infarction is much worse for diabetics than non-diabetics. The time to recurrent myocardial infarction or fatal event was 5.3 years for diabetic men compared with 7.1 years in non-diabetic men in the Framingham Study.[13] In a Swedish study, in-hospital mortality for diabetic patients was 12 per cent compared with 8 per cent for non-diabetic subjects. At 5 years the overall mortality was 55 per cent versus 30 per cent in non-diabetics.[14]

Many studies have indicated that diabetics have a poorer prognosis following intervention procedures for coronary heart disease than non-diabetics.[15] In the recent Bypass Angioplasty Revascularisation Investigation,[16] the 5-year post-coronary artery bypass graft survival rate was 80.6 per cent in the diabetic subgroup compared with 89.3 per cent in non-diabetic subjects. A particularly poor outcome was noticed in diabetics after percutaneous transluminal coronary angioplasty, the 5-year survival rate being 65.5 per cent compared with 86.3 per cent in the non-diabetic group.

Cerebrovascular disease

Diabetic patients have a 2–4-fold increased relative risk of cerebrovascular disease.[1] In the Multiple Risk Factor Intervention Trial (MRFIT), diabetic men had an increased risk of fatal, non-haemorrhagic stroke of 3.8 per cent (95 per cent confidence interval, 2.7–5.3).[17] Similarly in the Nurses' Health Study the age-adjusted risk of stroke for diabetic women versus non-diabetic women was 4.1 per cent (95 per cent confidence interval, 2.8–6.1).[18] Similar findings have been found in other populations, including the Rancho Barnado study, the Honolulu Heart Program and large prospective cohorts followed in Finland.[19–21]

Peripheral vascular disease

The presence of peripheral vascular disease, whether assessed by the presence of claudication, absence of foot pulses, or lower extremity amputations, is markedly increased in diabetics.[22] The risk of amputation is increased 10–15-fold and the presence of intermittent claudication in a large Finnish population was 3–4 times increased in diabetic men and 5–7 times in diabetic women.[23] Similar findings have been reported from the Framingham Study.[24] The typical medial artery calcification or Monkenberg's sclerosis appears to be an important risk predictor in diabetic patients and in a large Finnish cohort was associated with shortened survival rates and increased cardiovascular mortality.[25]

Proteinuria, nephropathy and risk of cerebrovascular disease

A well-recognised, but as yet unexplained, independent risk factor for cardiovascular events and mortality in diabetic patients is the presence of early nephropathy as indicated by the presence of proteinuria.[26,27] Proteinuria is associated with adverse changes in recognised cardiovascular risk factors such as hypertension and dyslipidaemia,[26] but this does not fully explain the association. It has been suggested that proteinuria may be a mark of widespread endothelial dysfunction or other vascular damage, leading to accelerated atherosclerosis and cardiovascular disease.[28] An association between proteinuria and stroke has also been demonstrated in some but not all studies.[1] The risk of cardiovascular disease is increased already at the microalbuminuric stage.[26]

Lipids, lipoproteins and atherosclerosis

The increased risk of atherosclerosis-related diseases in the diabetic population may be due to an increased prevalence of traditional risk factors, specific diabetic risk factors, an increased impact of a given risk factor, or a combination of these factors – which is likely to be the case. There is no doubt that hyperglycaemia is a risk factor for atherosclerosis-related disease. This relationship is already evident at the impaired glucose tolerance stage, so there is a relatively low threshold at which glucose concentration begins to be a risk factor.[1] The mechanism of the relationship between glucose and CHD most probably relates to the formation of advanced glycosylation end-products which have the potential to be involved in the many stages of the atherogenic process including increased low-density lipoprotein (LDL) oxidation and trapping in the arterial wall, endothelial cell damage with increased permeability and cell adhesion, procoagulant effects, monocyte/macrophage chemotaxis and activation with cytokine and growth factor secretion and smooth muscle proliferation.[29]

An early study, the University Group Diabetes Program, which examined the relationship between glycaemic control with various agents and cardiovascular mortality was stopped prematurely because of the apparent excess of cardiovascular mortality in the group receiving the sulphonylurea, tolbutamide.[30] This trial has been heavily criticised and to a large extent its findings have been ignored. However, it is now known that sulphonylureas act by closing ATP-dependent potassium channels in the β cell, leading to depolarisation, entry of calcium into the cell and insulin secretion.[31] Similar ATP-sensitive potassium channels are present in the vasculature and are important in ischaemic preconditioning. It is conceivable that sulphonylureas may interfere with important ATP-sensitive potassium channel activity outside the β cell.[32] However, the United Kingdom Prospective Diabetes Study on type II diabetes shows that more intensive glycaemic control with either sulphonylureas or insulin substantially reduces microvascular endpoints, but has non-significant effects on macrovascular disease. Nevertheless there did not appear to be adverse effects of sulphonylureas compared to insulin.[33] In the Diabetes Control and Complications Trial in type I diabetes there were insufficient numbers of events to examine the impact of tight glycaemic control with multiple insulin injections on macrovascular disease in type I diabetics;[34] however, there was a trend to reduction.

The physician caring for diabetic patients makes every attempt to achieve as good glycaemic control as possible to reduce the risk of the microvascular complications of retinopathy, nephropathy and neuropathy. However, with the drugs currently available for the treatment of type II diabetes and the progressive nature of the disease, it is unlikely that the degree of glycaemic control will be sufficient to decrease CHD risk[33] associated with increased glucose levels because of the low threshold at which risk begins to increase. For these reasons, a concerted effort to reduce the classical risk factors for atherosclerosis might prove to be more rewarding in reducing the burden of cardiovascular disease. The St Vincent Declaration has called for efforts along these lines.[35] In support of this recommendation the 12-year follow-up of the subjects screened in the MRFIT project has demonstrated the importance of conventional risk factors for cardiovascular death in a large diabetic population.[36] In all, 5163 individuals screened for the MRFIT study were known to have diabetes. At the 12-year follow-up, diabetic patients demonstrated a three-fold increased absolute risk of cardiovascular death which was independent of age, race, income, serum cholesterol, systolic blood pressure and cigarette smoking. These data confirm the independent association of diabetes with vascular risk shown in previous smaller studies. Increasing serum cholesterol was associated with increased cardiovascular risk in both diabetic and non-diabetic men (Fig. 4.1). This was also true for blood pressure and cigarette smoking and when the three major risk factors were combined. The authors concluded that rigorous intervention to lower cholesterol, abolish cigarette smoking and control blood pressure would result in a major reduction in cardiovascular disease in diabetic patients.[36] This massive database linking increasing serum cholesterol to cardiovascular risk in diabetes is supported by extensive data involving other populations in the Framingham Study,[37] Finnish[38] and British populations.[39]

Cholesterol and low-density lipoprotein-cholesterol

As in non-diabetic populations, the link between cholesterol and cardiovascular risk relates to LDL-cholesterol. There is extensive knowledge as to how LDL concentrations are controlled[40] and also how LDL interacts with the arterial wall to produce the fatty streak, the early lesion of atherosclerosis.[41] LDL is derived from very low-density lipoprotein (VLDL) following the progressive hydrolysis of triglyceride by lipoprotein lipase and hepatic lipase. The particle serves to transport cholesterol to peripheral cells and carries approximately 70 per cent of plasma cholesterol. Excess LDL is removed by the liver through a specific high-affinity receptor. The receptor has been cloned and localised to the shortarm of chromosome 19.[42] Following binding to the receptor, the receptor/LDL complex is internalised by the process of absorptive endocytosis. The increasing cellular cholesterol content is important in regulating cholesterol homeostasis within the cell. It reduces synthesis of cholesterol through inhibiting the rate-determining enzyme HMG-CoA reductase and stimulates its own re-esterification through the enzyme acyl:cholesterol acyltransferase. Increasing cellular cholesterol also reduces synthesis of LDL receptors. The activity of LDL receptors

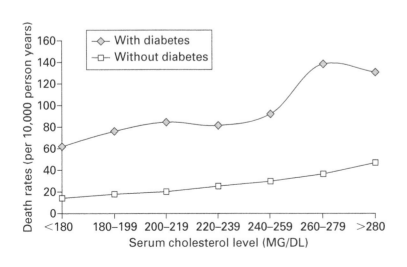

Figure 4.1

The Multiple Risk Factor Intervention Trial (MRFIT). Effect of diabetes on the relationship between the usual total cholesterol and 10 year death rate in men aged 35–57 years, with and without diabetes. (Adapted from reference 36.)

largely determines plasma LDL-cholesterol levels.

It has become clear that the monocyte macrophage plays an important role in foam cell formation and the fatty streak.[41] In experimental animals fed a high-cholesterol diet, the first identifiable lesion is the adherence of monocytes to the arterial endothelium. At a later stage these accumulate in the sub-endothelial space where they acquire the characteristics of macrophages and become lipid-laden foam cells. The accumulation of these cells leads to disruption of the overlying endothelium which allows platelet adhesion and aggregation, the release of powerful growth factors and further proliferation of the plaque.

Early studies showed that native LDL did not lead to foam cell formation when incubated with monocyte macrophages. However, chemically modified LDL was taken up avidly by these cells to produce foam cells.[42] It is likely that *in vivo* the modification of LDL resulting in its uptake by these cells is oxidation.[43,44] Oxidatively modified LDL can contribute to atherosclerosis in several ways, including direct cytotoxicity to endothelium and the stimulation of monocyte adhesion and chemotaxis. There are also important interactions between modified LDL and the coagulation system through increased expression of tissue factor and increased expression of plasminogen activator inhibitor 1 (PAI-1). Oxidised LDL also inhibits endothelial-derived relaxing factor and leads to enhanced expression of endothelin, a potent vasoconstrictor.

High-density lipoprotein

High-density lipoprotein (HDL)-cholesterol concentration is inversely related to vascular disease in diabetic populations, particularly in type II diabetics.[1] As measured by ultracentrifugation, HDL was the most powerful determinant for CHD in a large Finnish population of type II patients, low HDL being associated with a four-fold increase in risk of death from CHD.[45] The mechanism(s) by which HDL protects against atherosclerotic disease remains to be determined. The role of HDL in reverse cholesterol transport with the return of cholesterol from peripheral tissues including the arterial wall to the liver for excretion is an attractive hypothesis.[46,47] However, other hypotheses do not implicate HDL in a direct role and suggest that HDL cholesterol concentrations reflect the efficiency or otherwise of metabolism of triglyceride-rich lipoproteins and that this is the major relationship with vascular risk. Other important potential protective effects of HDL involve antioxidant and anti-inflammatory effects due to paraoxanase enzymes on the HDL complex which may limit oxidative modification of LDL. Furthermore, HDL may have antithrombotic effects through inhibiting platelet aggregation and stimulating prostacyclin production.

The relationship between increasing levels of plasma triglycerides and atherosclerotic-related disease remains controversial. There is no doubt that many studies have shown a strong relationship between triglyceride and CHD. However, when multivariate analysis was applied to the data and the relationship adjusted for other variables, particularly HDL cholesterol, cholesterol and obesity, the relationship disappeared.[48] Plasma triglycerides show more inherent biological variability than other lipid fractions, particularly cholesterol and HDL-cholesterol, and as a result come out less strongly in multivariate analysis. It is also inappropriate to separate plasma triglyceride from HDL-cholesterol in multivariate analysis, as these variables are intimately related metabolically. Much of the HDL fraction comes from the transfer of surface components from triglyceride-rich lipoproteins during hydrolysis.

Some authors have attempted to analyse the relationship of the cluster of high triglyceride, low HDL and high LDL to CHD risk. Data from the Framingham Study suggested that triglyceride was a risk factor when HDL-cholesterol was low.[49] In the placebo group of the Helsinki Heart Study[50] and in the PROCAM study,[51] increasing triglyceride did appear to be a risk factor when the LDL:HDL-cholesterol ratio was >5.

Although recent analysis of population-based prospective studies has pointed to an independent role for plasma triglycerides in non-diabetics even when the data were corrected for HDL-cholesterol,[52] it is likely that epidemiological studies will not provide definitive answers with regard to triglyceride. Perhaps a more useful approach is to learn more about the potential pathological mechanisms relating triglycerides to CHD.[53] It is known that some triglyceride-rich lipoproteins, particularly the remnants of chylomicrons and VLDL, are atherogenic. These accumulate in type III hyperlipidaemia, which is associated with premature and extensive atherosclerosis. Furthermore, hypertriglyceridaemia is associated with important alterations in other lipoprotein species, rendering them more atherogenic. With increasing plasma triglyceride, the distribution of LDL particles is shifted to smaller, more dense particles which are thought to be more atherogenic.[54] HDL levels are lower in the presence of hypertriglyceridaemia and it is likely that this is because of increased catabolism of HDL. Hypertriglyceridaemia is also associated with abnormalities which are likely to increase the risk of thrombosis. PAI-1 levels are increased leading to decreased fibrinolysis. In addition the serum protease, factor VII – an important component of the coagulation system – is also increased in hypertriglyceridaemia.[53]

Several studies of the relationship of triglycerides to cardiovascular risk in diabetes have pointed to a stronger relationship in diabetic patients.[1] However, to a large extent, HDL-cholesterol was not measured and therefore it is not possible to assess the independent nature of the association. In a substudy of the WHO Multinational Study, triglyceride levels were higher among those with major Q wave abnormalities on the electrocardiogram (ECG) and this association remained significant after adjustment for age, cholesterol and systolic blood pressure.[55] In the Paris prospective study triglyceride was associated with increased CHD risk in both diabetes and men with impaired glucose tolerance.[56] This relationship persisted after adjustment for total cholesterol, systolic blood pressure, body mass index and cigarette smoking. HDL-cholesterol was not measured in this study. In a large study of type II patients from Finland, high triglycerides were also a significant risk factor for stroke.[57]

Lipoprotein(a)

Lipoprotein(a) is a subpopulation of LDL to which an additional apoprotein, designated apoprotein(a), is attached by a disulphide bond.[58] Lipoprotein(a) concentrations vary widely between populations. In Europeans, the majority of individuals have low levels; however, there is a pronounced positive skew to the distribution, with some individuals having very high levels. This variation appears to be mainly genetically determined. Little is known about the physiology of lipoprotein(a), but it does appear that rate of production is a major determinant of plasma concentration. Apoprotein(a) has close structural homology with plasminogen and it has been speculated that this lipoprotein provides an important link with coagulation.[59] Lipoprotein(a) binds to the plasminogen receptor and may interfere with the normal action of plasminogen. Many case control studies have demonstrated a relationship between high levels of lipoprotein(a) and CHD risk.[60] It is also a risk factor for restenosis after angioplasty and coronary artery bypass grafting. It is likely that the relationship between lipoprotein(a) and cardiovascular risk is only present in populations with Western-type cholesterol levels.

Conflicting findings have appeared in the literature with regard to lipoprotein(a) concentrations in both type I and type II diabetes,[61–68] and more prospective studies of a possible relationship between lipoprotein(a) concentrations and CHD are required. In type I patients a relationship with proteinuria has been described,[63,64] but a relationship with glycaemic control has not been reported consistently.[63,65] In type II patients there does not appear to be an alteration in lipoprotein(a) concentrations.[66–68] In one prospective study, as part of the Wisconsin Epidemiology Survey, no relationship was found between lipoprotein(a) levels and CHD risk.[69]

Lipid abnormalities in type I diabetes

Total lipid and lipoprotein concentrations in type I patients will depend on the degree of glycaemic control, the degree of obesity and the presence or absence of nephropathy.[70–73] Patients with good glycaemic control have similar lipid and lipoprotein concentrations to non-diabetic control subjects. In the patients taking part in the Diabetes Control and Complications Trial it was only LDL-cholesterol concentrations in women that were slightly higher than in matched non-diabetic populations.[74] In type I patients with poor glycaemic control the concentrations of VLDL and LDL increase due to increased production of apoB-containing lipoproteins in the liver and their decreased clearance by lipoprotein lipase secondary to insulin deficiency. Chylomicronaemia can occur in severe insulin deficiency with eruptive xanthomata and the risk of pancreatitis. Instigation of appropriate insulin therapy rapidly corrects these abnormalities. Although total lipoprotein concentrations are similar to controls, there are potentially important qualitative changes in type I patients, particularly glycation of apoprotein B. Glycated LDL binds less well to the LDL receptor, tends to have a prolonged half-time in the circulation and is also more prone to oxidation.

Lipid abnormalities in type II diabetes

Quantitative and qualitative abnormalities of lipid and lipoproteins are more common in type II patients and collectively the abnormalities are often referred to as diabetic dyslipidaemia.[71,73,75,76] This clustering of lipid abnormalities includes moderate hypertriglyceridaemia with or without a moderate increase in total cholesterol and a reduced concentration of HDL-cholesterol. These abnormalities are strongly related to insulin resistance and prospective studies such as the San Antonio Heart Study suggest that elevated insulin concentrations precede the development of the other associated metabolic abnormalities.[77] The hypertriglyceridaemia is associated with an accumulation of remnant particles which are thought to be highly atherogenic and enhanced postprandial lipaemia. Furthermore, hypertriglyceridaemia in type II patients is a major determinant of the presence of small dense LDL particles.

It has been recognised for many years that LDL is not homogeneous and there are distinct subspecies which vary in size, density and lipid content.[78,79] LDL particle diameter and the relative content of lipid decrease as LDL density increases. LDL-II tends to be the most abundant subspecies and women have proportionately more LDL-I than men who have proportionately more LDL-III. LDL sub-fractions are optimally separated by density gradient ultracentrifugation, but this is not practical in large epidemiological studies. However, it is possible to separate LDL parti-cles by gradient gel electrophoresis. With this technique Austin and colleagues[54] have defined two distinct subclasses designated pattern A and pattern B. Pattern B was found to be asso-ciated with a three-fold increased risk of myocardial infarction. Small dense LDL is also related to coronary atherosclerosis demonstra-ted in angiographic studies (Fig. 4.2).[80]

The pathogenesis of the dyslipidaemia of type II diabetes is not yet fully understood. However, it is possible to explain many of the abnormalities on the basis of current knowl-edge.[76] In the presence of insulin resistance and hyperinsulinaemia there will be decreased inhibition of hormone-sensitive lipase in adipose tissue leading to an increased flux of non-esterified fatty acids to the liver. This is a major stimulus to VLDL production which is increased, particularly large VLDL. Kinetic studies have shown that large VLDL is con-verted to small, dense LDL. In the postpran-dial state, hepatic output of VLDL continues and this competes for the hydrolytic activity of lipoprotein lipase with exogenously derived lipid carried by chylomicrons. Postprandial lipaemia is prolonged with increased lipid transport between lipoprotein particles via cholesterol ester transfer protein, leading to relative triglyceride enrichment of both LDL and HDL which are then substrates for hepatic lipase. This leads to relative lipid depletion of both LDL and HDL, leading to small dense HDL and small dense LDL. Small dense HDL is catabolised more rapidly, lead-ing to low HDL-cholesterol concentrations.

There is increasing evidence of the impor-tance of small dense LDL in atherosclerosis; however, the exact mechanisms of this rela-tionship are not fully understood. Small dense LDL is a poorer ligand for the LDL receptor, therefore it will tend to be diverted into more atherogenic pathways. Small dense LDL is more susceptible to oxidation, and oxidised LDL is central to many of the processes involved in atherosclerosis. Small dense LDL also penetrates the arterial wall more effec-tively and binds to glycosaminase glycans more effectively in the arterial wall.

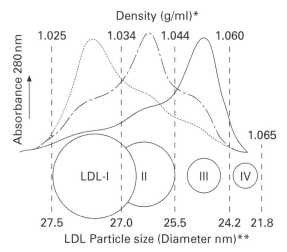

Figure 4.2
*Distribution of human plasma LDL subclass density and particle size. *LDL subclass density profiles were obtained by density gradient ultracentrifugation. Representative gradient profiles are shown for a healthy female (— —), healthy male (__ _ __) and patient with coronary artery disease (___). (Reproduced from reference 79.)*

Lipid and lipoprotein abnormalities in nephropathic patients

It is clear that alterations in lipid and lipoprotein concentrations occur in diabetic patients with nephropathy. Even at the early stage of microalbuminuria, lipoprotein abnormalities are evident with an increase in cholesterol and triglyceride and a decrease in HDL-cholesterol. Lipoprotein(a) concentrations are also increased in proteinuric diabetic patients. As renal impairment increases, more marked lipid and lipoprotein concentrations can occur. If the nephrotic syndrome develops there can be substantial increases in LDL-cholesterol with a smaller increase in VLDL. In chronic renal failure VLDL and therefore triglyceride concentrations rise, with a smaller increase in LDL and a decrease in HDL. These changes persist in patients receiving haemodialysis or chronic ambulatory peritoneal dialysis.

Management of diabetic dyslipidaemia

From the above discussion it is clear that it is important to include measures of lipid and lipoprotein concentrations as part of the annual assessment of diabetic patients. For clinical purposes, a fasting cholesterol, triglyceride and HDL-cholesterol are sufficient. From these data LDL-cholesterol can be calculated from the Friedewald equation:[81]

$$LDL\text{-cholesterol} = \text{total cholesterol} -$$
$$HDL\text{-cholesterol} - \frac{\text{triglyceride}}{2.19}$$

(all concentrations in mmol/l). This equation gives a reasonable approximation of LDL-cholesterol as long as total triglycerides are <4.5 mmol/l. However, in type II diabetics, because of the qualitative changes in VLDL, this equation may be less accurate than in non-diabetic patients.[82] Obtaining a fasting sample may be inconvenient, particularly in type I patients, where random samples may suffice. In type II patients it is generally best to obtain a fasting sample, as this allows more accurate measurement of HDL, but if the random triglyceride is <2.5 mmol/l then fasting triglyceride will generally provide a satisfactory result.

In the management of lipid abnormalities in diabetes, other possible secondary causes of dyslipidaemia and coexistent primary lipid abnormalities should be considered. It is particularly important to exclude hypothyroidism as a cause of significant hypercholesterolaemia, but hypothyroidism may be associated

Risk	LDL cholesterol	HDL cholesterol	Triglyceride
High	≥130	<35	≥400
Borderline	100–129	35–45	200–399
Low	<100	>45	<200

Table 4.1
Category of risk based on lipoprotein levels in adults with diabetes. Values are given as mg/dl. For women the HDL cholesterol levels should be increased by 10 mg/dl.

	Lifestyle modification		Drug therapy	
	Initiation	LDL goal	Initiation	LDL goal
With CVD, PVD or CHD	≥100 mg/dl	<100 mg/dl	≥100 mg/dl	<100 mg/dl
Without CVD, PVD or CHD	≥100 mg/dl	<100 mg/dl	≥130 mg/dl*	<100 mg/dl

Table 4.2
*Lifestyle modification refers to diet and exercise. *For these patients, a variety of treatment strategies are recommended, including more aggressive lifestyle management and statin therapy.[84]*

with any lipid abnormality. Diabetic patients, particularly type II, commonly have concurrent hypertension and consideration should be given to the possible adverse effects of some antihypertensive agents – not only on the dyslipidaemia but also on insulin resistance.

Goals of therapy

The American Diabetes Association (ADA) have recently issued a new 'position statement' on the management of dyslipidaemia in adults with diabetes. [83,84] Because of the high risk of CHD, an aggressive policy for identification and treatment of dyslipidaemia has been advocated. They have categorised the level of CHD risk for people with type 2 diabetes, according to lipoprotein levels, as shown in Table 4.1. It is recommended that because of the frequent fluctuations in glycaemic control and its effects on lipoproteins, the lipid profile should be measured and the risk re-assessed annually.

The ADA has defined 'optimal' LDL cholesterol levels for adults with diabetes as <100 mg/dl (2.60 mmol/l), optimal HDL cholesterol levels are defined as >45 mg/dl

(1.15 mmol/l) and desirable triglyceride levels are <150 mg/dl (1.7 mmol/l). Because women without diabetes generally have higher HDL cholesterol levels than men, the statement suggests it may be desirable to recommend even higher optimal HDL levels in diabetic women.

The guidance prioritizes LDL cholesterol lowering and the treatment initiation thresholds and therapeutic goals are shown in Table 4.2. These recommendations are consistent with the recent guidance from the National Cholesterol Education Programme (NCEP III) for LDL cholesterol lowering in adults.[85] It can be seen that priority is given to lowering LDL-cholesterol. From the above discussion it should be clear that although LDL-cholesterols are similar in diabetic and non-diabetic subjects, qualitative changes in LDL make it more atherogenic within the diabetic population. Furthermore, available information from intervention trials on diabetic subgroups points to the benefits of lowering LDL-cholesterol in preventing the development of CHD and reducing subsequent events in those with established disease.[86–89] The second priority is to increase HDL-cholesterol by lifestyle measures – particularly weight reduction, cessation

1. LDL CHOLESTEROL LOWERING:
   - First Choice:
   - HMG-CoA Reductase Inhibitor (STATIN)
   - Second Choice:
   - Bile Acid Binding Resin (RESIN) or Fenofibrate

2. HDL CHOLESTEROL RAISING:
   - First Choice:
   - Lifestyle Intervention

3. TRIGLYCERIDE LOWERING:
   - Glycaemic control is first priority
   - Fibrates: Gemfibrozil or Fenofibrate
   - Statins can be moderately effective in high dose in patients who have co-existing elevated LDL cholesterol

4. COMBINED HYPERLIPIDAEMIA:
   - First Choice:
   - Improved glycaemic control + High dose statin
   - Second Choice:

Glycaemic control + statin + fibrate* (specialist care)

Table 4.3
Order of Priorities for Treating Diabetic Dyslipidaemias. Adapted from the ADA position statement.[83]
*The combination of statins with fibrates (i.e. gemfibrozil or fenofibrate) may carry an increased risk of myositis.

of cigarette smoking, improved glycaemic control and increasing physical activity. The third priority is to treat hypertriglyceridaemia by weight reduction and improving glycaemic control. If these measures fail then fibrate therapy may be necessary.

In contrast to data with statins, there is less evidence from clinical trials on which to base recommendations for fibrate therapy. These are discussed later.[90] The fourth priority is to treat mixed hyperlipidaemia, which is really the province of the specialist, and may require combined therapy of a statin and a fibrate. This combination of drugs is very effective, but because of the increased risk of side-effects, particularly myopathy, careful monitoring is required.

Table 4.3, taken from the recent ADA position statement[84] summarizes the order of priorities for the management of dyslipidaemia in adults with diabetes.

Glycaemic control and lifestyle measures

There is no doubt that improving glycaemic control in type I and type II patients with appropriate therapy will improve the lipid profile, particularly by reducing the VLDL concentrations. However, diabetic patients established on best available therapy for that individual often continue to show lipid abnormalities.[91] This is not surprising, because diabetic dyslipidaemia is an important part of the insulin resistance syndrome and available drugs do not have a major impact on insulin sensitivity. Early studies with sulphonylureas suggested that HDL concentrations were reduced, but these findings were not substantiated by further studies. Small but potentially beneficial effects on lipid and lipoprotein concentrations have been observed with metformin, which decreases hepatic glucose output.[92,93] There may be considerable potential to see beneficial effects on diabetic dyslipidaemia with the new class of antidiabetic agents, the thiazoladine diones, and early studies have shown a decrease in plasma triglycerides and an increase in HDL-cholesterol.[94] However, LDL-cholesterol levels have remained unchanged or increased slightly with no change in apoB, suggesting that the distribution of LDL has been changed to larger more buoyant, less atherogenic particles.

Lifestyle measures, particularly weight reduction and increased physical activity, will have an impact on plasma lipids and lipoproteins – particularly plasma triglycerides.[95,96] There may be more modest reductions in LDL-cholesterol with slight increases in HDL. Although an important part of management in all diabetic patients, the amount of physical activity required to have these beneficial metabolic effects is difficult to achieve – often because of associated medical problems, particularly cardiovascular disease, and also because of poor long-term motivation and compliance with exercise regimes.

The usual dietary recommendations involve reduction in the amount of calories from saturated fat and replacement with complex carbohydrate, with a high fibre content. An alternative approach in type II patients is to receive more calories from fat, but incorporate mono-unsaturated fat.[97] This approach offers an important alternative which may be more palatable to some individuals and has beneficial effects on insulin sensitivity and lipoprotein levels. In individuals who take a high carbohydrate diet but do not increase the fibre content there may be less beneficial effect, particularly with regard to persisting hypertriglyceridaemia and small dense LDL particles.

Lipid-lowering medications
Statins

Current evidence supports the use of statins as first-line lipid lowering therapy in people with diabetes. The initial evidence was derived from retrospective sub-group analysis of cohorts of patients with diabetes in a series of primary and secondary prevention trials evaluating the efficacy of statin therapy. The secondary prevention trials in patients with pre-existing CHD have shown that statins reduce the risk of CHD morbidity and mortality in patients with diabetes and that the effects equate to approximately a 25% reduction in CHD per mmol reduction in LDL cholesterol, maintained over 5 years.[86–88, 98] The 4S study compared 20–40 mg daily of simvastatin with placebo and the average difference in total cholesterol was 1.7 mmol/l. CARE and LIPID compared pravastatin 40 mg daily, with placebo, and the average differences in cholesterol were 1.0 and 1.1 mmol respectively. The outcome of these interventions are summarized in Fig. 4.3.

Thus, the evidence for secondary prevention of cardiovascular events with statins in people with diabetes and pre-existing CHD was consistent and strong.

Further evidence emerged with subgroup analysis of diabetic patients within a primary prevention study with lovastatin versus placebo; AFCAPs/TexCAPS.[89] However, this

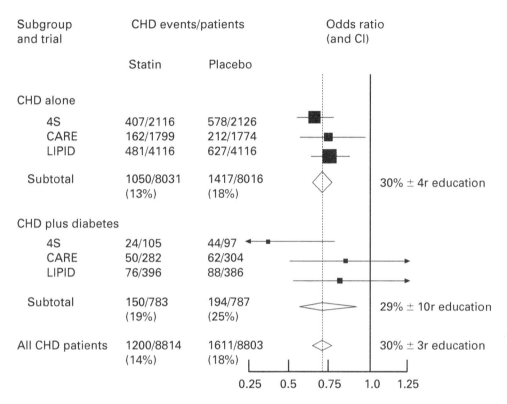

Figure 4.3
Observed effects on major CHD events in randomised controlled trials of cholesterol lowering with statin treatment among people with pre-existing CHD, subdivided by diagnosis of diabetes to baseline. Odds ratios (Ors) for CHD events in each trial are shown as black squares, with the area of the square proportionate to the number of events. The 99% confidence intervals (CIs) are shown as horizontal lines. The subtotal Ors are shown as open diamonds with 95% CIs. (Adapted from Armitage J and Collins R. Heart 2000, 84: 357–60.)

study contained only 239 patients with diabetes and although there was a trend to a 43% reduction in CHD, the study was substantially under-powered to definitively assess the role of statins in primary prevention against CHD and other vascular events in people with diabetes (Figs 4.4 and 4.5).

Powerful data for primary prevention with statins in diabetes emerged recently with the publication of the results from the Heart Protection Study (HPS) in the UK.[99] The HPS randomized 20,536 adults (aged 40–80 years) with coronary disease, other occlusive vascular disease or diabetes, to receive simvastatin 40 mg daily or matching placebo, for a duration of 5 years. Of the patients, three-quarters were men. The average study compliance with simvastatin was 85% and the average use of non-study statin in the placebo group was 17%. Thus, the intention to treat comparison actually assessed the effect of about two-thirds of patients actually taking a statin, yielding an average difference in LDL-cholesterol of 1 mol/l.

Study	Drug	No.	Baseline LDL-C, mg/dl (mmol/l)	LDL-C Lowering
Primary prevention				
AFCAPS/TexCAPS	Lovastatin	239	150 (3.9)	25%
Secondary prevention				
CARE	Pravastatin	586	136 (3.6)	28%
4S	Simvastatin	202	186 (4.8)	36%
LIPID	Pravastatin	782	150* (3.9)	25%

Figure 4.4
Sub-group analysis of diabetic cohorts within primary and secondary cardiovascular disease prevention trial using statins. Baseline cholesterol and cholesterol lowering.

Study	Drug	No.	CHD risk reduction (overall)	CHD risk reduction (diabetes)
Primary prevention				
AFCAPS/TexCAPS	Lovastatin	239	37%	43%
Secondary prevention				
CARE	Pravastatin	586	23%	25% ($p = 0.05$)
4S	Simvastatin	202	32%	55% ($p = 0.002$)
LIPID	Pravastatin	782	25%	19%
4S-Extended	Simvastatin	483	32%	42% ($p = 0.001$)

Figure 4.5
Sub-group analysis of diabetic cohorts within primary and secondary cardiovascular disease prevention trial using statins. CHD risk reduction with statin therapy in all patients and those with diabetes at baseline.

In the HPS all cause mortality was significantly reduced by statin treatment mainly due to a highly significant reduction in coronary death, which was reduced by about 25%. Fatal and non-fatal stroke was also reduced by about 25%. (Figs 4.6 and 4.7). The proportional reduction in the event rates was similar in each subcategory of patient studied, including those with coronary disease, stroke, peripheral vascular disease or diabetes.

The HPS included 5,963 patients with diabetes (10% type 1 and 90% type 2) aged 40–80 years. Previous myocardial infarction was reported at study entry in 1,125 (19%) of the diabetic cohort. There was some other history of CHD in a further 853 (14%). A total of 3,982 patients had no prior history of coronary disease (67%) and 2,913 (49%) had no history of any cardiovascular disease at baseline. 19% of patients with type 1 diabetes and

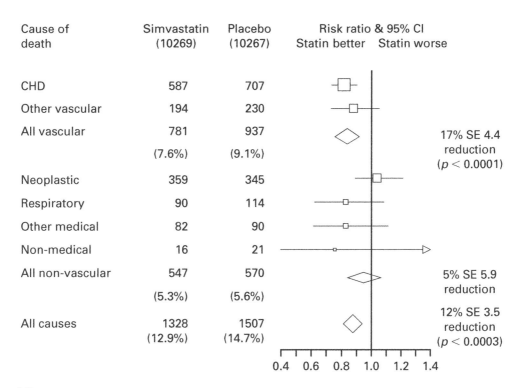

Cause of death	Simvastatin (10269)	Placebo (10267)	Risk ratio & 95% CI Statin better Statin worse	
CHD	587	707		
Other vascular	194	230		
All vascular	781	937		17% SE 4.4 reduction (p < 0.0001)
	(7.6%)	(9.1%)		
Neoplastic	359	345		
Respiratory	90	114		
Other medical	82	90		
Non-medical	16	21		
All non-vascular	547	570		5% SE 5.9 reduction
	(5.3%)	(5.6%)		
All causes	1328	1507		12% SE 3.5 reduction (p < 0.0003)
	(12.9%)	(14.7%)		

Figure 4.6
Effects of simvastatin on death in the Heart Protection Study.[99]

43% of those with type 2 had treated hypertension. The mean age was 52.6 years (type 1) and 63.2 years (type 2).

Overall, the risk reduction was approximately 25% in simvastatin treated people with diabetes when compared to placebo allocated participants. This is similar to the risk reduction for the entire study. However, the absolute risk reduction was clearly greater in those with diabetes and prior coronary disease because of the higher baseline risk. The risk reduction in HPS with regard to baseline cardiovascular disease status is shown in Table 4.4.

Importantly, the proportional reduction in risk in the HPS was not influenced by the pre-treatment cholesterol or triglyceride concentrations. This is illustrated in Table 4.5. Thus, the HPS shows unequivocally that lowering LDL-cholesterol from 3.0 mmol/l (116 mg/dl) to 2.0 mmol/l (77 mg/dl) reduces vascular risk by about 25%. The aforementioned ADA guidelines and ATP III recommendations suggest that LDL-cholesterol levels of people at risk i.e. people with diabetes, should be reduced to below 100 mg/dl (2.6 mmol/l).[84,85] In HPS, about 3,500 patients presented with an LDL-cholesterol that was already below this 'target' level and among them, the risk reduction due to statin therapy was as great as that seen in people presenting with a much higher baseline LDL-cholesterol (Table 4.5).

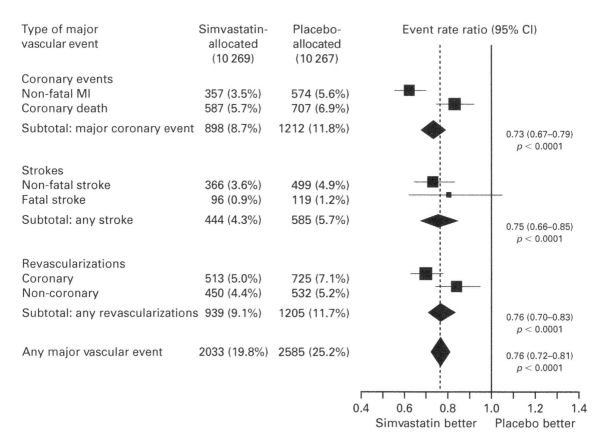

Figure 4.7
Effects of simvastatin allocation on first major coronary event, stroke and revascularization (defined prospectively as 'major vascular events'). Analyses are of the numbers of participants having a first event of each type during follow-up (with non-fatal and fatal events also considered separately) so there is some non-additivity between different types of event. MI=myocardial infarction.[99]

These observations suggest that current guidelines may lead to undertreatment of people at high risk who present with an LDL-cholesterol at or around the current LDL-cholesterol targets. Moreover, these benefits observed in the HPS occurred irrespective of the use of other cardiovascular protective interventions i.e. aspirin, ACE-inhibitors, β-blockers and other antihypertensive therapies.

Another important finding from the HPS was the safety and good tolerability of statin therapy. Liver and muscle enzymes were measured throughout the study and there was difference in the number of patients discontinuing therapy in the simvastatin versus placebo-allocated patients, due to elevated liver enzymes or myopathy. Put simply, simvastatin was safe, well tolerated and very effective at reducing risk.

The HPS has been an important milestone in defining the role of statin therapy in people with and without diabetes. Further studies are

Prior disease	Simvastatin	Placebo	Risk reduction
Diabetes + prior MI or other CHD	325/972 (33.4%)	381/1009 (37.8%)	12%
Diabetes + no prior CHD	276/2006 (13.8%)	367/1976 (18.6%)	26%
Diabetes + CHD or no prior CHD	601/2978 (20.2%)	748/2985 (25.1%)	20%
All patients	2033/10,269 (19.8%)	2585/10,267 (25.2%)	24%

Table 4.4
The effect of simvastatin on the first major vascular event in participants in the Heart Protection Study with diabetes, according to their baseline vascular disease status. All patients refer to the overall study result. Data from reference 99.

Pre-treatment LDL-cholesterol mmol/l (mg/dl)	Simvastatin allocated	Placebo allocated	Risk reduction	
2.6 (100)	282 (16.4%)	358 (21.0%)	22%	p<0.0006
3.0 (116)	598 (17.6%)	756 (22.2%)	21%	p<0.0001
5.0 (193)	360 (17.7%)	472 (23.1%)	23%	p<0.0001

Table 4.5
Risk reduction in HPS according to pre-treatment LDL-cholesterol level. (From reference 99.)

currently ongoing that further clarify the role of statins in patients with diabetes with and without hypertension but without pre-existing coronary heart disease (Table 4.6).

Fibrate therapy
Surprisingly, given the length of time that the drugs have been available for clinical use, there is limited information available regarding the potential use of 'fibrates' for the treatment of diabetic dyslipidaemia. A small number of diabetics were included in the Helsinki Heart Study in which there was a trend to cardiovascular risk reduction with gemfibrozil, but the numbers were too small to be of statistical significance.[90]

The Diabetes Atherosclerosis Intervention Study (DAIS) recently reported.[100] This study was conducted in patients with type 2 diabetes who had mild lipid abnormalities characteristic of type 2 diabetes. The primary objective of the study was to assess whether correcting such lipid abnormalities with micronized fenofibrate (200 mg daily) would alter the progression of coronary artery disease as determined by computer assisted angiographic

Study	Patients	Cholesterol lowering therapy	Approximate number of CHD events in diabetic patients without pre-existing CHD	Estimated study end-date
ALLHAT	Type 2 with hypertension	Pravastatin 40 mg daily versus usual care	250/3500	2002
ASCOT	Type 2 with hypertension and 2 other risk factors	Atorvastatin 10 mg daily versus placebo	200/4000	2003
ASPEN	Type 2 with one risk factor	Atorvastatin 10 mg daily versus placebo	300/4000	2003
CARDS	Type 2 with one risk factor	Atorvastatin 10 mg daily versus placebo	300/3000	2004

Table 4.6
Ongoing trials of statin therapy of ~ 5 years duration in which at least 100 coronary heart disease (CHD) events are expected in people with diabetes. ALLHAT (Antihypertensive and Lipid Lowering treatment to prevent Heart Attack Trial), ASCOT (Anglo-Scandinavian Cardiovascular Outcomes Trial), ASPEN (Atorvastatin study for the Prevention of End-points in NIDDM), CARDS (Collaborative Atorvastatin in Diabetes Study).

assessment of coronary lesions. This was a prospective, randomized, placebo controlled double blind study in med and women aged 40–65 years with a mean follow-up of 39 months. All patients had at least one visible coronary lesion on angiography and 50% had a prior history of clinical CHD, with 33% having had a previous coronary intervention. A total of 731 patients were screened for inclusion and 418 met the cardiac and metabolic entry criteria. The changes in lipid levels during the trial are shown in Fig 4.8. There was no effect of fibrate therapy on blood pressure.

The DAIS study showed that fenofibrate significantly reduced the progression of coronary lesions in patients with type 2 diabetes (Fig. 4.9). The trial was not powered to detect differences in clinical end-points but these were recorded and adjudicated. There was a consistent but non-significant trend to fewer deaths, fewer myocardial infractions and fewer coronary interventions in the fenofibrate treated group. Overall this meant a non-significant trend to fewer clinical end-points in the fenofibrate froup (38 versus 50).

The findings of the DAIS study suggest that in addition to the importance of LDL-cholesterol, the common and seemingly mild lipid disturbances with regard to HDL-Cholesterol and triglyceride levels in people with type 2 diabetes are worthy of intervention with

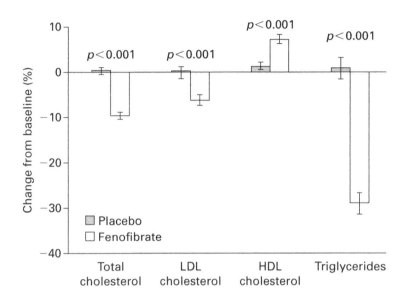

Figure 4.8
Changes in lipid levels in patients in the DAIS study allocated to treatment with fenofibrate or placebo. (From reference 100.)

fibrate therapy. Moreover, such intervention is likely to reduce the risk of coronary disease. In this regard, further information regarding the importance of fibrate therapy will come from a major ongoing primary prevention trial co-ordinated from Australia, using fenofibrate in type 2 diabetes. (Fenofibrate Intervention and Event Lowering in Diabetes (FIELD))

There is also the intriguing possibility of added benefit from combining fibrates and statins. The literature of statin:fibrate combination therapy is limited. A recent study of 120 patients with type 2 diabetes were treated for 24 weeks with either atorvastatin (20 mg/day) or fenofibrate (200 mg/day) alone or in combination to determine the effects of treatment on LDL and HDL-cholesterol and triglycerides. All treatments were well tolerated. The combination therapy of statin and fibrate was the most effective at reducing LDL-cholesterol (−46%) and trigycerides (−50%) as well as elevating HDL-cholesterol (+22%).[101] Whether this kind of impressive modification in the diabetic dyslipidaemic profile will ultimately translate into improved

cardiovascular protection over and above that seen with statins alone seems likely but needs to be evaluated in longer term outcome trials.

Summary

It is clear that dyslipidaemia in the diabetic population contributes significantly to the huge burden of premature and extensive macrovascular disease in these patients. The emergence of powerful new data confirming the efficacy of lipid lowering with statins and emerging data with fibrates will enable much needed cost-benefit analyses to be performed. In the author's opinion, the existing evidence along with that promised from ongoing trials will confirm the overwhelming benefit of treating diabetic patients with lipid lowering therapy. So much so, that along with antihypertensive therapy, lipid lowering will become a primary therapeutic target. There is little doubt that the Heart Protection Study provides a basis from advocating even more aggressive lipid lowering than currently rec-

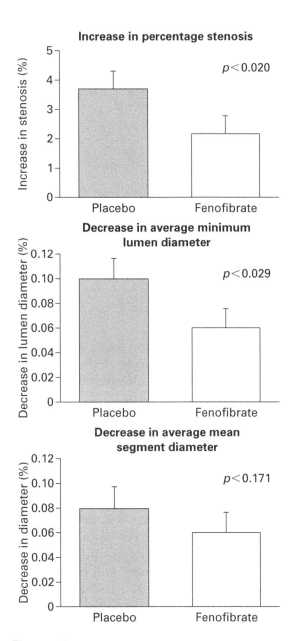

Figure 4.9
Angiographic changes in the fenofibrate and placebo groups. Error bars = SE. (From reference 100.)

ommended by international guidelines. The results from the HPS also question the concept of 'thresholds and targets' in that all patients treated with a statin appeared to benefit with a similar relative risk reduction irrespective of baseline cholesterol. Statin therapy was well tolerated and safe within HPS. However, this is not a cue for complacency on safety. The experience with cerivastatin, which was withdrawn due to safety concerns despite potent cholesterol lowering efficacy, provided a valuable lesson; notably, that safety is not a class effect.

The evidence for statins is compelling and growing. Current guidance recommends drug therapy with a statin when LDL cholesterol is >130 mg/dl in those with diabetes without other risk factors. The threshold for diabetes is >100 mg/dl when other risk factors are present. In both cases the goal is less than 100 mg/dl. Many physicians would have considered these thresholds and goals as being too aggressive prior to HPS. Since HPS, others have argued that high risk patients would benefit from statin therapy irrespective of the baseline cholesterol. Further data on the benefits of statins in people with hypertension will come from ALLHAT and ASCOT (see earlier).

The data with fibrates and the use of fibrates in combination with statins is less substantial than that for statins alone and requires further clarification, Nevetherless, this is from a mechanistic perspective, a logical combination as the two drug classes have complememtary actions on lipid profiles. Clinical outcome studies will be required to determine whether this therapeutic potential translates into clinical benefit. What is clear is that the statins evaluated in outcome trials, especially HPS, have proven to be safe, well tolerated and highly effective at reducing cardiovascular risk (including stroke) in people with diabetes – the challenge will be to implement these new findings in routine clinical practice.

References

1. Laakso ML, Lehto S. Epidemiology of macrovascular disease. *Diabetes Rev* 1997; **5**: 294–315.
2. Robertson WB, Strong JP. Atherosclerosis in persons with hypertension and diabetes mellitus. *Lab Invest* 1968; **18**: 538–51.
3. Crall FV Jr, Roberts WC. The extramural and intramural coronary arteries in juvenile diabetes mellitus. Analysis of nine necropsy patients aged 19–38 years with onset of diabetes before age 15 years. *Am J Med* 1978; **64**: 221–30.
4. Centre for Economic Studies in Medicine. Direct and indirect costs of diabetes in the United States in 1987. Alexandria, VA, American Diabetes Association. 1988.
5. Nathan DM, ed. Diabetes and the heart. *Lancet* 1997; **350** (Suppl 1): 1–32.
6. Raman M, Nesto RW. Heart disease in diabetes mellitus. In: Brownlee MA, King GL, eds. Chronic complications of diabetes. *Endocrinol Metab Clin North Am* 1996; **25**: 425–38.
7. Baroldi G, Falzi G, Mariana F. Sudden coronary death: a post-mortem study in 208 selected cases compared to 97 'control' subjects. *Am Heart J* 1979; **98**: 20–31.
8. Waller B, Palumbo P, Roberts W. Status of the coronary arteries at necropsy in diabetes mellitus with onset after age 30 years. *Am J Med* 1980; **69**: 498–506.
9. Granger C, Califf R, Young S, et al. Outcome of patients with diabetes mellitus and acute myocardial infarction treated with thrombolytic agents. *J Am Coll Cardiol* 1992; **21**: 920–5.
10. Mueller H, Cohen L, Braunwald E, and the TIMI investigators. Predictors of early morbidity and mortality after thrombolytic therapy of acute myocardial infarction. *Circulation* 1992; **85**: 1254.
11. Stein B, Weintraub W, King S. Influence of diabetes mellitus on early and late outcome after percutaneous transluminal coronary angioplasty. *Circulation* 1995; **91**: 979–89.
12. Karlson BW, Herlitz J, Hjalmarson A. Prognosis of acute myocardial infarction in diabetic and non-diabetic patients. *Diabetic Med* 1993; **10**: 449–54.
13. Abbott RD, Donahue RP, Kannel WB, Wilson PWF. The impact of diabetes on survival following myocardial infarction in men vs women. The Framingham Study. *JAMA* 1988; **260**: 3456–60.
14. Herlitz J, Malmberg K, Karlsson B, Ryden L, Hjalmarsson A. Mortality and morbidity during a five year follow up of diabetics with myocardial infarction. *Acta Med Scand* 1988; **24**: 31–8.
15. Webster MWI, Scott RS. What cardiologists need to know about diabetes. *Lancet* 1997; **350** (Suppl 1): 23–8.
16. The Bypass Angioplasty Revascularization Investigation (BARI) Investigators. Comparison of coronary bypass surgery with angioplasty in patients with multivessel disease. *N Engl J Med* 1996; **335**: 217–25.
17. Neaton JD, Wentworth DN, Cutler J, Stamler J, Kuller L. Risk factors for death from different types of stroke. Multiple Risk Factor Intervention Research Group. *Ann Epidemiol* 1993; **3**: 493–9.
18. Manson JE, Colditz GA, Stampfer MJ et al. A prospective study of maturity-onset diabetes mellitus and risk of coronary heart disease and stroke in women. *Arch Intern Med* 1991; **151**: 1141–7.
19. Barrett-Connor E, Khaw K-T. Diabetes mellitus: independent risk factor for stroke? *Am J Epidemiol* 1988; **128**: 116–23.
20. Abbott RD, Donahue RP, Kannel WB, Wilson PWF. The impact of diabetes on survival following myocardial infarction in men vs women. The Framingham Study. *JAMA* 1988; **260**: 3456–60.
21. Tuomilehto J, Rastenyte D, Jousilahti P, Sarti C, Vartainen E. Diabetes mellitus as a risk factor for death from stroke: prospective

study of the middle-aged Finnish population. *Stroke* 1996; **27**: 210–15.

22. LoGerfo FW, Gibbons GW. Vascular disease of the lower extremities in diabetes mellitus. In: Brownlee M, King GL, eds. Chronic complications of diabetes. *Endocrinol Metab Clin North Am* 1996; **25**: 439–45.

23. Lehto S, Rönnemaa T, Pyörälä K, Laakso M. Risk factors predicting lower extremity amputations in patients with NIDDM. *Diabetes Care* 1996; **19**: 607–12.

24. Brand FN, Abbott RD, Kannel WB. Diabetes, intermittent claudication and risk of cardiovascular events: the Framingham Study. *Diabetes* 1989; **38**: 504–9.

25. Lehto S, Niskanen L, Suohenen M, Rönnemaa T, Laakso M. Medial artery calcification: a neglected harbinger of cardiovascular complications in non insulin dependent diabetes mellitus. *Arterioscler Thromb Vasc Biol* 1996; **16**: 978–83.

26. De Fonso RA. Diabetic nephropathy: aetiologic and therapeutic considerations. *Diabetes Rev* 1995; **3**: 510–64.

27. Kuusisto J, Mykkänen L, Pyörälä K, Laakso M. Hyperinsulinaemic microalbuminuria: a new risk indicator for coronary heart disease. *Circulation* 1995; **91**: 831–7.

28. Deckert T, Feldt-Rasmussen BM, Borch-Johnsen K, Jensen T, Kofoed-Enevoldsen A. Albuminuria reflects widespread vascular damage. The Steno Hypothesis. *Diabetologia* 1989; **32**: 219–26.

29. Lyons TJ, Jenkins AJ. Glycation, oxidation, and lipoxidation in the development of the complications of diabetes: a carbonyl stress hypothesis. *Diabetes Rev* 1997; **5**: 365–91.

30. University Group Diabetes Program. A study of the effects of hypoglycaemic agents on vascular complications in patients with adult onset diabetes. *Diabetes* 1976; **25**: 1129–53.

31. Smits P, Thien T. Cardiovascular effects of sulphonylurea derivatives. *Diabetologia* 1995; **38**: 116–21.

32. Pogatsa G. Potassium channels in the cardiovascular system. *Diabetes Res Clin Pract* 1995; **28** (Suppl 1): S91–S98.

33. UK Prospective Diabetes Study (UKPDS) Group. Intensive blood glucose control with sulphonylureas or insulin compared with conventional treatment and risk of complications in patients with type 2 diabetes (UKPDS 33). *Lancet* 1998; **352**: 837–53.

34. DCCT Research Group. The effective intensive treatment of diabetes on the development and progression of long-term complications in insulin-dependent diabetes mellitus. *N Engl J Med* 1993; **329**: 877–986.

35. Krans HMJ, et al., eds. The St Vincent Declaration. Diabetes Care and Research in Europe. Geneva, World Health Organization: 1992.

36. Stamler J, Vaccaro O, Neaton JD, Wentworth D, for the Multiple Risk Factor Intervention Trial Research Group. Diabetes, other risk factors and 12 year cardiovascular mortality for men screened in the Multiple Risk Factor Intervention Trial. *Diabetes Care* 1993; **16**: 434–44.

37. Kannel WB, McGee DL. Diabetes and cardiovascular risk factors: the Framingham Study. *Circulation* 1979; **59**: 8–13.

38. Rönnemaa T, Laakso M, Kallio V, et al. Serum lipids, lipoproteins and apolipoproteins and the excessive occurrence of coronary heart disease in non insulin dependent diabetic patients. *Am J Epidemiol* 1989; **130**: 632–45.

39. Jarrett RJ, Shipley MJ. The Whitehall Study: comparative mortality rates and indicators of risks in diabetics. *Acta Endocrinol* 1985; **10** (Suppl 272): 21–6.

40. Brown MS, Goldstein JL. A receptor mediated pathway for cholesterol homeostasis. *Science* 1986; **232**: 34–47.

41. Ross R. The pathogenesis of atherosclerosis: a perspective for the 1990s. *Nature* 1993; **362**: 801–9.

42. Brown MS, Goldstein JL. Receptor-mediated control of cholesterol metabolism. *Science* 1986; **191**: 150–4.

43. Steinberg D, Parthasarathy S, Carew TE, et al. Beyond cholesterol: modifications of low density lipoprotein that increase its atherogenicity. *N Engl J Med* 1989; **320**: 915–24.

44. Witztum JL. The oxidation hypothesis of atherosclerosis. *Lancet* 1994; **344**: 793–5.

45. Laakso M, Lehto S, Pentillo I, Pyörälä K. Lipids and lipoproteins predicting coronary heart disease mortality and morbidity in

patients with non insulin dependent diabetes. *Circulation* 1989; **88**: 1421–30.

46. Barter P. High density lipoproteins and reverse cholesterol transport. *Curr Opin Lipidology* 1993; **4**: 210–17.

47. Miller NE. HDL vs triglycerides: which is important in cardiovascular disease? In: Woodford FP, Davignon J, Sniderman A, eds. Atherosclerosis X. Amsterdam, Elsevier Science, 1995: 743–8.

48. Hulley SB, Rosenman RH, Bawal RD et al. Epidemiology as a guide to clinical decisions: the association between triglyceride and coronary heart disease. *N Engl J Med* 1980; **302**: 1383–9.

49. Castelli WP. The triglyceride issue: a view from Framingham. *Am Heart J* 1986; **112**: 432–7.

50. Manninen V, Tenkanen H, Koskinen P, et al. Joint effects of triglycerides and LDL cholesterol and HDL cholesterol concentrations on coronary heart disease risk in the Helsinki Heart Study. Implications for treatment. *Circulation* 1992; **85**: 37–45.

51. Assmann G, Schulte H. Relation of high density lipoprotein cholesterol and triglycerides to incidence of atherosclerotic coronary artery disease (the PROCAM experience). *Am J Cardiol* 1992; **70**: 733–7.

52. Hokanson J, Austin MA. Plasma triglyceride level is a risk factor for cardiovascular disease independent of high density lipoprotein cholesterol level: a metaanalysis of population-based prospective studies. *J Cardiovasc Risk* 1996; **3**: 213–19.

53. Hamsten A, Karpe F. Triglycerides and coronary heart disease – has epidemiology given us the right answer? In: Betteridge DJ, ed. *Lipids: current perspectives*. London, Martin Dunitz, 1996: 43–68.

54. Austin MA, Breslow JL, Hennekens CH, Buring JE, Willott WC, Krauss RM. Low density lipoprotein subclass patterns and risk of myocardial infarction. *JAMA* 1988; **260**: 1917–21.

55. West KM, Ahuja MMS, Bennett PH, et al. The role of circulating glucose and triglyceride concentrations and their interactions with other risk factors; as determinants of arterial disease in nine diabetic population

samples from the WHO multinational study. *Diabetes Care* 1983; **6**: 361–9.

56. Fontbonne E, Eschwege E, Cambien F, et al. Hypertriglyceridaemia as a risk factor for coronary heart disease mortality in subjects with impaired glucose tolerance or diabetes. *Diabetologia* 1989; **32**: 300–4.

57. Lehto S, Rönnemaa T, Pyörälä K, Laakso M. Prediction of stroke in middle-aged patients with non insulin dependent diabetes. *Stroke* 1996; **27**: 63–8.

58. Seed M. In: Betteridge DJ, ed. *Lipids: current perspectives*. London, Martin Dunitz, 1996: 69–88.

59. Scott J. Lipoprotein(a). Thrombogenesis linked to atherogenesis at last? *Nature* 1989; **341**: 22–3.

60. Seed M, Doherty E, Stubbs P. Lipoprotein(a): a prothrombotic risk factor for coronary artery disease. *J Cardiovasc Risk* 1995; **2**: 206–15.

61. Schernthaner G, Kostner GM, Dieplinger H, et al. Apolipoproteins (A-I, A-II, B), Lp(a) lipoprotein and lecithin:cholesterol acyltransferase activity in diabetes mellitus. *Atherosclerosis* 1983; **49**: 277–93.

62. Austin A, Warty V, Janosky J, Arslanian S. The relationship of physical fitness to lipids and lipoprotein(a) levels in adolescents with IDDM. *Diabetes Care* 1993; **16**: 421–5.

63. Guillausseau PJ, Peynet J, Chanson P, et al. Lipoprotein(a) in diabetic patients with and without chronic renal failure. *Diabetes Care* 1992; **15**: 976–9.

64. Gall MA, Rossing P, Hommel E, et al. Apolipoprotein(a) in insulin dependent diabetic patients with and without diabetic nephropathy. *Scand J Clin Lab Invest* 1992; **52**: 513–22.

65. Haffner SM, Tuttle KR, Rainwater DL. Decrease of lipoprotein(a) with improved glycaemic control in IDDM subjects. *Diabetes Care* 1991; **14**: 302–7.

66. Heller FR, Jamart J, Honore P, et al. Serum lipoprotein(a) in patients with diabetes mellitus. *Diabetes Care* 1993; **16**: 819–23.

67. Kuusi T, Yki-Jarvinen H, Kauppinen-Makelin R, et al. Effect of insulin treatment on serum lipoprotein(a) in non insulin dependent diabetes. *Eur J Clin Invest* 1995; **25**: 194–200.

68. Haffner SM, Morales PA, Stern MP, Truber KM. Lp(a) concentrations in NIDDM. *Diabetes* 1992; **41**: 1267–72.

69. Haffner SM, Moss SE, Klein BE, Klein R. Lack of association between lipoprotein(a) concentrations and coronary heart disease mortality in diabetes: the Wisconsin Epidemiologic Survey of Diabetic Retinopathy. *Metabolism* 1992; **41**: 194–7.

70. Betteridge, DJ. Lipids, diabetes and vascular disease: the time to act. *Diabetic Medicine* 1989; **6**: 195–218.

71. Betteridge DJ. Diabetic dyslipidaemia: implications for vascular risk. In: Betteridge DJ, ed. *Lipids: current perspectives*. London, Martin Dunitz, 1996: 135–57.

72. Laakso M. Epidemiology of diabetic dyslipidaemia. *Diabetes Rev* 1995; **3**: 408–22.

73. Howard BV. Pathogenesis of diabetic dyslipidaemia. *Diabetes Rev* 1995; **3**: 423–32.

74. The DCCT Research Group. Lipid and lipoprotein levels in patients with IDDM. Diabetes Control and Complications Trial Experience. *Diabetes Care* 1992; **15**: 886–94.

75. Stern MP, Haffner SM. Dyslipidaemia in type 2 diabetes. *Diabetes Care* 1991; **14**: 1144–59.

76. Syvanne M, Taskinen M-R. Lipids and lipoproteins as coronary risk factors in non insulin dependent diabetes mellitus. *Lancet* 1997; **350** (Suppl 1): S120–S123.

77. Haffner SM, Valdez RA, Hazuda HP, Mitchell BD, Morales PA, Stern MP. Prospective analysis of the insulin resistance syndrome (syndrome X). *Diabetes* 1992; **41**: 715–22.

78. Krauss RM, Burke DJ. Identification of multiple subclasses of plasma low density lipoproteins in normal humans. *J Lipid Res* 1982; **23**: 97–104.

79. Betteridge DJ. LDL heterogeneity: implications for atherogenicity in insulin resistance and NIDDM. *Diabetilogia* 1997; **40**: S149–S151.

80. Griffin BA. Low density lipoprotein heterogeneity. In: Betteridge DJ, ed. *Baillière's Clinical endocrinology and metabolism*, vol 9, no. 5. London, Baillière Tindall, 1995: 687–703.

81. Friedewald WT, Levy R, Frederickson DS. Estimation of the concentration of low density lipoprotein in plasma without use of the preparative ultracentrifuge. *Clin Chem* 1972; **18**: 499–502.

82. Riboes-Prat J, Reverter JL, Senti M, et al. Calculated low density lipoprotein cholesterol should not be used for management of lipoprotein abnormalities in patients with diabetes mellitus. *Diabetes Care* 1993; **16**: 1081–6.

83. Haffner SM. Management of dyslipidaemia in adults with diabetes. *Diabetes Care* 1998; **21**: 160–78.

84. American Diabetes Association: Position Statement. Management of dyslipidaemia in adults with diabetes. *Diabetes Care* 2002; **25**(Suppl 1): S74–S77.

85. Executive summary of the third report of the National Cholesterol Education Panel (NCAP III) on detection, evaluation and treatment of high blood pressure in adults. *JAMA* 2001; **285**: 2486–97.

86. Pyörälä K, Pedersen TR, Kjeksus J, Faergerman O, Olsson AG, Thorgeirsson G. Cholesterol lowering with simvastatin improves prognosis of diabetic patients with coronary heart disease: a subgroup analysis of the Scandinavian Simvastatin Survival Study (4S). *Diabetes Care* 1997; **20**: 614–20.

87. Sacks FM, Pfeffer MA, Moye LA, et al. for the Cholesterol and Recurrent Events Trial Investigators. The effect of pravastatin on coronary events after myocardial infarction in patients with average cholesterol levels: Cholesterol and Recurrent Events Trial Investigators. *N Engl J Med* 1996; **335**: 1001–9.

88. Prevention of cardiovascular events and death with Pravastatin in patients with coronary heart disease and a broad range of initial cholesterol levels. The Long-term Intervention with Pravastatin in Ischemic Disease (LIPID) study group. *N Engl J Med* 1998; **339**: 1349–57.

89. Downs JR, Clearfeld M, Weis S, et al. for the AFCAPS/TexCAPS Research Group. Primary prevention of acute coronary events with lovastatin in men and women with average cholesterol levels: results of AFCAPS/Tex-CAPS. *JAMA* 1998; **279**: 1615–22.

90. Koskinen P, Mänttari M, Manninen V, Hutti-

nen JK, Heinonen OP, Frick MH. Coronary heart disease incidence in NIDDM patients in the Helsinki Heart Study. *Diabetes Care* 1992; **15**: 820–5.

91. Stern MP, Mitchell BD, Haffner SM, Hazuda HP. Does glycaemic control of type II diabetes suffice to control diabetic dyslipidaemia? A community perspective. *Diabetes Care* 1992; **15**: 638–44.

92. Nagi DK, Yudkin JS. Effects of metformin on insulin resistance, risk factors for cardiovascular disease and plasminogen activator inhibitor in NIDDM subjects. *Diabetes Care* 1993; **16**: 621–9.

93. Jeppersen J, Zhou M-Y, Che Y-DI, Reaven GM. Effect of metformin on postprandial lipaemia in patients with fairly to poorly controlled NIDDM. *Diabetes Care* 1994; **17**: 1093–9.

94. Kumar S, Boulton AJ, Beck Nielsen H, et al. Troglitazone, an insulin action enhancer, improves metabolic control in NIDDM patients. *Diabetologia* 1996; **39**: 701–9.

95. Schneider SH, Morgado A. Effects of fitness and physical training on carbohydrate metabolism and associated cardiovascular risk factors in patients with diabetes. *Diabetes Rev* 1995; **3**: 378–407.

96. Kelley DE. Effects of weight loss on glucose homeostasis in NIDDM. *Diabetes Rev* 1995; **3**: 366–77.

97. Garg A, Grundy SM. Treatment of dyslipidaemia in patients with NIDDM. *Diabetes Rev* 1997; **3**: 433–45.

98. Goldberg RB, Mellies MJ, Sacks FM et al. for the CARE Investigators. Cardiovascular events and their reduction with pravastatin in diabetic and glucose-intolerant myocardial infarction survivors with average cholesterol levels. Subgroup analysis in the cholesterol and recurrent events (CARE) trial. *Circulation* 1998; **98**: 2513–19.

99. Heart Protection Study Collaborative Group. MRC/BHF Heart Protection Study of cholesterol-lowering with simvastatin in 20,536 high risk individuals: a randomised placebo-controlled trial. *Lancet* 2002; **360**: 7–22.

100. Diabetes Atherosclerosis Intervention Study Investigators. Effect of febofibrate on the progression of coronary heart disease in type 2 diabetes: The Diabetes Atherosclerosis Intervention Study, a randomised study. *Lancet* 2001; **357**: 905–10.

101. Athyros V, Demitriadis DS, Papageorgiou AA et al. Atorvastatin and mirconized fenofibrate alone and in combination in type 2 diabetes with combined hyperlipidaemia. *Diabetes Care* 2002; **25**: 1198–202.

5

Disturbances in 24-hour blood pressure regulation in diabetic subjects

Philip Weston and King Sun Leong

Introduction

Diabetes mellitus is associated with an increased risk of hypertension and an increase in cardiovascular mortality. In keeping with many other biological systems blood pressure is subject to circadian variations and abnormalities in the circadian rhythm can have profound consequences on the patient's morbidity and mortality. Thus, a single clinic blood pressure measurement is a poor representation of an individual's blood pressure. With the development of non-invasive 24-hour blood pressure monitoring a better idea of a subject's blood pressure profile is possible and an abnormal diurnal blood pressure rhythm is recognised as an independent cardiovascular risk factor.

This chapter will introduce the concept of 24-hour blood pressure monitoring, and discuss the abnormalities seen in blood pressure profiles of diabetic subjects and the consequences of these changes. Finally, the clinical implications of these abnormalities will be discussed.

Ambulatory blood pressure monitoring

Non-invasive ambulatory blood pressure monitoring (Figs 5.1a, b) has developed over the past 30 years. There is now extensive literature on the clinical usefulness of the technique

and there are a variety of commercially available monitors that are reliable, convenient and accurate. The technique allows three types of information to be acquired: first, an average blood pressure; second, diurnal blood pressure changes and third, the short-term variability of blood pressure. As will be described below, ambulatory blood pressure monitoring has become a useful clinical and research tool in the care of diabetic patients.

Circadian blood pressure variation ('dippers and non-dippers')

Since the first automated intra-arterial blood pressure recording in unrestricted man,[1] circadian fluctuation of blood pressure, with higher levels during the day and lower levels during the night, has been well described in both normal and hypertensive subjects. A detailed study of 24-hour blood pressure profiles in hypertensive subjects reported that blood pressure was highest at 10 am then progressively fell through the day, reaching its lowest levels during sleep at 3 am.[2] Blood pressure then rose and from 6 am it increased rapidly, even more so after waking at 7 am.[2]

The simplest method of assessing circadian changes in blood pressure is by the difference between mean day-time and mean night-time pressures (either diastolic or more usually

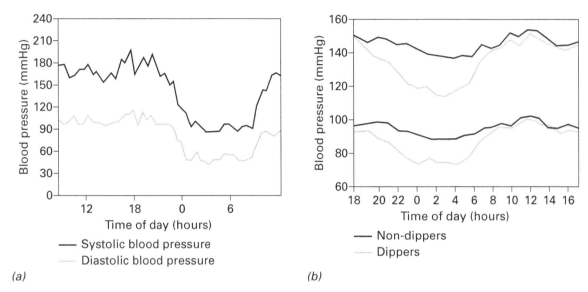

Figure 5.1
(a) A typical 24-hour ambulatory 24-hour blood pressure profile in a hypertensive type non-diabetic patient with a normal nocturnal dip of > 10%. (b) An example of ambulatory blood pressure readings from two hypertensive diabetic patients, one with a nocturnal dip, the other with a markedly disturbed profile and a 'non-dipper'.

systolic blood pressure). A decrease of >10 per cent from day to night mean blood pressure is the norm and patients are classified as being 'dippers', whilst a fall of <10 per cent is seen in 'non-dippers'.[3,4] Approximately 17 per cent of non-diabetic hypertensive patients can be classified as non-dippers[3] and other pathophysiological conditions, such as endogenous glucocorticoid excess and hyperthyroidism as well as some causes of secondary hypertension, are associated with an absent fall of blood pressure at night.[5,6] Reduced day–night variation of blood pressure has also been reported in accelerated hypertension, eclampsia and congestive cardiac failure.[7] Imai and colleagues suggested that the lack of diurnal variation of blood pressure under these conditions could be due to cerebral ischaemia which activates a compensatory mechanism preventing a fall in nocturnal blood pressure and thus

a further reduction in cerebral blood flow at night.[7] Whilst controversial, this hypothesis received some support from the observation that an excessive nocturnal fall in blood pressure critically lowers the perfusion to organs such as the heart and brain.[8]

Sleep is the primary determinant of the nocturnal fall in blood pressure. Non-rapid eye movement (REM) sleep is associated with a fall in blood pressure and a reduction in blood pressure variability, whilst REM sleep increases blood pressure variability and is associated with a slight rise in average blood pressure readings.[9] More recent data obtained from non-invasive blood pressure measurement and microneurographic recordings of muscle sympathetic nerve activity have shown a reduction in heart rate, blood pressure and sympathetic nerve activity during non-REM sleep,[10,11] whilst REM sleep is associated with a marked increase in sympathetic activity and a rise in heart rate and blood pressure, often to levels seen whilst awake. Further evidence for the role of the autonomic nervous system in the circadian modulation of blood pressure comes from a variety of clinical settings. Thus, in patients with primary autonomic failure there is a reduction in the circadian variation of blood pressure[12] and the normal circadian pattern may well be reversed, with blood pressure increasing at night and falling on waking. Similarly in tetraplegic patients, who have impaired autonomic reflexes, and in patients following cardiac transplant, circadian fluctuations of blood pressure are inhibited.[13] Richards and colleagues[14] related fluctuations in blood pressure to sympathetic activity, as assessed by plasma noradrenaline levels, over a 24-hour period and found a close coupling – giving further support for a major role of the sympathetic nervous system in controlling blood pressure levels.

24-Hour blood pressure profiles in diabetic subjects

The earliest documented abnormality of circadian blood pressure variability in diabetic patients is a loss of the normal nocturnal fall in blood pressure with normal blood pressure variability during the daytime.[15–18] The earliest studies of circadian blood pressure variation in diabetic subjects stressed the importance of autonomic dysfunction in the loss of the nocturnal fall in blood pressure. This relationship was first observed by invasive direct intra-arterial blood pressure measurement,[19] and confirmed using a non-invasive ambulatory blood pressure monitoring system.[20,21] In the study by Wiegmann and associates,[20] no measure of autonomic function was made, but they showed that in type I diabetic subjects

ambulatory blood pressure significantly exceeded control values at all time-points measured, despite patients being identified as 'normotensive' on clinic sphygmomanometer readings. The concept of blood pressure load or burden was also introduced at this time, i.e. the number of readings above a certain 'average' value. Using an arbitrary average value of 135/85 mmHg, 50 per cent of readings in the diabetic population were found to be higher than this value. Furthermore, compared to day-time readings, the mean night-time blood pressure values were not significantly lower in the type I diabetic population, unlike blood pressure readings in the control group. The albumin excretion rate was 18.2 μ/min/m^2 for the diabetic group and although no assessment of albumin excretion was made in the control population the changes in circadian blood pressure variation were said to be independent of kidney function. Felici and colleagues[21] found that there was a loss of the normal nocturnal decline in blood pressure in a population of type II and type I diabetic patients with clinical evidence of autonomic dysfunction. However, their population of diabetic subjects was mixed, with over half being hypertensive on clinic blood pressure readings. Furthermore, no detailed assessment of diabetic nephropathy was made, with patients included in the study if their creatinine clearance was >20 ml/min/m^2.

Liniger and colleagues[15] assessed the relationship between 24-hour ambulatory blood pressure profiles and autonomic function as assessed by the cardiovascular reflex tests. They found that 75 per cent of type I diabetic patients with abnormal cardiovascular reflex tests had an impairment of the normal circadian pattern of blood pressure. Moreover, in half of this group, the systolic blood pressure rose at night, whilst in the others night-time blood pressure did not differ from day-time levels. They postulated that as autonomic damage became more severe (as assessed by an increasing autonomic neuropathy 'score') so the circadian changes in blood pressure became more abnormal. The patients in whom systolic blood pressure rose at night, all had a systolic blood pressure fall on standing. On closer examination of the small number of patients in each group, there was a significantly higher 24-hour protein excretion in the type I diabetic group with abnormal circadian blood pressure profiles compared with those with a normal night-time dip in blood pressure, as well as a higher serum creatinine, although this was not statistically significant. In a more recent study, the relationship between 24-hour blood pressure and autonomic function has become a little clearer. Phong Chau and colleagues[18] found that a mixed group of type I and type II diabetic patients with abnormal cardiovascular reflex tests had a significant reduction in night-time blood pressure change compared with a control population matched for age and clinic blood pressure. Furthermore, they found an increased variability of systolic blood pressure during the day in those patients with autonomic dysfunction, although this did not reach statistical significance. The association between diabetic nephropathy and circadian changes in blood pressure was also investigated, revealing that those patients with autonomic dysfunction who had microalbuminuria had a further reduction in the change of systolic blood pressure at night.

A similar loss of the diurnal variation of blood pressure has been observed in a non-diabetic population with renal disease,[22] leading to the suggestion that the loss of circadian change in blood pressure in the diabetic population is secondary to diabetic renal disease. In particular, an attenuated fall of nocturnal blood pressure in type I diabetic patients with microalbuminuria has been reported. For example, a study investigating type I diabetic patients who were normotensive on clinic blood pressure readings (<140/90 mmHg) showed an increased ambulatory blood pressure at night in those with microalbuminuria as compared with a control population without microalbuminuria.[23] No formal assessment of autonomic function was made, but a review of the study data shows that the nocturnal heart rate was significantly higher in the microalbuminuric group – possibly an early marker of autonomic dysfunction. Other workers have reported a similar loss of circadian variation of blood pressure and have postulated that the early renal damage results in abnormal circadian blood pressure changes.[17,24] Consequently, there has been some uncertainty as to whether the abnormal circadian blood pressure pattern is actually dependent on the presence of neuropathy or nephropathy. In one study in young type I diabetic patients, microalbuminuria was associated with slightly increased blood pressure levels compared with normoalbuminuric subjects, but there were no differences in circadian blood pressure variation unless autonomic neuropathy was present.[16] Furthermore, the same group found that the loss of the nocturnal fall in blood pressure was related to an abnormal sympathetic predominance at night, suggesting a possible pathogenic link between autonomic dysfunction and impaired circadian fluctuations of blood pressure. The inter-relationship between autonomic neuropathy and 24-hour blood pressure profiles has been further explored by Torffvit and colleagues,[25] who showed that all patients with clinical diabetic nephropathy (defined as a positive urine dipstix for albumin) had evidence of autonomic neuropathy. Moreover, those patients with diabetic nephropathy showed an impairment of circadian blood pressure change.

In summary, impaired circadian changes of blood pressure are well documented in diabetic subjects. There appears to be a close association between reduced night-time fall in blood pressure and autonomic dysfunction and this may be an inverse linear relationship; the worse the autonomic dysfunction the lower the decline in night-time blood pressure. In those patients with severe autonomic dysfunction, blood pressure may even rise at night (cycle inversion). Patients with microalbuminuria also have impaired circadian changes of blood pressure, but it appears that autonomic dysfunction may be the causative factor. It is thus safe to assume that diabetic patients with a blunted nocturnal fall in blood pressure have some degree of autonomic dysfunction.

Significance of the abnormal circadian pattern of blood pressure

Cross-sectional and retrospective studies indicate that damage to target organs is more closely linked to 24-hour blood pressure profiles than random clinic blood pressures.[26] Hypertensive patients who are non-dippers have an increased prevalence of strokes,[3] atherosclerosis[27] and left ventricular hypertrophy.[4]

The situation in diabetic subjects is less clear. Liniger and colleagues[15] found a significantly higher incidence of fatal and severe non-fatal cardiovascular events in the small number of patients who had a nocturnal rise in blood pressure (i.e. those with severe autonomic dysfunction). It should be remembered, however, that there is a higher risk of cardiovascular events in diabetic subjects with autonomic dysfunction.[28,29] A more recent study of 23 microalbuminuric, type I diabetic patients showed no significant increase in left ventricular mass index or cardiovascular disease,[30] although only small numbers of non-dippers were studied and no assessment of autonomic function was made in this group. Another study looking at left ventricular mass in normotensive patients with diabetic autonomic neuropathy demonstrated an increase in left ventricular mass index despite normal renal function.[31]

Does abnormal blood pressure load result in or result from diabetic nephropathy?

It has been documented that if albumin excretion is normal in type I diabetic patients then the prevalence of hypertension is the same as in the control population.[32] However, if persistent microalbuminuria is present there is a dramatic increase in the prevalence of hypertension and this increase is even more pronounced in overt diabetic nephropathy.[33] Initially, these results were taken to suggest that elevated blood pressure was secondary to renal abnormalities and some support for this was received from longitudinal studies.[34,35] However, these studies did not utilise 24-hour ambulatory blood pressure recordings, but relied on repeated clinic blood pressures. In contrast, other workers have reported recently that raised blood pressure precedes the development of microalbuminuria, although blood pressure was again measured by conventional sphygmomanometry.[36] As discussed earlier, ambulatory blood pressure recording clearly has advantages over single clinic readings, allowing assessment of the circadian change in blood pressure, as well as better reflecting the risk of developing end-organ damage in non-diabetic patients.[3,4] However, the debate continues as to whether increases in 24-hour blood pressure (particularly at night) pre-date the development of microalbuminuria or are a consequence of early renal disease. Poulsen and colleagues reported that clinic and 24-hour ambulatory blood pressure were normal until after the development of microalbuminuria in a longitudinal study of type I diabetic patients initially without microalbuminuria.[37] Interestingly, those patients who eventually progressed on to microalbuminuria had a diminished reduction in nocturnal diastolic blood pressure, although this could be related to the duration of diabetes, which was greater in this group. In another study, type I diabetic patients with microalbuminuria were noted to have a blunted nocturnal fall in blood pressure, although the mean 24-hour blood pressure was normal.[17] A subpopulation of patients without microalbuminuria in this study showed a reduced decline in nocturnal blood pressure, and the authors suggested that the blood pressure dysregulation and microalbuminuria were independent of each other. Further studies again confirmed the finding that patients with microalbuminuria had a higher mean 24-hour blood pressure than those without microalbuminuria.[38,39] However, in these studies, patients without microalbuminuria had raised ambulatory blood pressure readings intermediate between non-diabetic subjects and those patients with microalbuminuria. There was an increase in left ventricular mass index in both diabetic groups and it was suggested that arterial pressure rises before the development of overt microalbuminuria. In the study by Page and colleagues,[39] the 'non-microalbuminuric' group had a significantly higher mean urinary albumin excretion of 19.5 mg/24 hours – higher than the 'non-microalbuminuric' in the other studies. Such 'incipient microalbuminuria' may influence blood pressure profiles.

In summary, as microalbuminuria develops in type I diabetic patients there is an increase in blood pressure. The current studies do not answer the question as to whether an initial rise in blood pressure triggers or is triggered by an increase in urinary albumin excretion, but there is little doubt that the two phenomena are closely linked. Abnormalities of the circadian blood pressure change, and thus an increase in the blood pressure load may be important in determining the development of diabetic nephropathy.

Other possible mechanisms for abnormal circadian blood pressure rhythms

Just as blood pressure has a circadian rhythm, 24-hour power spectral analysis of heart rate variability has documented a circadian oscillation in autonomic activity with a predominance of sympathetic tone during the day and a predominance of vagal tone at night;[40] i.e. it parallels the changes in circulating catecholamines and vasoactive hormones.[14] In a mixed population of type I and type II diabetic patients with abnormal clinical tests of autonomic function, Spallone and colleagues showed that this autonomic circadian rhythm was impaired.[16] As discussed above, abnormalities of 24-hour blood pressure variability have also been described in diabetic subjects with abnormal bedside cardiovascular reflex tests.[16,18] These abnormalities have been postulated to be due to the impaired circadian rhythm of autonomic function and an abnormal nocturnal sympathetic predominance. Reviewing the data of Phong-Chau and co-workers reveals that they did find an increase in day-time systolic blood pressure variability, although this did not reach statistical significance ($P = 0.06$).[18] Another group, using an increased frequency of blood pressure recordings during the day time, have shown an increased variability of systolic blood pressure in a population of type II diabetic patients with no historical evidence of autonomic dysfunction.[41]

Variability of blood pressure at rest is dependent on the sensitivity of the intact arterial baroreflex.[42] It is possible, therefore, that increased variability of day-time systolic blood pressure is due to the well-documented reduction in baroreceptor-cardiac reflex sensitivity seen in type I diabetic patients.[43] Baroreflexes buffer changes in arterial pressure,[44] and failure of the baroreflex results in a loss of this buffering mechanism and thus increased variability in blood pressure.[45] Baroreceptor-cardiac reflex sensitivity is lower in patients with essential hypertension than in normotensive controls.[46] Traditionally, it has been held that baroreceptor-cardiac reflex sensitivity declines as a consequence of essential hypertension, rather than impaired baroreceptor-cardiac reflex sensitivity causing hypertension. However, recently the converse has been suggested – that hypertension develops as a result of impaired baroreceptor-cardiac reflex sensitivity.[47] Studies in humans with carotid baroreceptor denervation, in some cases, have shown an initial increase in blood pressure variability and a later persistent blood pressure elevation.[45] It is possible, therefore, that in diabetic subjects, the impaired arterial baroreflex mechanisms may be responsible for the reduced nocturnal decline in systolic blood pressure.

Evidence to support this suggestion comes from our own work. In a group of type I diabetic patients with normal bedside tests of autonomic function there was evidence of an increased variability in day-time blood pressure, as shown by an increase in the standard deviation over the 24-hour period (Table 5.1). In addition, this study utilised the cumulative sums (Cusums) method of assessing circadian blood pressure variation.[48] This method is time-independent and has been shown to be more reproducible when assessing the diurnal changes in blood pressure.[49] The type I diabetic patients had a reduced diurnal variation in blood pressure, as assessed by the Cusum-derived circadian alteration of magnitude (CDCAM), compared with the control group. CDCAM showed a significant negative correlation with duration of diabetes and HbA_1. In addition, there was a positive correlation with

	Controls (n = 65)	Diabetics (n = 65)	P‡
Clinic SBP	122 ± 13	126 ± 12	0.1
Mean 24-hour SBP	119 ± 9	126 ± 17	0.07
Day-time SBP	125 ± 11	128 ± 21	0.2
Night-time SBP	109 ± 5	115 ± 12	<0.05
D–N	18 ± 4.1	14 ± 3.7	0.07
CDCAM	26.8 ± 8.4	18.5 ± 9.9	<0.03

SBP, systolic blood pressure;
D–N, day–night difference in systolic blood pressure;
CDCAM, Cusum-derived circadian alteration of magnitude.

Table 5.1
Systolic blood pressure (mmHg) data of control and IDDM groups (mean ± SD).

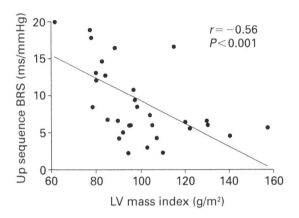

Figure 5.2
Relationship between left ventricular mass index and baroreceptor-cardiac reflex sensitivity derived from sequence analysis.

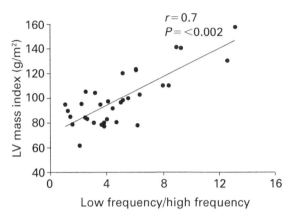

Figure 5.3
Relationship between sympathovagal balance and left ventricular mass index.

the low frequency (sympathetic activity)/high frequency (parasympathetic activity) ratio and CDCAM (Fig. 5.2). Furthermore, a significant positive correlation between left ventricular mass index and sympathovagal balance was observed (Fig. 5.3).

It is possible, therefore, that the diabetic group in this study may be at an increased risk of developing persistent hypertension and that the earliest evidence for this is the reduced nocturnal decline in systolic blood pressure. Subjects with symptomatic diabetic autonomic neuropathy have been shown to have abnormal ventricular systolic function on radionuclide ventriculography in the absence of ischaemic heart disease.[50] Furthermore, in type I diabetic patients with poor metabolic control, echocardiographic evidence of abnormal left ventricular function has been observed and associated with adrenergic hypersensitivity.[51] As discussed earlier, autonomic dysfunction has been associated with increased left ventricular mass index.[31] Similarly, deficits in the baroreceptor-cardiac reflex are highly correlated with the level of cardiac hypertrophy in

animal models.[52] In our work, there was a significant increase in left ventricular mass index in the type I diabetic patients as baroreceptor-cardiac reflex sensitivity declined. Furthermore, left ventricular mass index was positively correlated with sympathovagal balance. It is possible therefore that the increase in left ventricular mass index is due to the increase in blood pressure load associated with a reduced diurnal rhythm of systolic blood pressure, which in turn may be due to a relative sympathetic overactivity.

Factors other than circadian changes in autonomic function and baroreflex abnormalities may be responsible for the diurnal change in systolic blood pressure. These include the renin-angiotensin-aldosterone axis[53] and atrial natriuretic peptide.[54] Related to this, recent work suggests that latent overhydration may play a role in the nocturnal hypertension seen in diabetic patients.[24,55] When extracellular volume was measured in a population of type I diabetic patients with diabetic nephropathy (GFR ≤40 ml/min/m²) who had an impaired reduction of night-time blood pressure it was found to be significantly higher than in a group of 'dipping' type I patients with nephropathy. No assessment of autonomic function was made, as it was assumed that all patients would have some degree of neuropathy. It was stated that there was no correlation between day or night heart rate and the night/day blood pressure ratio. However, significant numbers of patients in the group were treated with beta-blockers. The assumption that fluid overload contributes to the lack of a nocturnal dip in systolic blood pressure does not exclude a role for the autonomic nervous system. As mentioned previously, the autonomic nervous system has an integral role in fluid balance homeostasis, through synergy with the renin-angiotensin system.

In non-diabetic normotensive subjects, smoking has been shown to acutely increase day-time blood pressure[56] and these changes persist in chronic smokers. Despite the fact that smoking increases the complication rate in diabetic subjects,[57] no association between smoking and abnormalities in ambulatory blood pressure has been described. Indeed, Hansen and colleagues have shown no changes in 24-hour blood pressure profiles in normoalbuminuric type I diabetics who smoked compared to non-smoking type I patients.[30]

Summary

In summary, 24-hour ambulatory blood pressure monitoring is a useful clinical and research tool in diabetic subjects. Abnormalities of circadian blood pressure change are the earliest detectable abnormalities in diabetic subjects' blood pressure profiles and this is detectable in 'normotensive' type I and type II patients. The loss of the nocturnal fall in blood pressure is an independent risk factor for cardiovascular and cerebrovascular disease. There are several possible explanations for the changes in circadian blood pressure, but impaired autonomic function seems integral to this abnormality. It is interesting to speculate that impaired baroreceptor-cardiac reflex sensitivity, possibly due to an impairment of parasympathetic function and a relative sympathetic predominance, may result in an increased blood pressure load at night. Twenty-four hour ambulatory blood pressure monitoring is patient-friendly and should be used more frequently in diabetic subjects to identify those patients at risk of end-organ damage.

References

1. Bevin AT, Honour AJ, Stott FH. Direct arterial pressure recording in unrestricted man. *Clin Sci* 1969; **36**: 329–34.
2. Miller-Craig MW, Bishop CN, Rafferty EB. Circadian variation of blood pressure. *Lancet* 1978; **i**: 795–7.
3. O'Brien E, Sheridan J, O'Malley K. Dippers and non-dippers (letter). *Lancet* 1988; **2**: 397.
4. Verdecchia P, Schillachi G, Guerrieri M, et al. Circadian blood pressure changes and left ventricular hypertrophy in essential hypertension. *Circulation* 1990; **81**: 528–36.
5. Littler WA, West MJ, Honour AJ, Sleight P. The variability of arterial blood pressure. *Am Heart J* 1978; **95**: 180–6.
6. Imai Y, Abe K, Miura Y. Hypertensive episodes and circadian fluctuations of blood pressure with phaeochromocytoma: studies of long term blood pressure monitoring based on a volume oscillometric method. *J Hypertens* 1988; **6**: 9–15.
7. Imai Y, Abe K, Munakata M, et al. Circadian blood pressure variations under different pathophysiological conditions. *J Hypertens* 1990; **8** (Suppl 7): S125–S132.
8. Stanton A, O'Brien E. Noninvasive 24 hour ambulatory blood pressure monitoring: current status. *Postgrad Med J* 1993; **69**: 255–67.
9. Mancia G, Zanchetti A. Cardiovascular regulation during sleep. In: Orem J, Barnes CD, eds. *Physiology in sleep*. New York, Academic Press, 1980: 1–55.
10. Okada H, Iwase S, Mano T, Sugiyama Y, Watanabe T. Changes in muscle sympathetic nerve activity during sleep. *Neurology* 1991; **41**: 1961–6.
11. Somers VK, Dyken ME, Mark AE, Abboud FM. Sympathetic nerve activity during sleep in normal subjects. *N Engl J Med* 1993; **328**: 303–7.
12. Mann S, Altman DG, Rafferty EB, Bannister R. Circadian variation of blood pressure in autonomic failure. *Circulation* 1988; **68**: 477–83.
13. Reeves RA, Shapiro AP, Thompsen ME, Johnsen A-M. Loss of nocturnal decline in blood pressure after cardiac transplantation. *Circulation* 1986; **73**: 401–8.
14. Richards AM, Nicholls MG, Espiner EA, Ikram H, Cullens M, Hinton D. Diurnal patterns of blood pressure, heart rate and vasoactive hormones in normal man. *Clin Exp Hypertens* 1986; **A8**: 153–66.
15. Liniger C, Favre L, Assal J-Ph. Twenty four hour blood pressure and heart rate profiles of diabetic patients with abnormal cardiovascular reflexes. *Diabetic Med* 1991; **8**: 420–7.
16. Spallone V, Bernardi L, Ricordi L, et al. Relationship between the circadian rhythms of blood pressure and sympathovagal balance in diabetic autonomic neuropathy. *Diabetes* 1993; **42**: 1745–52.
17. Lurbe A, Redon J, Pascual JM, Tacons J, Alvarez V, Batlle DC. Altered blood pressure during sleep in normotensive subjects with type 1 diabetes. *Hypertension* 1993; **21**: 227–35.
18. Chau PN, Bauduceau B, Vilar J, Gautier D. Relationship between autonomic dysfunction and BP variability in subjects with diabetes mellitus. *J Hum Hypertens* 1993; **7**: 251–5.
19. Hornung RS, Mahler RF, Rafferty EB. Ambulatory blood pressure and heart rate in diabetic patients: an assessment of autonomic function. *Diabetic Med* 1989; **6**: 579–85.
20. Wiegmann TB, Herron KG, Chonko AM, Macdougall ML, Moore WV. Recognition of hypertension and abnormal blood pressure burden with ambulatory blood pressure recordings in type 1 diabetes mellitus. *Diabetes* 1990; **39**: 1556–60.
21. Felici MG, Spallone V, Maiello MR, et al. Twenty-four hours blood pressure and heart rate profiles in diabetics with and without autonomic neuropathy. *Funct Neurol* 1991; **6**: 299–304.
22. Baumgart P, Walger P, Gerke M, Dorst KG, Wetter H, Rahn KH. Nocturnal hypertension

in renal failure, haemodialysis and after renal transplantation. *Hypertension* 1989; **7** (Suppl 6): S70–S71.

23. Benhamou PY, Halimi S, Gaudemaris RD, et al. Early disturbances of ambulatory blood pressure load in normotensive type 1 diabetic patients with microalbuminuria. *Diabetes Care* 1992; **15**: 1614–19.

24. Hansen KW, Mau-Pedersen M, Marshall SM, Christiansen JS, Mogensen SM. Circadian variation in blood pressure in patients with diabetic nephropathy. *Diabetologia* 1992; **35**: 1074–9.

25. Torffvit O, Agardh C-D. Day and night variations in ambulatory blood pressure in type 1 diabetes mellitus with nephropathy and autonomic neuropathy. *J Int Med* 1993; **233**: 131–7.

26. Mancia G, Parati G. Experience with 24-hour ambulatory blood pressure monitoring in hypertension. *Am Heart J* 1988; **116**: 1134–40.

27. Shimada K, Kawamoto A, Matsubayashi K, Nishinga M, Kimura S, Ozawa T. Diurnal blood pressure variations and silent cerebrovascular damage in elderly patients with hypertension. *J Hypertens* 1992; **10**: 875–8.

28. Ewing DJ, Clarke BF. Diagnosis and management of diabetic autonomic neuropathy. *Br Med J* 1982; **285**: 916–18.

29. Sampson MJ, Wilson S, Karagiannis P, Edmonds P, Watkins PJ. Progression of diabetic autonomic neuropathy over a decade in insulin dependent diabetics. *QJ Med* 1990; **75**: 635–46.

30. Hansen KW, Sorensen K, Christensen PD, Pedersen EB, Christiansen JS, Mogensen CE. Night blood pressure: relation to organ lesions in type 1 diabetic patients. *Diabetic Med* 1995; **12**: 42–5.

31. Gambardella S, Frontoni S, Spallone V, et al. Increased left ventricular mass in normotensive diabetic patients with autonomic neuropathy. *Am J Hypertens* 1993; **6**: 97–102.

32. Nørgaard K, Feldt-Rasmussen B, Borch-Johnsen K, Saelan H, Deckert T. Prevalence of hypertension in type 1 (insulin dependent) diabetes mellitus. *Diabetologia* 1990; **33**: 407–10.

33. Mogensen CE, Hansen KW, Osterby R, Damsgaard EM. Blood pressure elevation versus abnormal albuminuria in the genesis and prediction of renal disease in diabetes. *Diabetes Care* 1992; **15**: 1192–204.

34. Rudberg S, Persson B, Dalquist G. Increased glomerular filtration rate as a predictor of diabetic nephropathy. *Kidney Int* 1992; **41**: 822–8.

35. Mathiesen ER, Ronn B, Jensen T, Storm B, Deckert T. Relationship between blood pressure and urinary albumin excretion in the development of microalbuminuria. *Diabetes* 1990; **30**: 245–9.

36. Microalbuminuria Collaborative Study Group. Risk factors for the development of microalbuminuria in insulin dependent diabetic patients: a cohort study. *Br Med J* 1993; **306**: 1235–9.

37. Poulsen PL, Hansen KW, Mogensen CE. Ambulatory blood pressure in the transition from normo- to microalbuminuria. *Diabetes* 1994; **43**: 1248–53.

38. Moore WV, Donaldson DL, Chonko AM, Ideus P, Wiegmann TB. Ambulatory blood pressure in type 1 diabetes mellitus. *Diabetes* 1992; **41**: 1035–41.

39. Page SR, Manninig G, Ingle AR, Hill P, Millar-Craig MW, Peacock I. Raised ambulatory blood pressure in type 1 diabetes with incipient microalbuminuria. *Diabetic Med* 1994; **11**: 877–82.

40. Furlan R, Guzzetti S, Crivellaro W, et al. Continuous 24-hour assessment of the neural regulation of systemic arterial pressure and RR variabilities in ambulant subjects. *Circulation* 1990; **81**: 537–47.

41. McKinlay S, Foster C, Clark A, Clark S, Denver E, Coats AJS. Increased blood pressure variability during 24h blood pressure monitoring as an early sign of autonomic dysfunction in non-insulin dependent diabetics. *J Hum Hypertens* 1994; **8**: 887–90.

42. Siché JP, Longere P, DeGaudemaris R, Riachi M, Compart V, Mallion JM. Variability in arterial blood pressure at rest depends on the sensitivity of the baroreflex. *J Hypertens* 1993; **11** (Suppl 5): S176–S177.

43. Weston PJ, Panerai RB, McCullough A, et al. Assessment of baroreceptor-cardiac reflex sensitivity using time domain analysis in patients with IDDM and the relation to left ventricular mass index. *Diabetologia* 1996; **39**: 1385–91.

44. Ferguson DW, Abboud FM, Mark AL. Relative contribution of aortic and carotid baroreflexes to heart rate control in man during steady state and dynamic increases in arterial pressure. *J Clin Invest* 1985; **76**: 2265–74.

45. Robertson D, Hollister AS, Biaggioni I, Netterville J, Mosequeda-Garcia R, Robertson RM. The diagnosis and treatment of baroreflex failure. *N Engl J Med* 1993; **329**: 1449–55.

46. Bristow A, Honour AJ, Pickering GW, Sleight P, Smith HS. Diminished baroreflex sensitivity in high blood pressure. *Circulation* 1969; **39**: 48–54.

47. Ramirez AJ, Berteinieri G, Belli L, et al. Reflex control of blood pressure and heart rate by arterial baroreceptors and by cardiopulmonary receptors in unanaesthetised cats. *J Hypertens* 1985; **3**: 327–35.

48. Stanton A, Cox J, Atkins N, O'Malley K, O'Brien E. Cumulative sums in quantifying circadian blood pressure patterns. *Hypertension* 1992; **19**: 93–101.

49. Weston PJ, Robinson JE, Watt PAC, Thurston H. Reproducibility of the circadian blood pressure fall in healthy young volunteers. *J Hum Hypertens* 1996; **10**: 163–6.

50. Zola B, Khan JK, Juni JE, Vinik AI. Abnormal cardiac function in diabetic patients with autonomic neuropathy in the absence of ischaemic heart disease. *J Clin Endocrinol Metab* 1986; **63**: 208–14.

51. Maraud L, Gin H, Roudaut R, Aubertin J, Bricaud H. Echocardiographic study of left ventricular function in type 1 diabetes mellitus: hypersensitivity of β-adrenergic stimulation. *Diabetes Res Clin Pract* 1991; **11**: 161–8.

52. Minami N, Head GA. Relationship between cardiovascular hypertrophy and cardiac baroreflex function in spontaneously hypertensive and stroke-prone rats. *J Hypertens* 1993; **11**: 523–33.

53. Delea C. Chronobiology of blood pressure. *Nephron* 1979; **23**: 91–7.

54. Colantonio D, Pasqualetti P, Casale R, Natali G. Is atrial natriuretic peptide important in the circadian rhythm of arterial blood pressure? *Am J Cardiol* 1988; **63**: 1116.

55. Mulec H, Blohme G, Kullenberg K, Nyberg G, Bjorck S. Latent overhydration and nocturnal hypertension in diabetic nephropathy. *Diabetologia* 1995; **38**: 216–20.

56. Giopelli A, Giolgi DM, Omboni S, Parati G, Mancia G. Persistent blood pressure increase induced by heavy smoking. *J Hypertens* 1992; **10**: 495–9.

57. Chaturvedi N, Stephenson JM, Fuller JH. The relationship between smoking and microvascular complications in the EURODIAB IDDM complications study. *Diabetes Care* 1995; **18**: 785–92.

6

The unique vulnerability of diabetic subjects to hypertensive injury
Bryan Williams

Introduction

Diabetes mellitus is associated with a substantially increased risk of premature death from cardiovascular disease. In addition, diabetes is commonly complicated by microvascular disease. Hypertension is a recognized risk factor for macrovascular and microvascular disease and hypertension is very common in diabetic subjects.[1] The exact prevalence of hypertension in diabetes has been the subject of much debate because "hypertension" is arbitrarily defined and various definitions have been used.[2] If one utilizes a definition of hypertension of $\geq 140/90$ mmHg, a threshold consistent with that suggested by the Joint National Committee Guidelines in the USA, the WHO/ISH guidelines and the British Hypertension Society,[3] then the prevalence of hypertension in type I diabetes approximates to 25%, whereas in type II diabetes it is over 80%.[4] The ratio of type II to type I diabetes is about eight to one, thus the vast majority of diabetic subjects with hypertension have type II diabetes.

Few would argue that hypertension is a major risk factor for macrovascular and microvascular disease in diabetes. However, until the recent publication of major intervention trials such as the hypertension optimum treatment (HOT) study[5] and the United Kingdom Prospective Diabetes Study (UKPDS),[6]

the true potency of hypertension as a remediable risk factor was underestimated. In the author's view, the efficacy of antihypertensive therapy in protecting against vascular disease and its consequences in diabetic subjects should not have come as such a surprise. One of the striking features of target organ damage in diabetic subjects (macrovascular and microvascular) is its strong resemblance to the pathological change observed in severe and/or prolonged hypertension. This has prompted me to examine whether diabetic subjects might be especially vulnerable to hypertensive injury either via abnormal regulation of blood pressure, inefficient physiological protection against haemodynamic injury, and/or a deleterious interaction between pressure and the metabolic milieu. This hypothesis is explored below.

Hypertension and cardiovascular risk

The Framingham study has emphasized that at any level of blood pressure, the risk of cardiovascular disease is magnified by the presence of co-existing risk factors (see Chapter 2). Diabetes potently magnifies this risk by virtue of the unenviable clustering of cardiovascular risk factors that frequently occurs in diabetic subjects.[8] Elevated glucose concentrations *per se* have been independently implicated in the pathogenesis of cardiovascular injury.[7,9] Characteristic lipid disturbances also occur in diabetes, notably, increased circulating levels of triglycerides and decreased levels of HDL-cholesterol.[8] Although LDL-cholesterol levels are not usually markedly elevated and indeed often normal in diabetic subjects, this should not be reassuring. LDL-cholesterol is abnormal in diabetes, in particular, there is a disproportionate increase in the level of small dense LDL particles which are more atherogenic.[10] Moreover, the LDL is more likely to be oxidized and/or glycated, all of which would further increase its atherogenic potential.

Disturbances to thrombolytic pathways also occur in diabetes, typically increased circulating levels of fibrinogen, increased platelet adhesiveness and increased plasminogen activator-1 (PAI1) levels.[8] This combination of abnormalities predisposes to increased thrombosis and reduced thrombolysis. The biochemical basis of these abnormalities has been extensively studied and the popular consensus is that many of these abnormalities are linked to the insulin resistance that characterizes type II diabetes and frequently occurs in type I diabetes as well.[11,12]

In addition to these metabolic disturbances, diabetic subjects are also more likely to develop left ventricular hypertrophy (LVH) (see below). LVH is one of the most potent independent predictors of an adverse cardiovascular outcome, particularly stroke.[13]

The importance of this cardiovascular risk factor clustering in diabetic subjects is that it predicts a higher cardiovascular risk for diabetic subjects at *any level of blood pressure* when compared to non-diabetic subjects. In so doing, it provides a compelling argument for advocating lower blood pressure thresholds for intervention with antihypertensive therapy in diabetic subjects when compared to the general population. A logical conclusion that has not, until recently, been applied to national and international guidance on hypertension management in diabetes.

"Pressure:metabolic synergy"

Beyond the epidemiological associations between blood pressure and cardiovascular risk in diabetic subjects, there is also a considerable body of more basic evidence to support a deleterious interaction between elevated pressure and metabolic factors. It is beyond the scope of this chapter to consider this concept in detail but a few examples of a "pressure:metabolic synergy" are highlighted. For example, increased endothelial permeability to macromolecules is one of the earliest events in the pathogenesis of atherosclerosis.[14] Elevated glucose concentrations markedly increase endothelial permeability to macromolecules[15] and increased blood pressure and/or the associated shear stress might be expected to accentuate this process. Moreover, in cell culture systems, elevated glucose concentrations and mechanical forces independently promote vascular smooth muscle growth and cardiac myocyte hypertrophy.[16] This kind of interaction in vivo could, at least in part, account for the increased left ventricular hypertrophy noted in diabetic subjects when compared to non-diabetics with equivalent levels of systemic blood pressure.[17]

Abnormalities in blood pressure regulation

Blood pressure measured in the doctor's office provides only a "snap-shot" of the true blood pressure load over 24 hours. In otherwise healthy non-diabetic subjects, blood pressure measurements over 24 hours reveal a circadian rhythm characterized by a nocturnal fall or "dip" in pressure during sleep. This blood pressure dip reduces overall 24-hour blood pressure load. The autonomic nervous system plays a key role in the regulation of blood pressure and the maintenance of the normal circadian rhythm.[18] The nocturnal dip in blood pressure is characterized by a relative reduction in sympathetic nervous system activity. Consequently patients with clinical evidence of autonomic neuropathy (diabetic and non-diabetic) are characterized by a failure in this nocturnal dip in blood pressure.[19]

There is ample evidence of disturbed blood pressure regulation in patients with diabetes, even in those with "normal" clinic blood pressures. Disturbances in 24-hour blood pressure load, characterized by a reduced nocturnal blood pressure load, have been reported in otherwise "normotensive" diabetic subjects with microalbuminuria[20] and these disturbances appear to progress and are more easily detected once overt diabetic nephropathy develops in patients with type 1 or type 2 diabetes. More disturbingly perhaps are the findings in a series of studies by Weston et al (see Chapter 5) from our laboratories.[21] He has shown that subtle disturbances in nocturnal blood pressure regulation are established in seemingly healthy "normotensive" type I diabetic subjects within 2 years of diagnosis in the absence of any overt evidence of diabetic complications or autonomic neuropathy. These disturbances to blood pressure regulation are associated with a small but significant increase in the ratio of sympathetic:parasympathetic nervous system activity, particularly at night.[21] There was also an increase in nocturnal heart rate in diabetic patients when compared to controls, consistent with a disturbed sympathetic:parasympathetic balance resulting in a net increase in sympathetic activity. Importantly, this early and subtle autonomic dysfunction relative sympathetic overactivity is undetectable by conventional bedside autonomic function testing.

These subtle developments have important implications. They confirm that even when traditional office blood pressures are normal, the 24-hour blood pressure load experienced by diabetic subjects is already elevated when compared to the non-diabetic population. This increase in load is primarily due to an increase in nocturnal blood pressure. This disturbance in autonomic function is proportionate to the disturbance in glycaemic control and progresses over time. This will inevitably result in a progressive rise in blood pressure and a progressive evolution of target organ damage. Figure 6.1 outlines the stages of this evolution and the clinical consequences.

The disturbances in blood pressure regulation in patients with established microalbuminuria or proteinuria are so substantial that these patients will invariably experience disproportionate elevations of their 24-hour blood pressure load relative to their clinic blood pressures. On this basis, the concept of a "normotensive" patient with microalbuminuria or proteinuria is a serious misnomer in that these patients have elevated 24-hour blood pressures, even if their clinic blood pressure is normal. Moreover, they all have evidence of target organ damage which is at least in part haemodynamically mediated.

Accelerated vascular ageing

With normal ageing, the larger conduit blood vessels progressively stiffen and lose their natural elasticity and compliance.[22] This is due to various mechanisms, including; an age-related decline in endothelial dysfunction the progressive accumulation of vascular wall matrix proteins, and the modification of vascular collagens by the development of cross links via

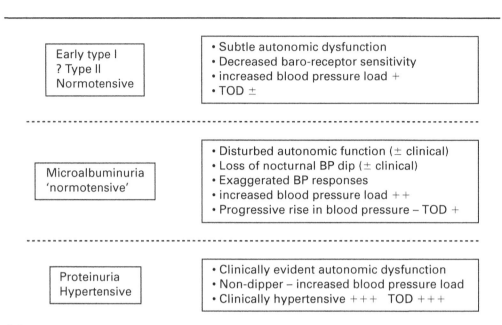

Figure 6.1
A proposed scheme for the evolution of blood pressure changes in diabetes mellitus in relation to the development of microalbuminuria.

the formation of advanced glycation end-products (AGEs).[23] Ageing, mechanical strain, sympathetic nervous system activity and activation of the renin–angiotensin–aldosterone system may all play a role in promoting vascular matrix accumulation.[24] Moreover, elevated glucose concentrations have also been shown to promote matrix synthesis in vitro.[25] With regard to the formation of AGEs, their presence within the vascular wall is evident early in the development of age-associated increases in vascular wall stiffness. The formation of AGEs is accelerated in diabetes and as such, this highlights a mechanism for accelerated ageing and stiffness of the vasculature in patients with diabetes.[26] Consistent with this hypothesis that "diabetes is a state of accelerated vascular ageing", we have recently shown that aortic pulse wave velocity (PWV) (carotid:femoral) is significantly increased in

patients with type 2 diabetes when compared to age matched non-diabetic controls (Fig. 6.2).[27] This is consistent with the observations of others[28] and has profound clinical significance. Increased aortic stiffness increases the vascular load on the heart and the coupling efficiency between the heart and vasculature.[29,30] For example, the increase in PWV leads to early pulse wave reflection within the circulation and augmentation of central aortic systolic blood pressure. The consequence of this haemodynamic disturbance is that it increases systolic work and pressure, culminating in a premature widening of the pulse pressure. This premature stiffening of the aorta in diabetes explains the earlier development of systolic hypertension in diabetic subjects when compared to the non-diabetic population[22] (Fig. 6.3). It also renders the systolic blood pressure more difficult to control.[31]

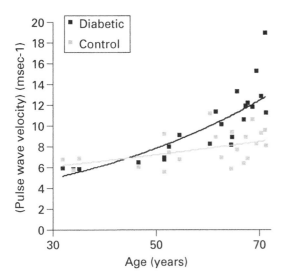

Figure 6.2
Increased pulse wave velocity in people with type 2 diabetes. Carotid femoral PWV in people with type 2 diabetes and an age-matched non-diabetic control population. The mean arterial blood pressure was similar in both groups. (O'Brien DG, Lacy PS, Williams B, Ref. 27 and unpublished data.)

The increased central arterial blood pressure that accompanies arterial stiffness and the increased systolic workload will in turn contribute to the premature development of LVH. Recently, a preliminary report of a 10-year follow-up on a cohort of type 2 diabetic patients showed that PWV measured at baseline was one of the strongest predictors of subsequent cardiovascular death and total mortality.[32]

It has long been my view that diabetes should be considered as a condition characterized by accelerated ageing of the vasculature. The impact of this accelerated vascular ageing process is compounded by any increase in systemic blood pressure and thus forms an important component of this unique vulnerability hypothesis.

Impaired microvascular protection

One of the hallmarks of the diabetic state is the predisposition to microvascular injury. This injury has a strong haemodynamic basis because it can be limited by manoeuvres that reduce microvascular pressure.[33] This conclusion is further supported by the results of the UKPDS study, which revealed that a relatively small therapeutic reduction of systemic blood pressure (−10/5 mmHg) could dramatically protect against the development and progression of microvascular disease in type II diabetes, particularly retinal disease.[6] This dramatic benefit implies impaired protection of the microcirculation from systemic blood pressure. This observation is particularly pertinent when one considers that the baseline blood pressures of the patients in the UKPDS study were not at a level that would ordinarily be associated with microvascular injury in non-diabetic subjects. This further implies that even mild to moderate hypertension predisposes to devastating microvascular injury in diabetes. The only potential explanation for this observation is that the mechanisms that normally protect the microcirculation against haemodynamic injury are impaired in diabetic subjects.

The microcirculation is ordinarily protected from systemic blood pressures by microcirculatory autoregulation.[34] Increased tissue perfusion pressures promote the constriction of afferent arterioles thereby maintaining constant pressures within delicate capillary beds. This afferent arteriolar response to pressure is primarily due to a myogenic reflex. Increased perfusion pressure leads to increased stretch of afferent arteriolar smooth muscle which in turn responds by constricting the lumen of the afferent arteriole and limiting the rise in distal capillary pressure. This process may be

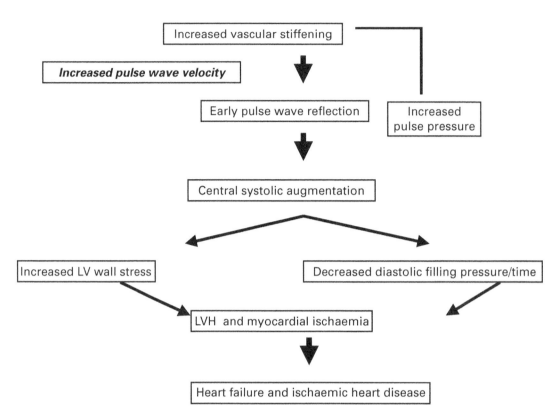

Figure 6.3
The consequences of accelerated conduit artery stiffening resulting in an increase in pulse wave velocity, early wave reflection, increased systolic left ventricular wall stress, increased systolic blood pressure and pulse pressure and ultimately increased left ventricular mass. The latter is compounded by "pressure:metabolic synergy" i.e. the trophic effects of the metabolic syndrome. The result is an early onset and increased prevalence of myocardial ischaemia and heart failure.

impaired at the cellular level by elevated glucose concentrations.[35] Impairment of this intrinsic microvascular response to hypertension would lead to increased microvascular perfusion pressures and capillary injury. Such impairment is likely to be a major factor in the pathogenesis of microvascular injury in diabetes. In support of this hypothesis, previous studies have shown that microcirculatory pressures are indeed elevated in diabetic subjects,[36,37] thereby implying that blood flow

autoregulation is impaired in diabetes. Moreover, numerous studies have demonstrated that microcirculatory blood flow in the retina and kidney is disproportionately increased in diabetes when compared to the non-diabetic state.[38,39] Further reports have confirmed an acute breakdown in retinal blood flow autoregulation in animals exposed to acute hyperglycaemia.[40] Moreover the studies of Patel (see Chapter 8) have elegantly confirmed that retinal blood flow autoregulation is markedly impaired in people with diabetes when challenged by a rise in systemic blood pressure. Moreover, the magnitude of the autoregulatory deficit was proportional to the degree of hyperglycaemia. This important observation is another example of the diabetic state setting the stage for injury which is ultimately mediated by haemodynamic stress.

Thus, one of the most fundamental mechanisms accounting for microvascular injury in diabetes is impairment of blood flow autoregulation culminating in a "pressure passive" microcirculation that is uniquely vulnerable to increased systemic blood pressure (Fig. 6.4). This hypothesis explains why the diabetic microcirculation experiences microvascular hypertension even when systemic blood pressures are "normal" or only mildly elevated. In so doing it suggests that the microcirculation should benefit substantially from even small

reductions in systemic blood pressure and that if microcirculatory protection is to be optimized then blood pressure targets on therapy should be as low as possible.

Conclusions

People with diabetes mellitus and hypertension cannot be considered as just another subset of the general hypertension population. This chapter has highlighted numerous mechanisms that render the diabetic patient with hypertension particularly susceptible to premature macrovascular disease and uniquely susceptible to microvascular disease (Fig. 6.5). The potency of systemic hypertension to promote macrovascular and cardiac disease is greatly enhanced by the coexistence of multiple cardiovascular risk factors, disturbances to blood pressure regulation resulting in

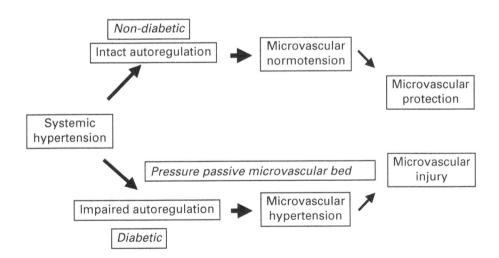

Figure 6.4
The vulnerability of the diabetic microcirculation to microvascular barotrauma and injury as a consequence of impaired blood flow autoregulation. Blood flow autoregulation protects the non-diabetic hypertensive subject from microvascular injury when systemic blood pressures are elevated. In people with diabetes, autoregulation is impaired; thus exposing the microcirculation to increased perfusion pressures, culminating in microangiopathy.

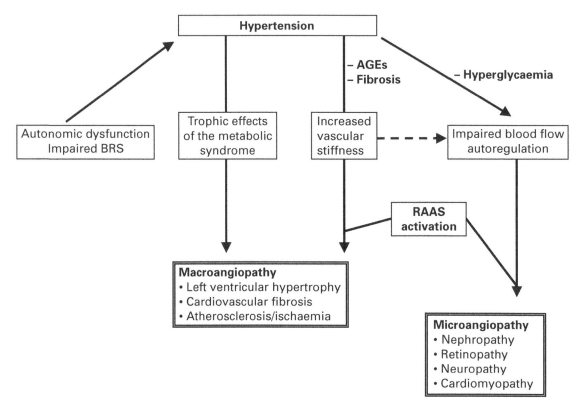

Figure 6.5

The multiple mechanisms conspiring to render people with diabetes uniquely vulnerable to hypertensive injury. The development of autonomic dysfunction and early impairment of BRS disturbs blood pressure regulation, increasing "blood pressure load". The adverse impact of the increase in blood pressure is compounded by the trophic effects of the metabolic syndrome, vascular stiffening, impaired blood flow autoregulation and inappropriate activation of the RAAS. (BRS = Baroreceptor sensitivity, AGEs = Advanced glycation end-products, RAAS = Renin-angiotensin-aldosterone system.)

increased 24-hour blood pressure load and accelerated ageing of large vessels thereby increasing haemodynamic and cardiac stress. At the cellular level, hyperglycaemia appears to act in concert with increased pressure to promote endothelial dysfunction and cardiovascular structural and functional changes, a process I have termed "pressure:metabolic synergy". The unique susceptibility to microvascular injury is another example of this synergy, in that it develops against the background of impaired blood flow autoregulation which appears to be directly related to the quality of glycaemic control. In effect, diabetes sets the stage for the development of premature and devastating cardiovascular injury and renders the patient uniquely vulnerable to even mild increases in blood pressure. Once the stage is set, blood pressure is a major perpetrator of the resulting injury.

References

1. Turner RC, Millns H, Neil HAW et al. Risk factors for coronary artery disease in non-insulin dependent diabetes: United Kingdom Prospective Diabetes Study. *BMJ* 1998; **316:** 823–8.
2. Cooper ME. Pathogenesis, prevention and treatment of diabetic nephropathy. *Lancet* 1998; **352:** 213–19.
3. Joint National Committee on prevention, detection, evaluation and treatment of high blood pressure (JNC VI). *Arch Intern Med* 1997; **157:** 2413–46.
4. EuroDiab Data base. Personal communication, H. Colhoun, University College, London, 1998.
5. Hansson L, Zanchetti A, Carruthers SG et al. Effects of intensive blood pressure lowering and low dose aspirin in patients with hypertension: principle results of the Hypertension Optimal Treatment (HOT) randomised trial. *Lancet* 1998; **351:** 1755–62.
6. UK Prospective Diabetes Study Group. Tight blood pressure control and risk of macrovascular and microvascular complications in type 2 diabetes. *BMJ* 1998; **317:** 703–13.
7. Kannel WB, McGee DL. Diabetes and glucose tolerance as risk factors for cardiovascular disease: The Framingham Study. *Diabetes Care* 1978; **2:** 120–6.
8. Williams B. Insulin resistance: a conspiracy of cardiovascular risk factors. *Diabetes Care* 1995; **3:** 4–5.
9. Stamler R, Stamler J, Lindberg HA et al. Asymptomatic hyperglycaemia and coronary heart disease risk in middle aged men in two employed populations in Chicago. *J Chronic Dis* 1979; **32:** 805–15.
10. Betteridge DJ. Diabetic dyslipidaemia – implications for vascular risk. In: Betteridge DJ, ed. *Lipids: Current Perspectives.* London: Martin Dunitz, 1996, 135–57.
11. Reavan GM. Role of insulin resistance in human disease. Banting Lecture 1988. *Diabetes* 1988; **37:** 1595–607.
12. Williams B. Insulin resistance: the shape of things to come. *Lancet* 1994; **344:** 521–4.
13. Kannel WB, Sorlie P. Left ventricular hypertrophy in hypertension: prognostic and pathogenic implications – The Framingham Study. In: Strauer BE, ed. *The Heart in Hypertension.* Berlin: Springer, 1981, 223–42.
14. Ross R. The pathogenesis of atherosclerosis: a perspective for the 1990s. *Nature* 1993; **362:** 801–9.
15. Williams B, Schrier RW. Glucose-induced PKC activity increases the permeability of bovine endothelial cell monolayers to albumin. *J Am Soc Nephrol* 1992; **3:** 556.
16. Yasunari K, Masakazu K, Kano H et al. Possible involvement of phospholipase D and protein kinase C in vascular growth induced by elevated glucose concentration. *Hypertension* 1996; **28:** 159–68.
17. Devereux KB, Roman MJ, Paranicas M et al. Impact of diabetes on cardiac structure and function: the strong heart study. *Circulation* 2000; **101:** 2271–6.
18. Somers VK, Dyken ME, Mark AE, Abboud FM. Sympathetic nerve activity during sleep in normal subjects. *N Engl J Med* 1993; **328:** 303–7.
19. Mann S, Altman DG, Rafferty EB, Bannister R. Circadian variation of blood pressure and autonomic failure. *Circulation* 1988; **68:** 477–83.
20. Page SR, Manning G, Ingle AR, Hill P, Millar-Craig MW, Peacock I. Raised ambulatory blood pressure in type 1 diabetics with incipient microalbuminuria. *Diabetic Med* 1994; **11:** 877–82.
21. Weston PJ, Panerai RB, McCullough A et al. Assessment of baroreceptor-cardiac reflex sensitivity using time domain analysis in patients with IDDM and the relation to left ventricular mass index. *Diabetologia* 1996; **39:** 1385–91
22. Kelly RP, Hayward C, Aviolo A, O'Rourke M. Non-invasive determination of age-related changes in the human arterial pulse. *Circulation* 1989; **80:** 1652–9.
23. Bucala R, Cerami A. Advanced glycosylation: chemistry, biology and implications for

diabetes and aging. *Adv Pharmacol* 1992; **23:** 1–24.

24. Williams B. Mechanical influences on vascular smooth muscle cell function. *J Hypertension* 1998; **16:** 1921–9.

25. Danne T, Spiro MJ, Spiro RG. Effect of high glucose on type IV collagen production by cultured glomerular epithelial, endothelial and mesangial cells. Diabetes 1993; **42:** 170–7.

26. Vlassara H, Fuh H, Makita Z, Kringkrai S, Cerami A, Bucala R. Exogenous advanced glycation end-products induce complex vascular dysfunction in normal animals: a model for diabetic and aging complications. *Proc Natl Acad Sci USA* 1992; **89:** 12043–7.

27. O'Brien DG, Lacy PS, Williams B. Pulse wave analysis fails to demonstrate increased vascular stiffness in diabetic patients. *J Human Hypertension* 2001, in press.

28. Woolham Gl, Shner PL, Valbona BS, Hoff HE. The pulse wave velocity as an early indicator of atherosclerosis in diabetic subjects. *Circulation* 1962; **25:** 533–9.

29. Lakatta E-G. Cardiovascular regulatory mechanisms in advanced age. *Physiol Rev* 1993; **73:** 413–67.

30. O'Rourke MF, Gallagher DE. Pulse wave analysis. *J Hypertension* 1996; **14** (Suppl 5): S147–S157.

31. Brown MJ, Castaigne A, de-Leeuw PW, Mancia G, Palmer CR, Rosenthal T, Ruilope LM. Influences of diabetes and type of hypertension on response to antihypertensive treatment. *Hypertension* 2000;, **35:** 1038–42.

32. Cruickshank JK, Gosling RG, Wright J, Riste L, Dunn G. Aortic pulse wave velocity predicts mortality in type 2 diabetes. *J Human Hyp* 2000; **14:** 11–12.

33. Zatz R, Brenner BM. Pathogenesis of diabetic microangiopathy: the hemodynamic view. *Am J Med* 1986; **80:** 443–6.

34. Johnson PC. Autoregulation of blood flow. *Circ Res* 1986; **59:** 483–95.

35. Williams B, Schrier RW. Effect of elevated extracellular glucose concentrations on transmembrane calcium ion fluxes in cultured rat VSMC. *Kidney Int* 1993; **44:** 344–51.

36. Bensten N, Larsen B, Lassen NA, Chronically impaired autoregulation of cerebral blood flow in long term diabetics. *Stroke* 1975; **6:** 497–502.

37. Faris I, Nielsen HV, Henricksen O, Parving HH, Larsen NA. Impaired autoregulation of blood flow in skeletal muscle and subcutaneous tissues in long term type I diabetic patients with microangiopathy. *Diabetologia* 1983; **25:** 486–8.

38. Sinclair SH, Grunwald JE, Riva CE et al. Retinal vascular autoregulation in diabetes mellitus. *Ophthalmology* 1982; **89:** 748–50.

39. Parving HH, Kastrup J, Smidt UM et al. Impaired autoregulation of glomerular filtration in type I diabetics with nephropathy. *Diabetologia* 1984; **27:** 547–52.

40. Atherton A, Hill DW, Keen H, Young HS, Edwards EJ. The effect of acute hyperglycaemia on the retinal circulation of the normal cat. *Diabetologia* 1980; **18:** 233–7.

II Target Organ Damage

7

Hypertension, microvascular function and diabetes mellitus

John E Tooke and Angela C Shore

Hypertension as a risk factor for microangiopathy

Although diabetic microangiopathy is undoubtedly multifactorial in origin, numerous studies have demonstrated a relationship between hypertension and the risk of development of microangiopathy. Most compelling are recent data from the UKPDS showing that tight blood pressure control retards the development of microangiopathic complications in patients with type II diabetes.[1] The Pima Indian study demonstrated that over a 5-year period the incidence of retinal exudates in diabetic subjects with systolic pressures >145 mmHg[2] was more than twice that of subjects whose systolic pressure was <125 mmHg of mercury. As far as diabetic nephropathy is concerned, controversy has raged as to whether hypertension is an initiating factor or develops concurrently with the appearance of increased protein leak. The latter view is currently favoured,[3] although there are conflicting data suggesting that patients prone to nephropathy more commonly have a family history of hypertension.[4,5] However, the link with hypertension and nephropathy is emphasised by the fact that hypotensive therapy delays the progression of the nephropathic process.[6]

There are several different interpretations of the data suggesting that the hypertension is a significant risk factor for microangiopathy.

High blood pressure and diabetes could result in synergistic mechanisms resulting in microvascular damage; alternatively there could be a common pathogenetic antecedent that results in both diabetes and hypertension. As the ensuing sections illustrate, both scenarios are plausible possibilities.

The first part of this chapter will consider the impact of diabetes on microvascular function; then the impact of high arterial blood pressure in normoglycaemic individuals will be considered. Finally the available information about the combined effects of high blood pressure and dysglycaemia will be reviewed.

Microvascular function in diabetes mellitus

Type I diabetes

Microvascular function is involved with the transport and exchange of nutrients and waste products between blood and tissue fluid. The microcirculation is also involved in tissue defence and repair and additionally various organ beds have specialised functions such as heat dissipation by the skin and excretion of waste products by the kidney. The key determinants of the transport and exchange function are capillary pressure, flow and permeability. Until relatively recently there has been a dirth of techniques for directly measuring these quantities in human diabetes. In the

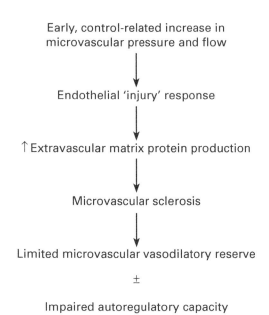

Early, control-related increase in microvascular pressure and flow

↓

Endothelial 'injury' response

↓

↑Extravascular matrix protein production

↓

Microvascular sclerosis

↓

Limited microvascular vasodilatory reserve

±

Impaired autoregulatory capacity

Figure 7.1
The haemodynamic hypothesis of the pathogenesis of diabetic microangiopathy in type I diabetes

last decade or so this situation has been rectified[7] and there is now cumulative evidence for a pattern of disturbance in microvascular function that antedates the emergence of clinical complications.

Clinical observation and estimations of total organ blood flow suggested to Parving and colleagues the so-called haemodynamic hypothesis of the pathogenesis of diabetic microangiopathy[8] (Fig. 7.1). This suggested that early in (type I) diabetes paradoxical increases in capillary pressure and flow occurred which had an injurious effect on the microvascular endothelium, stimulating the production of extravascular matrix proteins. This build up of relatively indistensible material limits the ability of the microvessel to dilate

and compromises autoregulation, i.e. the change in vessel diameter that normally accommodates changes in perfusion pressure. The apparent protection afforded to the kidney from the process of diabetic nephropathy by unilateral renal artery[9] stenosis as well as the relative infrequency of diabetic retinopathy in the presence of ipsilateral carotid artery stenosis[10] supports the importance of perfusion pressure as a prime moving mechanism in the genesis of diabetic microangiopathy. Nonetheless, proof of the hypothesis has awaited the development of techniques capable of measuring capillary pressure directly. Glomerular capillary hypertension has been demonstrated in a diabetic rat model[11]. Sandeman et al. used an electronic servonulling technique to measure nailfold capillary pressure, and demonstrated raised mean capillary pressure in a cross-sectional study of type I diabetic patients compared with age- and sex-matched healthy controls.[12] Furthermore, in keeping with criteria for a prime moving mechanism, capillary pressure in the diabetic subjects correlated with the level of glycated haemoglobin at the time of pressure measurement. Furthermore, improvement in diabetic control by attention to diet, insulin and exercise for 3 months resulted in a reduction in capillary pressure to near normal values.

Further support for the haemodynamic hypothesis comes from the fact that the impairment of microvascular vasodilatory reserve in type I diabetic subjects becomes more marked with increasing duration of disease[13] and in the presence of other diabetic complications. Rayman and co-workers correlated the degree of basement membrane thickening with the degree of vasodilatory impairment.[14] Kastrup et al. demonstrated that peripheral autoregulatory failure correlated with the degree of arteriolar hyalinosis.[15]

Thus in type I diabetes there is direct exper-

Function	Type I	Type II*
Capillary pressure	Control-related increase	Normal
Capillary filtration	Control-related increase	Normal
Microvascular vasodilatory reserve	Duration-related reduction	Early, profound reduction

Normotensive patients.

Table 7.1
Differences in microvascular function in type I and II diabetes.

imental evidence for the haemodynamic hypothesis, suggesting a pivotal role for capillary hypertension in the pathogenesis of diabetic microangiopathy. It might be assumed that the mechanisms would be identical in type II diabetes until it is appreciated that the expression of vascular disease and the prevalence of hypertension differs from that observed in type I diabetes. For example, complications are commonly found at the diagnosis of type II diabetes, whereas a significant duration of type I diabetes has to elapse before complications are observed. Maculopathy is the common form of visual loss compared with proliferative retinopathy in the type I patient and the expression of neuropathy and nephropathy may also differ.

Type II diabetes

Direct measurements of capillary pressure flow and permeability have revealed a different pattern of abnormalities in type II diabetes[16] (Table 7.1). In normotensive type II diabetic patients, capillary pressure is indistinguishable from that observed in normal subjects, although there is an inverse correlation with the duration of diabetes.[17] This suggests that perhaps capillary pressure is elevated before the diagnosis is made (which often occurs many years after the emergence of hyperglycaemia). Measurements of capillary pressure in subjects with impaired fasting glucose but otherwise normal glucose tolerance reveal a minority of subjects with high values but no group difference when such subjects are compared with age- and sex-matched controls.[18] A further contrast with type I diabetes is that in type II diabetes, microvascular vasodilatory reserve is markedly impaired at the diagnosis of the condition.[19] Although this could represent years of undisclosed diabetes, an alternative hypothesis is that some feature of the insulin-resistant state that underlies type II diabetes could be having an impact on vasodilatory mechanisms with the resultant relative increase in arteriolar resistance. Such a mechanism could also account for the high prevalence of hypertension in such subjects. In

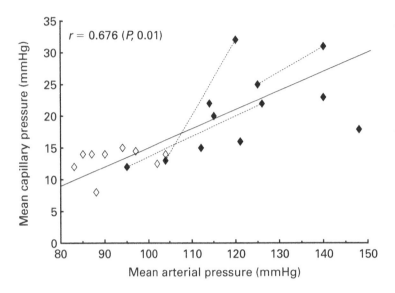

Figure 7.2
Nailfold capillary pressure values in non-diabetic subjects with essential hypertension (◆) and age- and sex-matched normotensive controls (◇). The effect of lowering systemic blood pressure is shown in three subjects (...).

keeping with this latter hypothesis, Jaap et al. demonstrated that microvascular vasodilatory reserve was impaired in subjects with impaired fasting glucose[20] and furthermore that the degree of impairment correlated with calculated insulin sensitivity.[21] Subsequent studies have shown microvascular vasodilatory reserve to be impaired in other insulin-resistant states.[22] Mechanistic studies suggest that the impairment is associated with a defect in endothelial-dependent vasodilatation,[23] supporting the concept that endothelial dysfunction may be the common antecedent to several of the features of the insulin resistance syndrome.[24]

Microvascular function in essential hypertension

Although typically essential hypertension is defined on the basis of elevated brachial artery pressure, it is a complex process involving all parts of the circulation as well as the kidney. Superficial scrutiny of the complications of hypertension points to involvement of the microcirculation, notably the renal consequences and hypertensive retinopathy. The conventional view of hypertension is that pressure elevation represents a sustained increase in peripheral vascular resistance which is predominantly sited at arteriolar level. Williams et al. measured nailfold capillary pressure in untreated patients with essential hypertension and normotensive controls matched for age, sex and menstrual cycle phase and demonstrated a significant elevation in capillary pressure in the hypertensive subjects[25] (Fig. 7.2). This suggests that at least some of the increased peripheral resistance must be sited at capillary or post-capillary level to account for the pressure rise. Indeed there is evidence that capillary density is reduced in essential hypertension[26] and venous compliance is also reduced.[27] Although oedema is not a feature of essential hypertension, increased transcapillary escape rate of albumin is consistent with increased convective transport across the capillary wall.[28]

There is abundant evidence that the resistance vessels undergo remodelling in the presence of sustained hypertension with an increase in wall to lumen ratio.[29] This might be expected to reduce vasodilatory reserve and indeed this has been demonstrated using similar techniques to those employed in diabetic studies.[30] It is clear therefore from the above that the pattern of haemodynamic change observed in the microcirculation in essential hypertension bears considerable similarity to the change observed in type I diabetes.

The impact of raised arterial blood pressure on microvascular function in diabetic subjects

Responses to a physiological increase in arterial pressure

Arterial blood pressure varies considerably with activity and posture. In normal subjects an increment in arterial blood pressure induced by isometric exercise is not transmitted to the capillary bed, capillary pressure remaining constant during the ramp in arterial pressure[31] (Fig. 7.3a). Although the mechanisms are unclear this can be considered as an example of capillary pressure autoregulation. In subjects with type I diabetes this control mechanism appears to break down such that capillary pressure rises paralleling the increase in arterial blood pressure (Fig. 7.3b).

Capillary pressure and diabetic patients with nephropathy and hypertension

Type I patients with microalbuminuria (incipient diabetic nephropathy) are more prone to many of the other complications of diabetes. Capillary pressure in these subjects is particu-

larly raised and significantly so compared with age- and sex-matched type I patients of similar disease duration and similar levels of glycaemic control who remain free of significant microangiopathic complications.[32] Indeed in the latter group capillary pressure equates to that observed in normal subjects. With the development of nephropathy arterial blood pressure tends to rise. However, this rise does not appear to result in a further increment in capillary pressure, although it remains significantly elevated. It has been suggested that this reflects arteriolar remodelling associated with the insulin resistance that accompanies the nephropathic state in much the same way as insulin resistance *per se* appears to impair precapillary vasodilatation.

Although there have been no systematic studies of capillary pressure in diabetic patients with essential hypertension, microvascular vasodilatory reserve has been assessed in such individuals.[33] The impairment observed is greater than that observed with diabetes alone, i.e. hypertension and a diabetic state appear to be synergistic (Fig. 7.4). Further evidence of the synergism of hypertension and type II diabetes comes from the increased cardiovascular risk in those subjects with both hypertension and diabetes compared with normotensive diabetics.[34]

Therapeutic implications

Until recently, few treatments other than glycaemic control have been shown to retard the development or progression of diabetic microangiopathy. One such treatment is hypotensive therapy, particularly ACE inhibition, which has been shown to delay the progression of diabetic nephropathy[35] as well as diabetic retinopathy.[36] It has been demonstrated in pilot studies that ACE inhibition will reduce capillary pressure in patients with

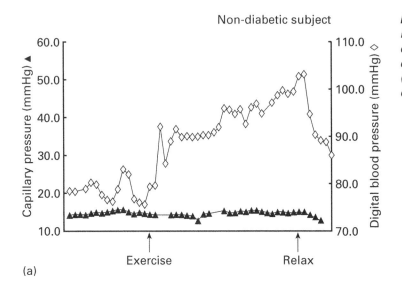

Non-diabetic subject

(a)

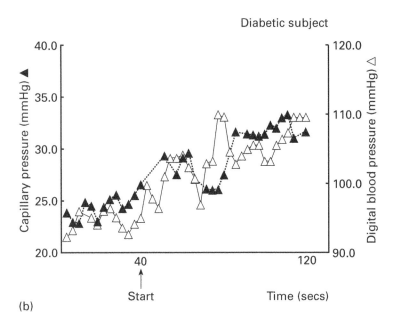

Diabetic subject

(b)

Figure 7.3
Nailfold capillary pressure and digital pressure during isometric exercise (contralateral handgrip) in (a) a healthy subject and (b) type I diabetic patient.

essential hypertension as well as capillary pressure in diabetic subjects with established nephropathy[37] and incipient nephropathy[38] (Fig. 7.5). Although such evidence points to a key role for arterial hypertension, a reduction in capillary pressure in incipient nephropathic patients occurred in subjects who were normotensive and was achieved without a significant reduction in their arterial blood pressure, suggesting that local microvascular control mechanisms may have been favourably influenced. Protracted treatment with hypotensive agents has been shown to achieve some remodelling of the circulation in hypertension, notably the

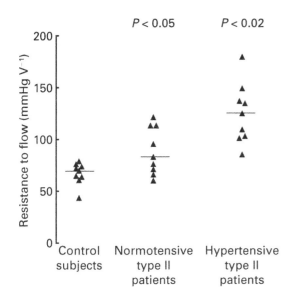

Figure 7.4
Minimal microvascular resistance in type II diabetics with and without hypertension and in healthy normotensive controls.

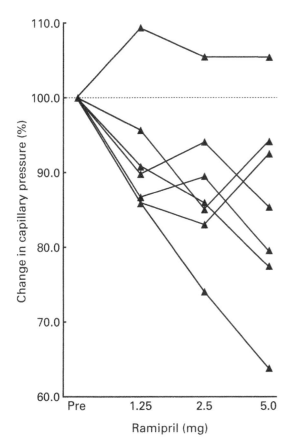

Figure 7.5
Dose ranging pilot study of the effects of the ACE inhibitor ramipril on nailfold capillary pressure in type I diabetic patients with incipient nephropathy.

changes in wall to lumen ratio.[39] Experimental work with ACE inhibitors in insulin-resistant states suggests that this class of agent may induce similar favourable changes.[40] However, the UKPDS has demonstrated that it is the lowering of blood pressure that is more important than agent class in preventing microangiopathy.[1]

Conclusions

Studies of microvascular haemodynamics in patients with diabetes and hypertension are revealing the functional abnormalities of this part of the circulation and their role in the genesis of diabetic complications. In the type I patient there is accumulating evidence that hypertension is a significant risk factor for the development of complications and it is likely that this represents aggravation of the control-related capillary hypertension characteristic of this form of the disease. In type II diabetes hypertension can be considered as integral to the remodelling of microvascular resistance which appears to antedate the emergence of hyperglycaemia. The concurrence of hypertension accelerates this remodelling process, resulting in profound limitation of microvascular vasodilatory reserve. Important studies of capillary pressure in subjects with micro-albuminuria and/or hypertension remain to be conducted, but the autoregulatory impairment observed in diabetes suggests that it is unlikely that the capillary bed will be completely protected from the increase in capillary pressure. The observed microvascular pathophysiological changes further rationalise the prompt and aggressive treatment of arterial hypertension in subjects with diabetes and suggest plausible mechanisms whereby these two major cardiovascular risk factors might inter-react.

References

1. UKPDS. Tight blood pressure control and risk of macrovascular and microvascular complications in type 2 diabetes UKPDS 38. *BMJ* 1998; **317**: 703–13.
2. Knowle WC, Bennett PH, Ballantine EJ. Increased incidence of retinopathy in diabetes with elevated blood pressure. *N Engl J Med* 1980; **302**: 645–50.
3. Jensen T, Borch-Johnsen K, Deckert T. Changes in blood pressure and renal function in patients with type 1 (insulin-dependent) diabetes mellitus prior to clinical diabetic nephropathy. *Diabetes Res* 1987; **4**: 159–62.
4. Barzilay J, Warram JH, Bak M, Laffel LMB, Canessa M, Krolewski AS. Predisposition to hypertension: risk factor for nephropathy and hypertension in IDDM. *Kidney Int* 1992; **41**: 723–30.
5. Krolewski AS, Canessa M, Warram JH, *et al*. Predisposition to hypertension and susceptibility to renal disease in insulin-dependent diabetes mellitus. *N Engl J Med* 1988; **318**: 140–5.
6. Mathiesen ER, Hommel E, Giese J, Parving H-H. Efficacy of captopril in postponing nephropathy in normotensive insulin dependent diabetic patients with microalbuminuria. *BMJ* 1991; **303**: 81–7.
7. Tooke JE. Methodologies used in the study of the microcirculation in diabetes mellitus. *Diabetes Metab Rev* 1993; **9**: 57–70.
8. Parving H-H, Viberti GC, Keen H, Christiansen JS, Lassen NA. Hemodynamic factors in the genesis of diabetic microangiopathy. *Metabolism* 1983; **32**: 943–9.
9. Berkman J, Rifkin H. Unilateral nodular diabetic glomerulosclerosis (Kimmelstiel-Wilson). Report of a case. *Metab Clin Exp* 1973; **22**: 715–22.
10. Behrendt T, Duane TD. Unilateral complications in diabetic retinopathy. *Trans Am Acad Opthalmol Otol* 1970; **74**: 28–32.
11. Hostetter TH, Troy JL, Brenner BM. Glomerular hemodynamics in experimental diabetes mellitus. *Kidney Int* 1981; **19**: 410–15.
12. Sandeman DD, Shore AC, Tooke JE. Relation of skin capillary pressure in patients with insulin-dependent diabetes mellitus to complications and metabolic control. *N Engl J Med* 1992; **327**: 760–4.
13. Rayman G, Williams SA, Spencer PD, Smaje LH, Wise PH, Tooke JE. Impaired microvascular hyperaemic response to minor skin trauma in type 1 diabetes. *BMJ* 1986; **292**: 1295–8.
14. Rayman G, Malik RA, Sharma AK, Day JL. Microvascular response to tissue injury and capillary ultrastructure in the foot skin of type 1 diabetic patients. *Clin Sci* 1995; **89**: 467–74.
15. Kastrup J, Norgaard T, Parving H-H, Henriksen O, Lassen NA. Impaired autoregulation of blood flow in subcutaneous tissue of long-term type 1 (insulin-dependent) diabetic patients with microangiopathy: and index of arteriolar dysfunction. *Diabetologia* 1985; **28**: 711–17.
16. Jaap AJ, Tooke JE. Pathophysiology of microvascular disease in non-insulin-dependent diabetes. *Clin Sci* 1995; **89**: 3–12.
17. Shore AC, Jaap AJ, Tooke JE. Capillary pressure in patients with NIDDM. *Diabetes* 1994; **43**: 1198–202.
18. Shore AC, Morris SJ, Stockman AJ, Tooke JE. Capillary pressure in subjects with fasting hyperglycaemia. *Diabetic Med* 1997; **14** (Suppl 1): S67.
19. Sandeman DD, Pym CA, Green EM, Seamark C, Shore AC, Tooke JE. Microvascular vasodilation in feet of newly diagnosed non-insulin-dependent diabetic patients. *BMJ* 1991; **302**: 1122–3.
20. Jaap AJ, Hammersley MS, Shore AC, Tooke JE. Reduced microvascular hyperaemia in subjects at risk of developing type 2 (non-insulin-dependent) diabetes mellitus. *Diabetologia* 1994; **37**: 214–16.
21. Jaap AJ, Shore AC, Tooke JE. Relationship of insulin resistance to microvascular dysfunction in subjects with fasting hyperglycaemia. *Diabetologia* 1997; **40**: 238–43.

22. Anastasiou E, Lekakis JP, Alevizaki M, *et al.* Impaired endothelium dependent vasodilation in women with previous gestational diabetes mellitus. *Diabetes Care* 1998; **21:** 2111–15.

23. Morris SJ, Jaap AJ, Shore AC, Tooke JE. Responses of the skin microcirculation to acetylcholine and sodium nitroprusside in subjects with fasting hyperglycaemia. *J Physiol* 1996; **491.P:** 14P.

24. Tooke JE, Goh KL. Endotheliopathy precedes type II diabetes. *Diabetes Care* 1998; **21:** 2047–9.

25. Williams SA, MacGregor GA, Smaje LH, Wasserman SM, Tooke JE. Capillary hypertension and abnormal pressure dynamics in patients with essential hypertension. *Clin Sci* 1990; **79** (Suppl 1): 5–8.

26. Williams SA, Tooke JE, MacGregor G. Rarefaction in skin capillaries in hypertension. *Clin Sci* 1986; **70:** 14P.

27. Safar ME, London GM. Arterial and venous compliance in sustained essential hypertension. *Hypertension* 1987; **10:** 133–9.

28. Parving H-H, Gyntelberg F. Transcapillary escape rate of albumin and plasma volume in essential hypertension. *Circ Res* 1973; **32:** 643–51.

29. Shore AC, Tooke JE. Microvascular function in human essential hypertension. *J Hypertens* 1994; **12:** 717–28.

30. Williams SA, Tooke JE. Noninvasive estimation of increased structurally-based resistance to blood flow in the skin of subjects with essential hypertension. *Int J Microcirc Clin Exp* 1992; **11:** 109–16.

31. Shore AC, Sandeman DD, Tooke JE. Effect of an increase in systemic blood pressure on nailfold capillary pressure in humans. *Am J Physiol* 1993; **265:** H820–H823.

32. Shore AC, Jaap AJ, Tooke JE. Capillary pressure in insulin dependent diabetic patients of long disease duration with and without microangiopathy. *Diabetic Med* 1992; **9** (Suppl 2): S11.

33. Jaap AJ, Shore AC, Tooke JE. Increased resistance to blood flow in the skin of hypertensive non-insulin dependent diabetic patients. *Diabetic Med* 1993; **10** (Suppl 3): S38.

34. Vaccaro O, Stamler J, Neaton JD. Sixteen-year coronary mortality in black and white men with diabetes screened for the Multiple Risk Factor Intervention Trial (MRFIT). *Int J Epidemiol* 1998; **27** 636–41.

35. Parving H-H. Effects of ACE inhibitors on renal function on incipient and overt diabetic nephropathy. *J Diabetic Complications* 1996; **10:** 133–5.

36. Parving H-H. Impact of blood pressure and antihypertensive treatment on incipient and overt nephropathy, retinopathy, and endothelial permeability in diabetes mellitus. *Diabetes Care* 1991; **14:** 260–9.

37. Sandeman DD, Shore AC, Tooke JE. Captopril reduces nailfold capillary pressure in type 1 diabetic patients with established nephropathy. *Diabetic Med* 1991; **8** (Suppl 1): 37A.

38. Shore AC, Donohoe M, Jaap AJ, Tooke JE. The effect of increasing doses of an angiotensin converting enzyme inhibitor on capillary pressure levels in patients with insulin-dependent-diabetes mellitus and microalbuminuria. *Diabetic Med* 1993; **10** (Suppl 1): A18.55.

39. Heagerty AM, Bund SJ, Aalkjaer C. Effects of drug treatment on human resistance arteriole morphology in essential hypertension: direct evidence for structural remodelling of resistance vessels. *Lancet* 1988; **2:** 1209–13.

40. Berne C, Pollare T, Lithell H. Effects of antihypertensive treatment on insulin sensitivity to ACE inhibitors. *Diabetes Care* 1991; **14:** (Suppl 4): 39–47.

8

Diabetic retinopathy and hypertension

Vinod Patel and Eva Kohner

Introduction

Diabetic retinopathy, as the commonest cause of blindness in the working population, remains an important public health concern.[1] In the most definitive epidemiological study to date, the yearly incidence of blindness due to diabetes mellitus was found to be 3.3 per 100 000 population.[2] This figure extrapolates to around 1600 cases for England and Wales each year. The other main site of microangiopathic insult in diabetic patients is the kidney. There the pathogenic mechanisms are becoming clear as it has now become apparent that hypertension and subsequent glomerular hyperfusion are central to the progression of diabetic glomerulopathy.[3,4]

Hypertension is thought to be an important risk factor in the pathogenesis and progression of diabetic retinopathy, although not all epidemiological studies have concluded this. In the first section of this chapter, epidemiological studies in relation to hypertension and diabetic retinopathy will be reviewed. The second section will cover the most important haemodynamic principles in relation to diabetic retinopathy and hypertension. The lesions of diabetic retinopathy and their relationship to hypertension will then be covered. Experimental and clinical evidence for a haemodynamic model for the pathogenesis of diabetic

retinopathy will be presented, including the EUCLID Study, which examined the role of ACE inhibition in retarding the progression of diabetic retinopathy.[5] The impact of blood pressure control on the development and progression of retinopathy in type 2 diabetes, as revealed by the United Kingdom Prospective Diabetes Study (UKPDS)[6] and the Appropriate Blood Pressure Control in Diabetes (ABCD)[7] study will also be discussed.

An understanding of the role of hypertension in the pathogenesis of diabetic retinopathy will serve to focus attention on the management of hypertension in diabetes and suggest avenues of research.

Epidemiology of diabetic retinopathy and hypertension

The most extensive epidemiological study of diabetic retinopathy to date has been the Wisconsin Epidemiological Study of Diabetic Retinopathy (WESDR).[8-12] This study divided the diabetic population into those diagnosed before the age of 30 (young onset) and those diagnosed after the age of 30 (older onset). In practice these two groups approximate, reasonably accurately, to type I and type II diabetes mellitus respectively.

The WESDR is based on a large population of diabetic subjects with assessment of diabetic retinopathy from seven field stereo-colour photographs of the retina. The prevalence of any diabetic retinopathy, in the 996 young-ones patients, was 17 per cent within 5 years duration of diabetes mellitus and 98 per cent at >15 years duration of diabetes. Proliferative diabetic retinopathy was not found in any young-onset subject with a duration of diabetes <5 years. This rose to 4 per cent at 10 years duration, 25 per cent at 15 years duration and 57 per cent at 30 years duration. The 4-year incidence of proliferative diabetic retinopathy was 11 per cent, based on the 713 subjects who did not have proliferative diabetic retinopathy at baseline. The prevalence of macular oedema was 29 per cent in the young-onset subjects after 20 years duration of diabetes. The 4-year incidence of macular oedema in this group was 8.2 per cent.

After 15 years duration of diabetes, the prevalence of any diabetic retinopathy in the 1370 older-onset diabetic subjects studied, was 85 per cent in subjects taking insulin and 63 per cent in those not on insulin treatment. Overall the prevalence of proliferative diabetic retinopathy was 16 per cent after 15 years duration of diabetes. At 4 years follow-up 7 per cent of the insulin-treated and 2 per cent of the non-insulin-treated subjects had developed proliferative diabetic retinopathy. The prevalence of macular oedema was similar to the young-onset diabetic subjects in the older-onset diabetic subjects (28 per cent) after 20 years duration of diabetes. The 4-year incidence of macular oedema was 8.4 per cent in the older-onset diabetics using insulin and 2.9 per cent in non-insulin diabetic subjects.

Elevated diastolic blood pressure was a significant risk factor for the development of severe diabetic retinopathy.[13,14] There was a 14.1-fold increase in severe retinopathy with a diastolic blood pressure of ≥70 mmHg.[13] This was independent of the presence of concomi-tant diabetic nephropathy, which might have been a confounding factor in other studies reporting the same result. Other studies found that a raised systolic blood pressure rather than the diastolic blood pressure was associated with the progression of diabetic retinopathy.[15,16] The WESDR found an association between systolic blood pressure and retinopathy in the younger-onset of diabetes group with no consistent association between blood pressure and retinopathy in the older-onset of diabetes group.[17]

The UKPDS study has demonstrated a significant trend for more severe retinopathy in patients with higher systolic and diastolic blood pressure. The incidence of new retinopathy was also significantly related to both diastolic and systolic blood pressure with the lowest tertile having a 13 per cent prevalence of new retinopathy at 6 years in comparison with 31 per cent in the highest tertile of blood pressure. A multivariate analysis showed systolic blood pressure to be the more important blood pressure parameter. The UKPDS also confirmed the importance of hypertension in the pathogenesis of diabetic retinopathy.[6]

In this study of type II diabetic subjects, a cohort of hypertensive patients were randomized to achieve two levels of blood pressure control; 'less good' and 'tighter control'. The achieved difference in blood pressure control was 10/5 mmHg. In the group with tighter blood pressure control there was a dramatic reduction in the incidence of microvascular disease, predominantly due to a decreased incidence in proliferative retinopathy. This was associated with a lesser loss of visual activity in those with tighter blood pressure control. Intriguingly, the impact of improved blood pressure control exceeded the benefit achieved by improved glycaemic control by almost 3:1, confirming the prime importance of hypertension in the pathogenesis of proliferative diabetic retinopathy.[6]

With respect to specific lesions of diabetic retinopathy the WESDR found a relationship between proliferative retinopathy and diastolic blood pressure.[8,9] A 5-year follow-up study in the Pima Native American Indians of Arizona found that the incidence of retinal hard exudates was two-fold greater in diabetic subjects with a systolic blood pressure of 145 versus a systolic blood pressure of ≤125.[15]

A 10-year prospective study of 104 type I and type II diabetic subjects without sight-threatening diabetic retinopathy revealed the following factors to be associated with progression to sight-threatening diabetic retinopathy: systolic blood pressure >135 mmHg, diastolic blood pressure no clear effect, mean arterial blood pressure >110 mmHg, retinal perfusion pressure >50 mmHg, pulse pressure (systolic-diastolic) >60 mmHg.[18] A recent study showed a clear association between diabetic retinopathy and hypertension. Furthermore it concluded that disturbed diurnal variation of blood pressure was a pathophysiological factor in the development of diabetic retinopathy.[19]

From these and other studies it can be concluded that hypertension is an important risk factor in the progression of a diabetic retina towards sight-threatening diabetic retinopathy.

Other clinical risk factors for diabetic retinopathy
Duration of diabetes mellitus

The WESDR study has demonstrated that the duration of diabetes is closely correlated to the prevalence of background retinopathy, maculopathy and proliferative retinopathy. Many

other studies are in general agreement with this conclusion.[20,21]

Glycaemic control

Physicians were ill at ease about concluding that diabetic complications, and particularly diabetic retinopathy, is related to poor glycaemic control. Initial doubts about the benefits of improved diabetic control were sown by the results of the various intervention studies comparing the effect of conventional treatment and those on a continuous subcutaneous insulin infusion (CSII). Those on CSII, with a lower HbA1%, had a higher rate of deterioration with respect to their diabetic retinopathy with more cotton wool spots and intraretinal microvascular abnormalities.[22] The Oslo study showed a similar worsening of retinopathy in the short-term, but their 7-year follow-up data showed a clear net beneficial effect of improved diabetic control with a reduced rate of progression of diabetic retinopathy.[23] Another study demonstrated that proliferative diabetic retinopathy only developed in patients with a mean HbA1% of over 10 per cent over a 10-year follow-up period.[24] In a follow-up study of 153 type I diabetic subjects over 4 years, in comparison with the diabetic group with excellent glycaemic control (HbA1% <8.3 per cent), there was an increased risk of progression to severe retinopathy with higher average HbA1% levels; 8.4–9.0 per cent × 5.3, 9.1–9.8 per cent × 16.4, 9.9–13.6 per cent × 26.1.[24] In the WESDR a significant relationship was found between the HbA1% and progression of retinopathy in both types of diabetes.[25] All doubts about the importance of glycaemic control have been laid to rest with the publication of the large randomised DCCT Study (Diabetes Control and Complications Study) which studied 1441 type I diabetic subjects over 6.5 years.[26] This compared intensive treatment reducing the HbA1c% to <7.0 per cent with more conventional treatment and an HbA1c% level of 9 per cent. Intensive control reduced the progression of diabetic retinopathy in the primary prevention cohort by 76 per cent and in the secondary prevention cohort by 54 per cent. Almost identical data were reported in a smaller Japanese study of type II diabetic subjects.[27,28] The UKPDS is the largest study to date which has examined the impact of intensified glycaemic control on many diabetes related end-points in patients with type 2 diabetes. Intensified glycaemic control resulting in a HBA1c decrease of 0.9%, reduced microvascular end-points by 25% ($P > 0.0099$) and retinopathy after 12 years of study by 21% ($P < 0.015$).[28]

Cholesterol level

Diabetic patients have a higher prevalence of hypercholesterolaemia. Data from the WESDR showed that 17 per cent of the young-onset and 30 per cent of the older-onset diabetic patients have serum cholesterol levels in the high-risk range for macrovascular disease as defined by the USA National Cholesterol Education Program guidelines (>6.1 mmol).[29]

Total serum cholesterol levels have been shown to be higher in patients with proliferative diabetic retinopathy than in background diabetic retinopathy and diabetic subjects without any retinopathy. A significantly higher mean serum cholesterol level and a higher diastolic blood pressure was found in type II diabetic subjects with exudative maculopathy.[30] On average the serum cholesterol level was 6.7 mmol in exudative maculopathy and 5.9 mmol in a matched diabetic control group without retinopathy. Both the above studies failed to demonstrated an association between diabetic retinopathy and triglyceride levels. Other studies also show hypercholesterolaemia to be associated with diabetic retinopathy.[18,21]

Other clinical risk factors

Diabetic patients with persistent microalbuminuria, corresponding to a 24-hour urinary albumin excretion rate of >300 mg, have an increased risk of proliferative diabetic retinopathy in comparison to those without microalbuminuria.[31] Autonomic neuropathy, as assessed from abnormalities of cardiovascular function, was found to be a significant risk factor for early onset proliferative diabetic retinopathy in type I diabetic subjects.[32] In relation to diabetic subjects without autonomic neuropathy, there was an increased risk of 34.6 with moderate abnormalities indicative of cardiovascular autonomic neuropathy and 77.5 with severe abnormalities. The mechanism of the effect of autonomic neuropathy may be haemodynamic. Abnormal autoregulation has been demonstrated to increase systemic blood pressure in diabetic subjects with autonomic neuropathy in comparison with diabetic subjects with no autonomic dysfunction.[33] The effect of smoking on the microvascular complications of diabetes remains controversial. Several reports concluded that it is a significant risk factor by a factor of around 2, whereas the results of the WESDR concluded that it was not.[34,35] The development of both severe exudative and proliferative diabetic retinopathy was found to be associated with heavy alcohol consumption.[36] The Pittsburgh Epidemiology of Diabetes Complications Study concluded that a modest degree of alcohol consumption may actually confer protection against diabetic complications including retinopathy.[37] The WESDR failed to confirm the association of diabetic retinopathy and heavy alcohol consumption, but provided further evidence for the protective effect of moderate alcohol consumption.[38]

Pregnancy

Multiple studies have concluded that pregnancy is associated with accelerated progression of diabetic retinopathy.[39] This effect is independent of any blood pressure and glycaemic changes. The WESDR found an increased risk of progression by a factor of 2.3.[40]

Haemodynamic considerations

As diabetic retinopathy is *prima facie* a condition of haemodynamic damage to the retinal circulation, it is important to examine the possible haemodynamic pathophysiological consequences of hypertension.

The relationship between flow and the essential factors affecting it is stated in Poiseuilles Law.[41]

$$\text{Flow} = \text{Pa} - \text{Pb} \frac{\pi . r^4}{8 \, n \, L}$$

Where: Pa − Pb = the pressure difference between the two ends of the tube or 'vessel'; n = viscosity; r = radius of the tube; L = length of the tube or 'vessel'. This formula holds true for a Newtonian fluid in a rigid tube and since vessels are compliant with blood consisting of a fluid with many components, its behaviour differs from Poiseuille flow. The most important difference is that the flow to vessel dimension relationship is not quadratic as stated above but cubic, this is often referred to as Murray's Law.[42] The law has been found to approximate microcirculatory flow generally, including the retinal circulation.[42] Clearly in hypertension retinal blood flow is going to increase in direct proportion to the perfusion pressure unless there is a protective regulatory response. This response is autoregulation and

is defined as the ability of a tissue to keep flow constant under conditions of varying perfusion pressure. Autoregulation is particularly important in the human retinal circulation as it lacks an autonomic innervation. In the normal human retinal circulation retinal blood is relatively constant until the mean arterial blood pressure is raised to 40 per cent above baseline.[43]

Retinal perfusion pressure

The retinal perfusion pressure is calculated from the following relationship:

$$[2/3 . \text{MAP}] - \text{IOP}$$

MAP = mean arterial pressure = 1/3. (systolic − diastolic) + diastolic; IOP = intraocular pressure. The 2/3 MAP function represents the drop in the systemic mean arterial pressure, calculated from the brachial artery measurement point to the level of the ophthalmic artery. Its validity and accuracy have been verified using Doppler ophthalmomanometry as an objective technique to measure the ophthalmic artery pressure.[44] The ophthalmic artery pressure and the brachial artery pressure were found to be highly correlated. The ratio of the ophthalmic artery pressure to the brachial artery pressure was found to be 0.68 SD 0.04, a figure that corresponds closely with the 2/3 factor used above in calculating the retinal perfusion pressure indirectly.

A consequence of the retinal perfusion/systemic perfusion relationship is that for a given increase in mean arterial blood pressure the increase in retinal perfusion pressure will be greater. For example, with blood pressure of 130/80 mmHg the MAP will be 96.7 mmHg. Assuming an intraocular pressure of 20 mmHg, the retinal perfusion pressure will be 44.4 mmHg. With an increase in blood pressure to 170/110 the MAP will be 130 mmHg, an increment of 34.4 per cent.

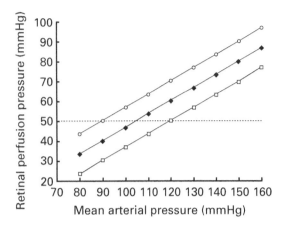

Figure 8.1
Inter-relationship of the MAP and the retinal perfusion pressure. For mean arterial blood pressure (MAP) values between 80 and 160 mmHg, the retinal perfusion values are shown for three intraocular pressure (IOP) levels. It is clear that a hypothetical 'dangerous' retinal perfusion value of 50 mmHg is reached at lower MAP levels at a lower IOP. (○), IOP = 10 mmHg; (◆), IOP = 20 mmHg; (□), IOP = 30 mmHg.

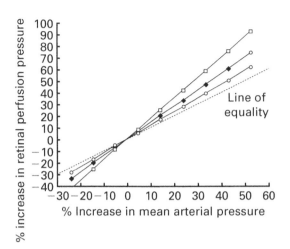

Figure 8.2
The inter-relationship of the MAP and retinal perfusion pressure. A plot of change in MAP and the resultant retinal perfusion pressure at three different IOP levels. From the line of equality it is apparent that the percentage increase in the retinal perfusion pressure is always higher than the percentage increase in MAP. (○), IOP = 10 mmHg; (◆), IOP = 20 mmHg; (□), IOP = 30 mmHg.

The retinal perfusion is now 66.6 mmHg, a far greater increment of 50 per cent. We speculate that this in part may explain the increased susceptibility of the retinal vasculature to hypertensive damage. This phenomenon is illustrated in Figs 8.1 and 8.2. These graphs also show that if there is a threshold retinal perfusion pressure above which retinal damage occurs, then this will happen at a relatively lower MAP in a diabetic subject with a low IOP. Our hypothesis has some evidence for it is provided by a pathophysiological 'experiment of nature', as diabetic subjects with a raised IOP were found to develop significantly less diabetic retinopathy in comparison to diabetic patients with normal or low IOP.[45,46]

If autoregulation fails then retinal blood flow will increase, leading to an increment in shear stress to the vessel wall as shear stress is directly proportional to flow.[41] Injury to the endothelium can result from shear stress alone with concomitant damage to pericyte and endothelial cells, as demonstrated in experimental hypertension.[47,48] Pericytes by virtue of their contractile properties are important in retinal vascular autoregulation. Pericyte damage impairs autoregulation, leading to a self-perpetuating cycle of damage to the retinal vasculature. Hypertension and increased retinal blood flow will also lead to capillary hypertension, as the hydrostatic pressure will be more easily transmitted to the smaller vessels if there is impaired autoregulation. The circumferential stress in a vessel is directly proportional to the perfusion pressure and radius.[41] Circumferential stress damage leads to both micro- and macro-aneurysm formation particularly as a consequence of the Laplace relationship.[41] This states that the tension in a vessel wall resisting the intraluminal distension pressure is inversely proportional to the radius. At a localised area of circumferential damage there is dilatation with a propensity towards aneurysm formation. The capillary hypertension and shear stress damage to the endothelial cells will result in a net increase in fluid leaving the retinal capillaries (Starling's forces). This would lead to retinal exudates and oedema, especially as there is no lymphatic drainage of the central nervous system tissues.

It is noteworthy that the lesions of hypertensive retinopathy, such as haemorrhages and cotton wool spots, are most concentrated around the optic disc and along the superior and inferior temporal arteries where the transmitted pressure is expected to be the greatest. These lesions are rarely found temporal to the macular region.

Pertinent to the diabetic retinal circulation is the observation that an increase in shear stress stimulates mitosis in endothelial cells and increases their turnover.[49] A similar study showed that increased shear stress can stimulate both the migration and proliferation of endothelial cells.[50]

Coefficient of autoregulation

It is useful to use a coefficient of autoregulation to measure the autoregulatory capacity of vascular beds under differing conditions and in different disease states. The classical Greek letter ϕ (phi) was adopted as the symbol as an allusion to the original Greek derivative for flow. It is defined as:

$$\phi = 1 - \frac{\% \text{ change in flow}}{\% \text{ change in perfusion pressure}}$$

When there is no change in flow for a given change in perfusion pressure, there is ideal autoregulation and ϕ will be 1. When the percentage increase in flow is comparable to the percentage increase in perfusion pressure, ϕ will tend towards 0. The expression '% change in flow/% change in perfusion' also represents the tangent of the angle created by the slope of the pressure-flow curve. A similar equation has been presented previously.[51]

Diabetic retinopathy: classification and clinical findings

Background diabetic retinopathy consists of the following lesions in the retina in the presence of diabetes mellitus: microaneurysms, dot and blot haemorrhages, hard exudates, cotton wool spots, intraretinal microvascular abnormalities, arterial and venous abnormalities (Table 8.1). It must be emphasised at the outset that background diabetic retinopathy encompasses a broad spectrum of findings ranging from mild to severe, ranging from only one of the above lesions present to all six occurring simultaneously. Preproliferative diabetic retinopathy is best regarded as a pattern of active and progressing non-proliferative retinopathy, often in the setting of clinical hypertension. Preproliferative diabetic retinopathy is defined by the Diabetic Retinopathy Study Group (1987) as the conglomeration of any three of the following lesions: intraretinal microvascular abnormalities, venous beading and/or reduplication, moderately severe retinal haemorrhages and/or microaneurysms and cotton wool spots. In current clinical practice preproliferative diabetic retinopathy is considered to be the triad of venous beading, intraretinal microvascular abnormalities and moderately severe retinal

Diabetic retinopathy grade	Lesions specifying grade	Lesions common to diabetic and hypertensive retinopathy	Hypertensive retinopathy grade
Non-proliferative retinopathy without macular involvement 'background'	Microaneurysms, haemorrhages, hard exudates, cotton wool spots (small numbers)	Microaneurysms: unusual in hypertension alone	Grade I: arteriolar narrowing
Non-proliferative retinopathy with macular involvement 'diabetic maculopathy'	Haemorrhages, hard exudates within one disc diameter of the centre of the macula	Haemorrhages: characteristically flame-shaped but can be dots and blots	Grade II: AV nipping
Pre-proliferative retinopathy	Venous irregularity (beading, reduplication, loops), multiple haemorrhages, multiple cotton wool spots, intraretinal microvascular abnormalities	Hard exudates: characteristically spokes around the macula (macular star if complete) rather than circinates	Grade III: haemorrhages, hard exudates,
Proliferative retinopathy	New vessels on the disc (NVD) or new vessels elsewhere (NVE)		Grade IV: papilloedema, haemorrhages, hard exudates
Advanced diabetic retinopathy	Vitreous haemorrhages, fibrous tissue, recent retinal detachment, rubeosis iridis		

Table 8.1
Lesions of diabetic and hypertensive retinopathy: refer proliferative retinopathy urgently for pan-retinal photocoagulation; diabetic maculopathy and pre-proliferative retinopathy need to be seen within a few weeks for consideration of laser photocoagulation.

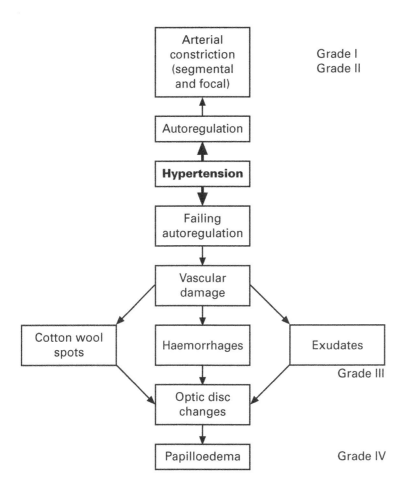

Figure 8.3
Hypertensive retinopathy and autoregulation.

haemorrhages. These lesions must be present in more than one quadrant.

Proliferative diabetic retinopathy and diabetic maculopathy represent the two main forms of sight-threatening diabetic retinopathy. Proliferative diabetic retinopathy can be subdivided into two groups by the position of new vessel formation. New vessel formation located on or within one disc diameter of the optic disc margin is called disc neovascularisation (NVD). Neovascularisation located more than one disc diameter from the optic disc margin is called retinal neovascularisation elsewhere (NVE) (Fig. 8.3). The main sight-threatening sequelae to retinal neovascularization are vitreous haemorrhage (Fig. 8.4) and retinal detachment and retinal fibrosis. Rubeosis iridis (new vessel formation of the iridal and adjacent circulations) is usually concomitant with retinal neovascularization. This is a devastating complication of diabetic eye disease, which apart from causing a painful eye, usually results in blindness of the affected eye.

Diabetic maculopathy, previously classified

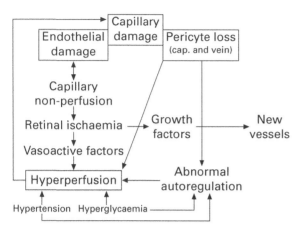

Figure 8.4
A haemodynamic model for the pathogenesis of diabetic retinopathy.

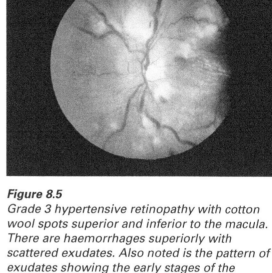

Figure 8.5
Grade 3 hypertensive retinopathy with cotton wool spots superior and inferior to the macula. There are haemorrhages superiorly with scattered exudates. Also noted is the pattern of exudates showing the early stages of the formation of a macular star, indicating macular oedema.

with background diabetic retinopathy merits separate consideration due to its potential for visual impairment and the need for the condition to be identified so that laser photocoagulation treatment can be given if necessary. Diabetic maculopathy, strictly speaking, is the presence of any lesion of diabetic retinopathy at the macula. Laser photocoagulation treatment may be required if 'clinically significant macular oedema' is detected. The latter was defined by the Early Treatment of Diabetic Retinopathy Study Research Group as retinal thickening within 500 μm of the macular centre or hard exudates within 500 μm of the macular centre if associated with thickening of the adjacent retina or retinal thickening at least one disc area in extent partly within one disc diameter of the macular centre.[52] These degrees of maculopathy constitute criteria for grid laser photocoagulation treatment (Figs 8.5–8.10).

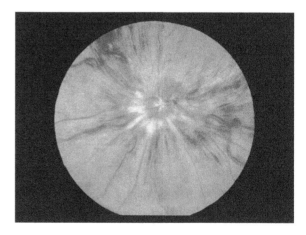

Figure 8.6
Central retinal vein occlusion. Severe haemorrhaging around the optic disc with swelling of the optic disc, the so-called 'blood and thunder' appearance. There are cotton wool spots at the 7 o'clock position at the edge of the field, indicating retinal ischaemia.

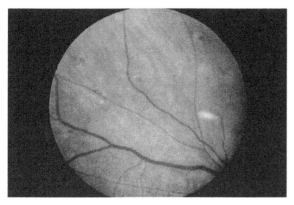

(a)

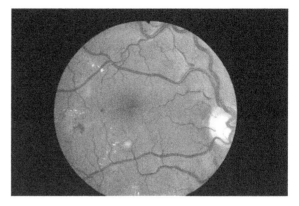

Figure 8.8
Non-proliferative diabetic retinopathy with early macular involvement. Microaneurysms, haemorrhages and hard exudates are evident on this plate. There is a cotton wool spot inferior to the macula. Within the central macular area there are a few hard exudates with a single microaneurysm. Photocoagulation may be indicated if there is significant macular thickening or oedema.

(b)

Figure 8.7
(a) and (b) Hypertensive retinopathy with choroidal infarcts: (a) shows multiple dark lesions – choroidal infarcts due to hypertensive changes in the choroid. A single clearly defined cotton wool spot is seen, which represents an area of focal retinal infarction

Method of examination for diabetic and hypertensive retinopathy

First visual acuity should be measured using a Snellen chart. External examination of the eye will reveals lesions such as xanthelesmata, corneal arcii and lens opacification. The pupils have to be dilated in the majority of patients. Tropicamide 1 per cent is usually sufficient, with black, Asian and other patients with dark irises additionally requiring phenylephrine 10 per cent drops. These are longer acting than tropicamide 1 per cent, but have stronger mydriatic action. Physicians have often been reluctant to use mydriatics for fear of precipitating acute angle glaucoma; this is so rarely encountered that this reason for not dilating a pupil is not tenable in clinical practice for any retinal assessment. Using a direct ophthalmoscope, starting at the optic disc, the superior and inferior temporal arcades should be examined. The macular area should be examined next, then moving onto the nasal arcades. Finally the periphery of the retina should be examined with particular attention to proliferative diabetic retinopathy and the presence of

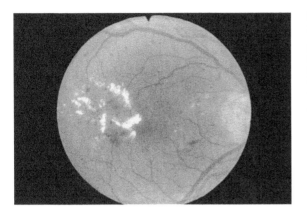

Figure 8.9
Diabetic maculopathy. There is extensive hard exudate formation adjacent to the macular area with multiple haemorrhages and microaneurysms. Focal laser photocoagulation will be required.

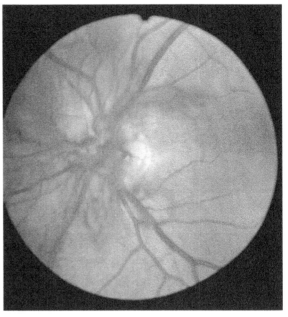

Figure 8.10
Proliferative diabetic retinopathy. New vessels emanating from the optic disc. These are spreading along the vascular arcades into all four quadrants. The normal retinal vessels are sharply focused, whilst the proliferative vessels are not. This is because the latter are growing forward into the vitreous away from the plane of the retina.

laser photocoagulation scars. The grade of diabetes and hypertension should be determined. Diabetic maculopathy with oedema is very difficult to appreciate without stereopsis such as can be obtained with indirect ophthalmoscopy or slit lamp examination with a suitable lens. Retinal oedema is often seen around exudates and is inferred if there is a darker hue to the retina around the exudates than elsewhere.

If facilities exist, slit lamp applanation tonometry should be done to measure the intraocular pressure, especially as it is an important determinant of the retinal perfusion pressure. Retinal photography is useful in clinical practice in selected cases and essential in research. Colour slide film or digital imaging are usually best for permanent records. If vessel diameter measurement is to be undertaken then it is advisable to take monochromatic fundus photographs with a red-free filter (around 530 nm). This allows maximal differentiation of the blood cell column from the vessel wall. Retinal photographs should be taken such as to ensure that most of the clinically relevant areas are photographed. As most of the lesions of diabetic and hypertensive retinopathy are around the optic disc and clinically of greatest relevance if the macula is affected, the following fields will suffice for most purposes.

1. A field centred on the optic disc.
2. A field centred on the macula

Fluorescein angiography is a useful additional investigation especially in research and to delineate microaneurysms, retinal leakage and areas of capillary non-perfusion.

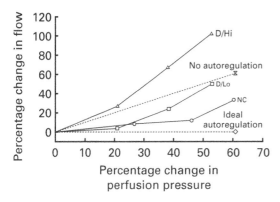

Figure 8.11
Percentage change in flow versus percentage change in perfusion pressure. NC, non-diabetic controls; D/Lo, diabetic subjects with low blood glucose; D/Hi, diabetic subjects with high blood glucose.

The lesions of diabetic retinopathy and hypertensive retinopathy

Both the colour photography and fluorescein appearances of non-diabetic hypertensive retinopathy and normotensive background diabetic retinopathy are often indistinguishable. The lesions of cotton wool spots, haemorrhages and cotton wool spots occur in diabetes at normotension because of abnormal autoregulation. It is then easy to envisage that progressive damage to retinal capillaries in diabetes leads to maculopathy, and with increasing retinal ischaemia to neovascularisation. A brief review of the lesions of diabetic retinopathy and hypertension is given, particularly to illustrate the similar pathophysiological events in the two conditions. Diabetic retinopathy should always be examined with hypertensive retinopathy in mind to allow early diagnosis and treatment of hypertension.

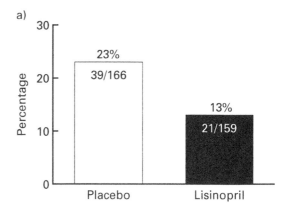

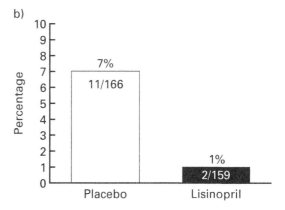

Figure 8.12
(a) Progression of retinopathy by at least one level; OR = 0.50 (0.28, 0.89), P = 0.02, reduction by 50 per cent.
(b) Progression to proliferative retinopathy; OR = 0.18 (0.04, 0.82), P = 0.03, reduction by 72 per cent.

The lesions of hypertensive retinopathy can be divided into those associated with the phase of autoregulation to the prevailing hypertension and those related to failed autoregulation (Fig. 8.3).

Arteriolar change and failure of autoregulation

The retinal arteries constrict to prevent increased retinal blood flow and subsequent damage to the retinal microcirculation. It is the intrinsic myogenicity of the arterial smooth muscle cells that is responsible for this protective response and is often referred to as the Bayliss response (Fig. 8.3). The normal ratio of the arterial to venous diameter is ≤3:4, less than this is arteriolar constriction. In experimental hypertension, a rapid rise in blood pressure resulted in arteriolar constriction, but with time the precapillary arterioles became occluded as vascular cells necrosed with increasing shear stress.[47] In the same study with a further increase in hypertension and failing autoregulation there was vascular dilatation and changes such as cotton wool spots, hard exudates and haemorrhages were observed. Focal degeneration of pericytes in experimental hypertension has been reported.[48] Retinal ischaemia heralds the lesions of hypertensive retinopathy consequent to a breakdown of the blood retinal barrier and failing autoregulation: retinal oedema, cotton wool spots and haemorrhages.

Arteriovenous crossing changes

At an arteriovenous crossing there is a common adventitial and glial sheath for the artery and vein. Arteriosclerosis and organisation of the common adventitial sheath leads to compression of the retinal vein. Various grades of arteriovenous crossing changes (AVC) have been described. In grade I AVC there is mild compression of the vein appreciated only as a reduction in venous red cell column visibility on either side of the artery. In grade II AVC there is a moderate degree of compression of the vein with tapering or nipping of the venous blood column (Gunn's sign). If the vein is above the artery then there is 'humping' of the vein anteriorly. In grade III AVC there is marked compression of the vein with a clear space on either side of the artery with no visible venous blood column traversing under the artery. Distal dilatation of the vein is often present. The course of the vein under the artery is sometimes displaced such that the vein is at right angles to the artery, this is expected if a low pressure vessel crosses one with a non-compliant wall under tension (Salus's sign). Grade IV AVC is traditionally not described, but a case can be made to call it the presence of complete or near complete obstruction of retinal vein flow resulting in a branch vein occlusion.

Exudative retinopathy

Retinal exudates appear as yellowish white deposits that vary in size from bare visualisation with the ophthalmoscope to larger confluent areas of exudation covering most of a retinal quadrant. Histologically there is an accumulation of free lipid material with lipid-containing retinal macrophages (microglia). Retinal leakage of plasma and other blood components only becomes marked when autoregulation breaks down. The vision of the patient may be reduced if there is exudation and oedema in the macular area. Prolonged macular exudation leads to the formation of a macular star and oedema. Early treatment of the hypertension at this stage leads to complete resolution of this lesion and any visual impairment, unless focal degenerative changes have occurred such as severe serious macular oedema in association with retinal detachment. In diabetic retinopathy the exudates can often be resolved into circinate rings, in the centre of which are leaking microaneurysms.

Haemorrhages

Haemorrhages are common to diabetes and

hypertensive retinopathy. The superficial haemorrhages are really part of the exudative phase and represent leakage of whole blood components through a disrupted blood retinal barrier. The blood presents as flame-shaped or splinter haemorrhages as they streak along the superficial nerve fibre layer. With the progression of severity of hypertension 'blot' haemorrhages are often seen. These are larger rounder blot-like lesions of the deeper layers of the retina where the extravasated blood has been able to diffuse around the intraretinal cells. Blot haemorrhages are secondary to retinal vascular occlusion and indicate advancing ischaemia of the retina. Haemorrhages can cause visual loss that is appreciated as localised scotoma if large or as more severe visual impairment if the haemorrhage is over the macula. Haemorrhage formation ceases when hypertension is effectively controlled, with their subsequent clearance over a period of 2–8 weeks. These are no visual sequelae unless the haemorrhage accompanies other complications such as retinal vein occlusion, when the sequelae of this condition, macular oedema and new vessel formation can occur. The latter can bleed extensively with retinal fibrous tissue formation leading to traction retinal detachment and blindness.

Cotton wool spots

The areas of endothelial and pericyte damage in the capillaries of the retinal circulation lead to areas of capillary dropout. Cotton wool spots representing areas of focal retinal ischaemia appear as dark areas of nonperfusion on fluorescein angiography surrounded by dilated capillaries. On direct ophthalmoscopy they appear as blurred greyish white areas with feathery blurred edges located superficially in the retina. Cotton wool spots are thought to be superficial nerve fibres with hypoxic damage resulting in accumula-

tions of orthograde and retrograde axoplasmic debris.[53] These axoplasmic accumulations in the distal and proximal ends of interrupted axons are due to deterioration of the normal capillary perfusion and oxygen delivery. With effective management of the hypertension, the cotton wool spots develop a yellowish granular appearance and eventually become almost indistinguishable from the normal surrounding retina.

Studies in experimental hypertension in rhesus monkeys have shown that cotton wool spots are areas of focal retinal capillary nonperfusion caused by occlusion of terminal retinal aterioles.[54] On fluorescein angiography there is obliteration of the majority of the capillaries with dilatation of some with abnormal intraretinal vascularisation (intraretinal microvascular abnormalities or IRMA). IRMAs are characteristic lesions of preproliferative diabetic retinopathy.

Microaneurysms

In hypertensive retinopathy microaneurysms are often seen around cotton wool spots; they are often noted in the normal retinal circulation as well. As the microaneurysm is usually the diameter of a small retinal vessel (around 12–50 mm) they are often missed on ophthalmological assessment. The fluorescein angiogram is particularly good for visualising patent microaneurysms. Thrombosis can occur, then they will not be apparent on the fluorescein angiogram. They are though to be a consequence of localised capillary weakness leading to localised dilatation. A consequence of the Laplace pressure–curvature relationship is that dilatation will progress with time and particularly if the perfusion pressure is increased leading to the formation of an aneurysm. Larger aneurysms or macroaneurysms are rare but striking, especially on fluorescein angiography. These are analogous to the Charcot Bouchard aneurysms that occur in the cerebral circulation, the disruption of which can result in cerebrovascular accidents.

Papilloedema

In clinical practice papilloedema usually refers to the appearance of the optic nerve head in conditions where there is raised intra-cranial pressure. It is therefore a misnomer when used to describe hypertensive optic disc oedema. True papilloedema can occur as a very late manifestation of hypertension if there is total failure of cerebral autoregulation with the presence of cerebral oedema, cerebral haemorrhages and subsequent elevation of intracranial pressure (hypertensive encephalopathy). The pathogenesis of papilloedema was studied in baboons made hypertensive by a modified Goldblatt procedure.[48] Initially there was blurring of the optic disc. Ischaemia of the optic disc head follows on from the early oedema, in part due to relative occlusion of the arterial supply. This study demonstrated that there was a delay in the transport and metabolism of axoplasmic components using tritiated-leucine autoradiography transport studies. The swelling of the optic nerve head is therefore similar in origin to cotton wool spots and not due to raised intra-cranial pressure. Haemorrhages often accompany the oedema of the optic disc head, making the appearance indistinguishable from true papilloedema.

Retinal vein occlusion

The association with hypertension is such that it may be considered to be a complication of hypertensive retinopathy. Systemic hypertension and diabetes have been found to be the single most important risk factor for central and branch retinal vein occlusion. There can be occlusion of the central retinal vein itself or of a branch of retinal vein. The site of retinal branch vein occlusion is often an arteriove-nous crossing that has resulted in complete occlusion of the normal retinal venous flow. The central retinal vein and central retinal artery travel together along the optic nerve in a single fascial sheath and it is thought that arteriosclerosis of the artery predisposes the vein to occlusion. Initially in the area of the vein occlusion there is haemorrhage, dilatation of the veins, retinal oedema and later cotton wool spots. Central retinal vein occlusion leads to severely impaired vision and even blindness, which is irreversible. In a branch retinal vein occlusion the relative hypoxia of the retina is a potent stimulus for neovascularisation to occur, as in diabetic retinopathy.

Pathogenic mechanisms in diabetic retinopathy

The earliest changes in the diabetic retinal circulation consist of thickening of the capillary basement membrane and loss of retinal pericytes.[55] Later there is increased retinal vessel permeability, which may advance to diabetic maculopathy and retinal neovascularisation (proliferative diabetic retinopathy) as a response to increasing retinal ischaemia. The exact causes of the early and late anatomical lesions of diabetic retinopathy are still far from clear and await further research and elucidation. In broad terms the mechanisms invoked in its pathogenesis can be divided into three main categories: biochemical, endocrine and haemodynamic.

Biochemical hypotheses

Hyperglycaemia leads to an increased uptake of glucose into the retinal pericytes and may cause cellular damage through two main biochemical consequences. First, there is activation of the polyol pathway leading to the accumulation of sorbitol in pericytes.[56] In normoglycaemic conditions the activity of the polyol pathway is very low, its normal function being to clear excess hexoses by converting them to hexose alcohols. In this pathway glucose and galactose, for example, are converted by the enzyme aldose reductase into sorbitol and galactitol respectively. The alcohols accumulate in cells and adversely affect cell metabolism. However, a large study of human diabetic subjects with early diabetic retinopathy, the Sorbinil Retinopathy Trial Research Group, found that there was no benefit from treatment with the aldose reductase inhibition over a 3-year period.[57] Similar negative results were reported using Ponalrestat, another aldose reductase inhibitor.[58]

The second main type of biochemical alteration implicated in the pathogenesis of diabetic retinopathy is formation of advanced glycation end-products (AGEs). The initial step is the condensation of glucose and the e-amino terminal of lysine residues of any protein. This leads to the formation of the unstable Schiff base which undergoes further reaction to form the stable Amadori product. The function of glycated proteins may be altered, particularly for example, in an enzyme that has lysine in its active site.[59] The Amadori products are capable of linking together such that complex cross-linking of proteins occurs at the lysine residues.[60] This is thought to be an important mechanism in the thickening of basement membranes in diabetes. An additional factor is that glycated proteins are less susceptible to proteolysis with a subsequent reduction in their turnover in the basement membrane.[61] Elevated glucose levels have been found to have a direct toxic effect on retinal pericytes in culture.[62] The responsiveness of retinal pericytes to endothelin 1 is reduced by hyperglycaemia.[63]

Endocrine factors

In 1953 Poulsen observed that a post-partum haemorrhage, resulting in infarction of the pituitary gland, was associated with regression of severe diabetic retinopathy. Interestingly diabetic retinopathy has been found to be absent in diabetic patients with growth hormone-deficient dwarfism.[64] Insulin-like growth factor 1(IGF-1) is secreted locally in most tissues under the control of pituitary growth hormone and it mediates most of the cellular actions of growth hormone. Diabetic patients with accelerating neovascularisation have elevated serum IGF-1 levels in comparison with diabetic subjects without retinopathy and non-diabetic control subjects.[65] Increased concentrations of IGF-I were also found in diabetic subjects with severe retinopathy, but this may reflect a breakdown in the blood–retinal barrier.[66] Recently inhibition of growth hormone secretion with a somatostatin analogue has been used to treat severe proliferative diabetic retinopathy in a small study, albeit with limited success.[67] High doses of octreotide, a somatostatin analogue, inhibit growth hormone secretion, but failed to have any significant effect on severe proliferative diabetic retinopathy in studies by other workers.[68] Since the original observation that vitreous fluid from diabetic subjects with neovascularisation stimulates bovine retinal vessel cells, many other growth factors have been implicated in the retinal cell proliferation.[69] The list includes acidic and basic fibroblast growth factor, vascular endothelial growth factor, transforming growth factor β and platelet-derived growth factor.

Haemodynamic alterations

It will be clear from the above discussion that there can be no single factor that is responsible for the development of diabetic retinopathy.

Factor	Effect on retinal blood flow	Comment
Hypertension	Increase	Aim <140/80 Aim pulse pressure <60 mmHg
Glycaemic control	Increase	Type 1 aim HbA1c% <7.0% Type 2 aim HbA1c% <7.0%
Duration of diabetes	Increase	
Pregnancy	Increase	Screen in each trimester of pregnancy
Hypercholesterolaemia	Unknown	Correct dyslipidaemia (according to local targets)
Smoking	Decrease? promotes critical ischaemia	Advise against for CHD risk alone
Alcohol	No change	Standard advice re alcohol consumption

Table 8.2
Clinical risk factors for diabetic retinopathy and effect on retinal blood flow.

Initial changes are likely to be specific biochemical changes related to an abnormally high glucose level. The retinal vessels are then subject to haemodynamic insults, the end result of which is retinal ischaemia. Retinal ischaemia leads to retinal oedema which presents as diabetic maculopathy. Various autocrine and endocrine factors then orchestrate in an attempt to alleviate the retinal ischaemia. The new vessels that are formed have an aberrant branching pattern and do not correct the retinal hypoxia. The sequel, proliferative diabetic retinopathy, can have devastating consequences for vision. The haemodynamic alteration in the diabetic and hypertensive retinal circulation will be examined in more detail.

A haemodynamic model for the pathogenesis of diabetic retinopathy: clinical and experimental studies

Retinal blood flow studies

Studies using the mean circulation time of fluorescein suggested increased retinal blood flow in diabetic retinopathy.[70] In another study using laser Doppler velocimetry and computerised retinal image analysis, retinal blood flow was found to be elevated in diabetic retinopathy.[71] This study showed hyperfusion in the diabetic retinal circulation in all groups with untreated diabetic retinopathy in comparison with non-diabetic controls and diabetic patients with no retinopathy. In comparison to diabetic subjects with no retinopathy, retinal blood flow was higher by 33.2 per cent in background, 69.4 per cent in pre-proliferative and 50.1 per cent in proliferative diabetic retinopathy. This was thought to represent failure of autoregulation even when the systolic and diastolic blood pressure are well within the limits defined for treatment of hypertension in diabetes. A haemodynamic model for the pathogenesis of diabetic retinopathy along the lines of the Brenner model for the pathogenesis of diabetic nephropathy and the Tooke model for diabetic microangiopathy was proposed (Fig. 8.4).[3,72] Clinical risk factors for the progression of diabetic retinopathy and their effect on retinal blood flow are shown in Table 8.2. Central to the retinopathy model is the observation that the earliest changes in diabetic retinopathy are thickening of the basement membrane and pericyte loss. Pericytes are very important in the regulation of blood flow, as they possess contractile properties, allowing changes in the vessel lumen to regulate blood flow.[55] At the capillary level in diabetes there is increased blood viscosity, decreased red cell deformability and increased platelet aggregation. Hyperfusion and capillary shear stress damage lead to decreased capillary blood flow and even thrombosis in the smallest vessels of the retinal circulation. It is worth noting that aspirin and ticlopidine both reduce the rate of microaneurysm formation in early retinopathy. This could be attributed to the platelet inhibitory anti-thrombotic effect of these drugs.[73,74]

The overall effect of basement membrane thickening, decreased capillary perfusion and the biochemical effects of hyperglycaemia is capillary closure. The resultant retinal ischaemia is a potent stimulus for an increase in retinal blood flow, indeed dilated capillaries in areas adjacent to capillary dropout are often seen on fluorescein angiography. It is generally accepted that retinal ischaemia leading to the production of angiogenic and vasoproliferative factors is the main stimulus for new vessel formation.[75]

Increased flow, increased viscosity and capillary closure – all of which occur in diabetes – tend to increase shear stress. Injury to the endothelium of a vessel can result from an increase in shear stress alone.[41] It has been postulated that increased glycation and thickening of the basement membrane results in 'locking' of the vessel.[72] This would tend to increase shear stress because the vessel diameter is unable to change. Hyperperfusion is also associated with increased capillary pressure, as the systemic blood pressure is more easily transmitted to the microcirculation in the presence of dilated vasculature.

The most important factors that lead to hyperperfusion in the diabetic retinal circulation are proposed to be hypertension and hyperglycaemia. The role of these two factors in promoting an abnormal haemodynamic milieu is examined below.

Retinal autoregulation to experimental hypertension in diabetic and control subjects

The effect of hypertension in retinal blood flow was studied in normal controls and diabetic subjects under conditions of normoglycaemia and hyperglycaemia.[43] Experimental hypertension was created using a continuous infusion of tyramine, a potent presynaptic reuptake inhibitor and releaser of nordrenaline. In non-diabetic subjects the retinal blood flow remained constant at a 15 per cent and 30 per cent increase in the systemic mean arterial blood pressure (MAP). Failure of autoregulation occurred at a 40 per cent increase in MAP in non-diabetic subjects with a 32.9 per cent increase in retinal blood flow. In normoglycaemic diabetic subjects retinal blood was autoregulated until a 30 per cent increase in MAP with a 49.9 per cent increase in retinal blood flow at 40 per cent increase in MAP. In contrast, in diabetic subjects under conditions

	Coefficient of autoregulation (Φ)		
	15%	30%	40%
Non-diabetic controls	0.76 (0.25–1.00)	0.91 (0.18–1.00)	0.38 (0.13–0.62)
Diabetes low glucose	1.00 (0.0–1.00)	0.53 (0.0–0.82)	0.10 (0.0–0.47)
Diabetes high glucose	0.05 (0.0–0.88)	0.08 0.0–0.22)	0.00 0.0–0.19

Table 8.3

Coefficient of autoregulation values at the MAP increases; results are expressed as the median and the interquartile range. 1.00 = ideal autoregulation; 0.00 = autoregulation.

of hyperglycaemia, there was failure of autoregulation at all levels of increase in MAP studied; 15 per cent MAP retinal blood flow increase 27.0 per cent, 30 per cent MAP retinal blood flow increase 66.9 per cent and 40 per cent MAP retinal blood flow increase 101.9 per cent.

A graph has been plotted with the percentage change in perfusion pressure along the x-axis and the percentage change in retinal blood flow along the y-axis for the groups studied (Fig. 8.11). The expected curves for ideal autoregulation and no autoregulation, as would occur if the retinal circulation behaved as a rigid tube and in accordance with Poiseuille's Law, are plotted for comparison. This graph suggests that the retinal circulation is not autoregulated at all in the presence of hyperglycaemia, with the system behaving according to Poisseuille's Law until a 20 per cent increase in perfusion pressure. Thereafter there is total failure of autoregulation. This point occurs at a 55 per cent increase in perfusion pressure in the normoglycaemic diabetic subjects and at around 70 per cent in the non-diabetic control subjects (if the curve was

extrapolated). The table of the coefficients of autoregulation shows autoregulation breaking down earlier in diabetic subjects than non-diabetic subjects with further impairment with hyperglycaemia (Table 8.3). This was the first application of the Coefficient of Autoregulation in the human circulation.

The mechanism whereby hyperglycaemia promotes abnormal retinal vascular autoregulation is unclear. Previously a 25 per cent increase in retinal volume blood flow was found during glucose infusion in normal cats using high speed cine fluorescence angiography.[76] Hyperglycaemia has been thought to lead to increased retinal lactic acid production, which acts as a stimulus to increase retinal blood flow through its vasodilatory action.[77] Another mechanism has been proposed whereby hyperglycaemia leads to increased blood flow.[78] Central to the explanation is that hyperglycaemia leads to an increase in the cytoplasmic ratio of free NADH to NAD^+. This is due to excess intracellular glucose being shunted through the sorbitol pathway, where the oxidation of sorbitol to fructose is coupled to the reduction of NAD^+ to

NADH. This process is particularly active in the retina as the influx of glucose into the cells of the central nervous system is proportional to the plasma concentration of glucose. The same redox imbalance, that of an increased $NADH/NAD^+$, is induced by hypoxia and transient ischaemia. This process has been given the elegant epithet 'hyperglycaemic-pseudohypoxia' by J.R. Williamson, the senior author of the above study. Elevated blood glucose levels in retinal pericytes have been found to induce resistance to contraction in response to endothelin-1.[63]

The above studies show that hypertension and hyperglycaemia act both as individual factors in promoting abnormal autoregulation with a marked effect when the two factors are present together.

The effect of hypertension and hyperglycaemia on retinal vascular reactivity

Retinal vascular reactivity to breathing an elevated oxygen concentration is a convenient method of assessing the degree of retinal vascular autoregulation to a metabolic stimulus. The normal response to hyperoxia is vasoconstriction, reducing retinal blood flow by 40 per cent. The specific effect of hyperglycaemia and hypertension on retinal vascular reactivity to hyperoxia was studied. Diabetic and non-diabetic subjects, with and without hypertension, were studied in order to test the hypothesis that hyperglycaemia and hypertension act individually and in concert to impair retinal vascular autoregulation.[79] Retinal blood flow itself was found to be higher in diabetic subjects in comparison to non-diabetic subjects.

The specific effect of a high blood glucose level was apparent from the result that oxygen reactivity was reduced to 21.7 per cent in normotensive diabetic subjects at a high blood glucose which improved to 32.1 per cent when the blood glucose level was normalised. The results in the hypertensive diabetic subjects were similar.

The conclusion was that retinal vascular reactivity was impaired in diabetic subjects both when they are normotensive and hypertensive in comparison to non-diabetic control subjects. Hyperglycaemia impairs retinal vascular reactivity even further. The hypothesis that hypertension and hyperglycaemia impair retinal vascular autoregulation has therefore been given further evidence.

Effect of ACE inhibitors

ACE inhibitors have specific beneficial effects in hypertensive diabetic patients with respect to the incidence and progression of diabetic nephropathy. The effect of ACE inhibitors on the diabetic retinal circulation has not been studied extensively. The effect of ACE inhibition and beta-blockade in retinal blood flow was studied in a group of 45 hypertensive diabetic subjects (both type I and II) using a randomised double-masked trial over a period of 12 months. Laser Doppler velocimetry and computerised image analysis were used to measure retinal blood flow.[80] The changes in blood pressure over 12 months were comparable. Retinal blood flow appeared to decrease in the perindopril group and increased with atenolol. Comparisons of the percentage changes in RBF (perindopril decrease of 7.2 per cent, atenolol increase of 15.3 per cent) were significant. There was an increase in RBF in 33.3 per cent of the subjects receiving perindopril and 70.6 per cent of those receiving atenolol.

This suggests that ACE inhibitor therapy may promote a haemodynamic milieu in the hypertensive diabetic retinal circulation that

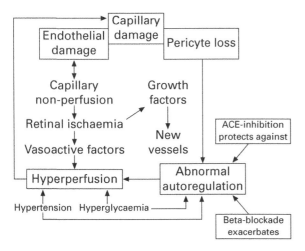

Figure 8.13
Hemodynamic model of the pathogenesis of diabetic retinopathy: effect of ACE inhibition and β-blockade.

serves to protect against the progression of diabetic retinopathy, whilst beta-blockade has the opposite effect (Fig. 8.13).

The above study may have provided a haemodynamic explanation of the results of the EUCLID Study (EURODIAB Controlled Trial of Lisinopril in Insulin-Dependent Diabetes Mellitus).[5] This was a large (n = 325), multicentre randomised double-masked placebo-controlled trial in type I normotensive diabetic subjects. Diabetic retinopathy progression was measured by a five-level scale (none, minimal non-proliferative, moderate non-proliferative, severe non-proliferative and post-laser photocoagulation or proliferative). Diabetic retinopathy progressed by at least one level was significantly reduced by lisinopril. There was progression in 13.2 per cent of the lisinopril subjects (21 of 159) and 23.4 per cent of the placebo subjects (39 of 166). Lisinopril also decreased progression by two or more grades by 73 per cent. Most significant was the finding that ACE inhibition

reduced progression to proliferative diabetic retinopathy by 72 per cent, although the number of subjects affected was small (lisinopril 2 of 159 progressed to proliferative retinopathy, placebo 11 of 166) (Figs 8.12a and 8.12b). These data suggest that 19 normotensive type I diabetic patients need to be treated with lisinopril 10 mg daily for 2 years to prevent one case of proliferative diabetic retinopathy.

The most important and well-characterised effect of ACE inhibitors is reduction in blood pressure. This is mediated via the inhibition of angiotensin-converting enzyme, thereby reducing the activity of angiotensin-II, a potent octapeptide vasoconstrictor. ACE inhibitors inhibit the breakdown of the vasodilator bradykinin and increase the formation of nitric oxide and prostacyclin. All these factors potentiate vasodilatation with additional antiplatelet action of nitric oxide and prostacyclin. ACE activity is particularly marked in the endothelium of the pulmonary vasculature, but now all the components of the renin-angiotensin system have been described in many other vascular beds including the coronary, brain, kidneys and testes. In diabetic subjects with retinopathy the plasma renin activity is elevated in comparison to both non-diabetic control subjects and diabetic subjects without retinopathy.[81] In a prospective study raised plasma prorenin levels predicted progression to microalbuminuria and retinopathy in a group of 196 type I diabetes patients.[82] Specific angiotensin-II receptors on human retinal vessels have been demonstrated.[83] A possible relationship between the impairment of the renin-angiotensin system and the pathogenesis of diabetic retinopathy may therefore be inferred. The role of angiotensin-II in neovascularisation remains unsubstantiated, but experimental evidence from the rabbit corneal pocket model has shown this substance to be a potent stimulator of neovascularisation.[84]

Evidence from the above studies suggests that there may be a role for the renin-angiotensin system in the retina in autoregulation and progression of diabetic retinopathy (Fig. 8.13).[85] The renin-angiotensin system may be particularly important in the retinal circulation as adrenergic innervation is lacking and therefore the most important components of the blood flow regulation would be the renin-angiotensin system, and the intrinsic myogenicity of the retinal vessels. The vascular effects of ACE inhibitors, particularly perindopril, have been studied in detail. Several studies have shown a decrease in the pulse wave velocity with ACE inhibition more and above other antihypertensive agents. Perindopril has also been shown to remodel the abnormal hypertensive vascular media/lumen ratio towards normal improving vessel compliance and blood flow regulatory ability.[86] Another effect of ACE inhibitors is to increase the capillary density at the tissue level, which may be particularly important as there is rarefaction of the human retinal circulation in hypertension. The improved capillary level haemodynamics would serve to reduce the ischaemic drive, resulting in retinal vascular hyperperfusion.

The pro-angiogenic actions of angiotensin II appear to be mediated via the AT_1 receptor and may depend on angiotensin II-induced expression of a potent angiogenic peptide; vascular endothelial growth factor (VEGF).[87–89] Levels of VEGF have been shown to be increased in the ocular fluid of human eyes with evidence of neovascularisation.[90] Moreover, in addition to angiotensin II, VEGF production is also upregulated by elevated extracellular glucose concentrations.[91] These observations prompt the hypothesis that specific angiotensin II receptor blockade may also be an effective means of limiting the development and progression of nephropathy. This hypothesis is currently being evaluated by the DIRECT study.[92]

Diabetic retinopathy and hypertension: a conclusion

Future research

Future research should be targeted towards preventing an abnormal haemodynamic milieu in the diabetic retinal circulation. Apart from the main studies cited above, the effects of the commonly used antihypertensive agents on retinal haemodynamics and autoregulation have not been determined to date. The panoply of agents used to treat hypertension in diabetes have widely differing modes of pharmacological action; ACE inhibition, diuretic, calcium channel antagonism, β-blockade, α-blockade, angiotensin II receptor antagonism, centrally acting imidazole re-uptake inhibitors, for example. Important differences may exist with agents conferring a beneficial or even detrimental effect with respect to retinal haemodynamics when used in the treatment of the hypertensive diabetic patient.

Latest trial evidence and concluding remarks

Two trials have recently addressed the impact of blood pressure control on retinopathy in patients with type 2 diabetes; the UKPDS and ABCD.

UKPDS

This large prospective randomised clinical trial included a large cohort (1,544) of patients who were hypertensive with a mean age of 56 years.[6] Of these, 1,148 were recruited into the 'hypertension in Diabetes study', embedded within the *UKPDS*.[6] The 1,148 hypertensive patients with type 2 diabetes were randomised to 'less tight' (<180/105 mmHg)(n = 390) or 'tight' (<150/85 mmHg)(n = 758) blood pressure control. The achieved difference in blood pressure control between the less tight and tight control groups was 10/5 mmHg over a median follow-up of 8.4 years.

Microvascular end-points were reduced by 37% in the group with tighter blood pressure control, largely due to a reduction in the risk of retinal photocoagulation and progressive retinopathy. There was an associated 47% reduced risk of deterioration of visual acuity. The impact of tighter blood pressure control on microvascular end-points was more than twice as great as that achieved by tight glycaemic control in the same study (see Chapter 17). This study confirmed that even modest reduction in blood pressure within the hypertensive range have a dramatic beneficial effect on retinopathy, supporting the 'haemodynamic hypothesis'.

ABCD study

The ABCD study was conducted in the USA and was a prospective randomised clinical trial designed to test the primary hypothesis that intensive versus moderate blood pressure control would prevent or slow the progression of nephropathy, neuropathy and retinopathy (i.e. microvascular complications) in people with type 2 diabetes, aged 40–74 years. The secondary hypothesis was that a long-acting CCB (nisoldipine Coat Core)-based therapy and an ACE-inhibitor-based therapy (Enalapril) would have equivalent effects on the prevention or progression of these diabetic complications. A total of 950 type 2 diabetic patients were randomised as two distinct cohorts; normotensive, (n = 480) and hypertensive (n = 470) (see Chapter 17).[93]

ABCD hypertensive cohort – impact of intensive versus moderate blood pressure control on retinopathy

The hypertensive cohort were randomised to achieve a diastolic blood pressure target of <75 mmHg (intensive group) or 80–90 mmHg (moderate group).[94] The mean blood pressures achieved in the intensive group was 132/78 mmHg and in the moderate group was 138/86 mmHg over a 5-year follow-up. Moreover, over the 5-year follow-up, there was no difference between the intensive and moderate blood pressure control groups with regard to the progression of retinopathy. Moreover, these results were similar irrespective of whether an ACE-inhibitor of CCB was used as the initial medication.

ABCD normotensive cohort – impact of intensive versus moderate blood pressure control on retinopathy

This cohort within ABCD examined whether lowering blood pressure in 'normotensive' type 2 diabetics (blood pressure <140/90 mmHg) offers any additional benefit with regard to microvascular complications.[6] The 480 normotensive type 2 diabetic patients were randomised to 'intensive' (10 mmHg below baseline diastolic blood pressure) versus 'moderate' blood pressure (diastolic blood pressure 80–90 mmHg). Patients randomised to moderate therapy were given placebo therapy, whereas those randomised to intensive therapy were randomised to either enalapril or nisoldipine. The mean follow up was 5.3 years and the mean blood pressure in the intensive group was 128/75 mmHg and in the moderate group was 137/81 mmHg. The more intensively treated group had significantly less progression of diabetic retinopathy at 2 years (13% versus 21%, $P < 0.046$) and after 5 years of follow-up (34% versus 46% $P < 0.019$). The number of patients developing new retinopathy after 5 years from no retinopathy at baseline was 39% in the intensive group and 42% in the moderate group. With regard to the development of proliferative retinopathy, 0% in the intensive group versus 3.9% in the moderate group. These conclusions apply whether the patients were treated with nisoldipine or enapalapril. This study shows that lowering blood pressure, even within the normotensive range has a marked effect of the development of nephropathy supporting the concept of impaired retinal autoregulation and demonstrating the importance of tight blood pressure control, well below the values often achieved in patients. This conclusion is consistent with a large study which showed that any form of diabetic retinopathy was significantly increased if systolic blood pressure was 132 mmHg when compared to 124 mmHg.[95]

Concluding remarks

The UKPDS and ABCD studies suggest that lowering blood pressure over a wide range, dropping well into the conventional 'normotensive range', is very effective in preventing and delaying the progression of retinopathy in type 2 diabetes. Moreover, blood pressure lowering per se appears to be more important than the drugs used to achieve it. Mindful of these observations, it would seem reasonable to support recent recommendations for a target blood pressure of <130/80 mmHg in an endeavour to prevent or delay progression of diabetic retinopathy.[96]

Acknowledgements

The authors acknowledge the help of Yolanda Warren and Kamini Ganapathi in the preparation of the manuscript.

References

1. Evans J, Rooney C, Ashwood F, Dattani N, Wormald R. Blindness and partial sight in England and Wales: April 1990, March 1991. *Health Trends* 1996; **28**: 1:5–12.

2. Moss SE, Klein R, Klein BEK. The incidence of vision loss in a diabetic population. *Ophthalmology* 1988; **95**: 1340–8.

3. Brenner BM, Meyer TW, Hostetter TH. Dietary protein intake and the progressive nature of kidney disease: the role of haemodynamically mediated glomerular injury in the pathogenesis of progressive glomerular sclerosis in ageing, renal ablation, and intrinsic renal disease. *N Engl J Med* 1982; **307**: 652–9.

4. Parving HH, Viberti GC, Keen H, Christiansen JS, Lassen NA. Haemodynamic factors in the genesis of diabetic microangiopathy. *Metabolism* 1983; **32**: 943–9.

5. Chaturvedi N, Sjolie A, Stephenson JM, et al., and the Euclid Study Group. Effect of lisinopril on prgression of retinopathy in normotensive people with type 1 diabetes. *Lancet* 1998; **351**: 28–31.

6. United Kingdom Prospective Diabetes Study Group. Tight blood pressure control and risk of macrovascular and microvascular complications in type 2 diabetes: UKPDS 38. *BMJ* 1998; **317**: 703–13

7. Schrier RW, Estacio RO, Esler A, Mehler P. Effects of aggressive blood pressure control in normotensive type 2 diabetic patients on albuminuria, retinopathy and strokes. *Kidney Int* 2002; **61**: 1086–97.

8. Klein R, Klein BEK, Moss SE, Davis MD, DeMets DL. The Wisconsin Epidemiologic Study of Diabetic Retinopathy: (II) Prevalence and risk of diabetic retinopathy when age at diagnosis is less than 30 years. *Arch Ophthalmol* 1984; **102**: 520–6.

9. Klein R, Klein BEK, Moss SE, Davis MD, DeMets DL. The Wisconsin Epidemiologic Study of Diabetic Retinopathy: (III) Prevalence and risk of diabetic retinopathy when age at diagnosis is 30 years or more. *Arch Ophthalmol* 1984; **102**: 527–32.

10. Klein R, Klein BEK, Moss SE, Davis MD, DeMets DL. The Wisconsin Epidemiologic Study of Diabetic Retinopathy: (IX) Four year incidence and progression of diabetic retinopathy when age at diagnosis is less than 30 years. *Arch Ophthalmol* 1989; **107**: 237–43.

11. Klein R, Klein BEK, Moss SE, Davis MD, DeMets DL. The Wisconsin Epidemiologic Study of Diabetic Retinopathy: (X) Four year incidence and progression of diabetic retinopathy when age at diagnosis is 30 years or more. *Arch Ophthalmol* 1989; **107**: 244–9.

12. Klein R, Moss SE, Klein BEK, Davis MD, DeMets DL. The Wisconsin Epidemiologic Study of Diabetic Retinopathy: (XI) The incidence of macular oedema. *Ophthalmology* 1989; **96**: 1501–10.

13. Janka HU, Warram JH, Rand LI, Krowelski AS. Risk factors for progression of background diabetic retinopathy. *Diabetes* 1989; **38**: 460–4.

14. Chase HP, Garg SK, Jackson WE, et al. Blood pressure and retinopathy in Type 1 diabetes. *Ophthalmology* 1990; **97**: 155–9.

15. Knowler WC, Bennett PH, Ballintine EJ. Increased incidence of retinopathy in diabetics with elevated blood pressure. *N Engl J Med* 1980; **302**: 645–50.

16. Chahal P, Inglesby DV, Sleightholm M, Kohner EM. Blood pressure and the progression of mild background diabetic retinopathy. *Hypertension* 1985; **7**: 1179–83.

17. Klein BE, Klein R, Moss SE, Palta M. A cohort study of the relationship of diabetic retinopathy to blood pressure. *Arch Ophthalmol* 1996; **114**: 109.

18. Patel V. *Diabetic Retinopathy: clinical and haemodynamic factors in the pathogenesis.* Koln, Germany, Verlag Eul 1995.

19. Poulsen PL, Bek T, Ebbehoj E, Hansen KW, Mogensen CE. 24th ambulatory blood pressure and retinopathy in normoalbuminuric

IDDM patients. *Diabetologia* 1988; **41:** 105–10.

20. Segal P, Treister G, Yalon M, Sandak R, Berezin M, Modan M. The prevalence of diabetic retinopathy: effect of sex, age, duration of disease, and mode of therapy. *Diabetes Care* 1983; **6:** 149–51.

21. Kostraba JN, Klein R, Dorman JS, et al. The epidemiology of diabetes complications study. IV. Correlates of background and proliferative retinopathy. *Am J Epidemiol* 1991; **133:** 381–91.

22. KROC Collaborative Study Group. Blood glucose control and the evolution of diabetic retinopathy and albuminuria. *N Engl J Med* 1984; **311:** 365–72.

23. Brinchmann-Hansen O, Dahl-Jorgensen K, Sandvik L, Hanssen KF. Blood glucose concentrations and progression of diabetic retinopathy: the seven year results of the Oslo Study. *BMJ* 1992; **304:** 19–22.

24. McCance DR, Hadden DR, Atkinson AB, Archer DB, Kennedy L. Long-term glycaemic control and diabetic retinopathy. *Lancet* 1989; **ii:** 824–8.

25. Klein R, Klein BE, Moss SE, Davis MD, DeMets DL. Glycosylated hemoglobin predicts the incidence and progression of diabetic retinopathy. *JAMA* 1988; **260:** 2864–71.

26. The Diabetes Control and Complications Trial Research Group. The effect of intensive treatment of diabetes on the development and progression of long-term complications in insulin-dependent diabetes mellitus. *N Engl J Med* 1993; **329:** 977–86.

27. Ohkubo Y, Kishikawa H, Araki E, et al. Intensive insulin therapy prevents the progression of diabetic microvascular complications in Japanese patients with non-insulin-dependent diabetes mellitus: a randomised prospective 6-year study. *Diabetes Res Clin Pract* 1995; **28:** 103–17.

28. United Kingdom Prospective Diabetes Study Group. Intensive blood glucose control with sulphonylureas or insulin compared with conventional treatment and risk of complications in patients with type 2 diabetes: UKPDS 33. *Lancet* 1998; **352:** 837–53.

29. Klein BE, Moss SE, Klein R, Surawicz TS. Serum cholesterol in the Wisonsin Epidemiologic Study of Diabetic Retinopathy. *Diabetes Care* 1992; **15:** 282–7.

30. Dodson PM, Gibson JM. Long term follow-up of and underlying medical conditions in patients with diabetic exudative maculopathy. *Eye* 1991; **5:** 699–703.

31. Kofoed-Enevoldsen A, Jensen T, Borch-Johnson K, Deckert T. Incidence of retinopathy in Type 1 (insulin-dependent) diabetes: association with clinical nephropathy. *J Diabetic Complications* 1987; **3:** 96–9.

32. Krolewski AS, Barzilay J, Warram JH, Martin BC, Pfeifer M, Rand LI. Risk of early-onset proliferative retinopathy in IDDM is closely related to cardiovascular autonomic neuropathy. *Diabetes* 1992; **41:** 430–7.

33. Lanigan LP, Clark CV, Allawi J, Hill DW, Keen H. Responses of the retina circulation to systemic autonomic stimulation in diabetes mellitus. *Eye* 1989; **3:** 39–47.

34. Muhlhauser I, Sawicki P, Berger M. Cigarette-smoking as a risk factor for macroproteinuria and proliferative retinopathy in Type 1 (insulin-dependent) diabetes. *Diabetologia* 1986; **29:** 500–2.

35. Moss SE, Klein R, Klein BE. Association of cigarette smoking with diabetic retinopathy. *Diabetes Care* 1991; **14:** 119–26.

36. Young RJ, McCulloch DK, Prescott RJ, Clarke BF. Alcohol: another risk factor for diabetic retinopathy. *BMJ* 1984; **288:** 1035–7.

37. Orchard TJ, Dorman JS, Maser RE, et al. Factors associated with avoidance of severe complications after 25 years of IDDM. Pittsburgh Epidemiological Study of Diabetes Complications Study I. *Diabetes Care* 1990; **13:** 741–7.

38. Moss SE, Klein R, Klein BE. Alcohol consumption and the prevalence of diabetic retinopathy. *Ophthalmology* 1992; **99:** 926–32.

39. Chen HC, Newsom RSB, Patel V, Cassar J, Mather H, Kohner EM. Retinal blood flow changes during pregnancy in women with diabetes. *Invest Ophthalmol Vis Sci* 1994; **35:** 3199–208.

40. Klein BEK, Moss SE, Klein R. Effect of pregnancy on progression of diabetic retinopathy. *Diabetes Care* 1990; **13:** 34–40.

41. Milnor WR. *Hemodynamics*. Baltimore, Williams and Wilkins, 1989: 140–1.

42. Riva CE, Grunwald JE, Sinclair SH, Petrig

BL. Blood velocity and volumetric flow rate in human retinal vessels. *Invest Ophthalmol Vis Sci* 1985; **26**: 1124–32.

43. Rassam SMB, Patel V, Kohner EM. The effect of experimental hypertension on retinal vascular autoregulation in humans: a mechanism for the progression of diabetic retinopathy. *Exp Physiol* 1995; **80**: 53–68.

44. Strauss AL, Kedra AW. Experiences with a new procedure for the measurement of the ophthalmic artery pessure: ophthalmo-manometry-Doppler. *Med Instrum* 1987; **21**: 255–61.

45. Beroniade VC, Lefebvre R, Falardeau P. Unilateral nodular diabetic glomerulosclerosis: recurrence of an experiment of nature. *Am J Nephrol* 1987; **7**: 55–9.

46. Gay AJ, Rosenbau, AL. Retinal artery pressure in asymmetric diabetic retinopathy. *Arch Ophthalmol* 1966; **75**: 758–62.

47. Garner A, Ashton N, Tripathi R, Kohner EM, Bulpitt CJ. Pathogenesis of hypertensive retinopathy, an experimental study in the monkey. *Br J Ophthalmol* 1975; **59**: 3–44.

48. Tso MOM, Jampol LM. Pathophysiology of hypertensive retinopathy. *Ophthalmology* 1982; **89**: 1132–45.

49. Davies PF, Remuzzi A, Gordon EJ, Dewey DF, Gimbrone MA. Turbulent fluid shear stress induces vascular endothelial cell turnover in vitro. *Proc Natl Acad Sci USA* 1986; **83**: 2114–17.

50. Ando J, Nomura H, Kamiya A. The effect of fluid shear stress on the migration and proliferation of cultured endothelial cells. *Microvasc Res* 1987; **33**: 62–70.

51. Norris CP, Barnes GE, Smith EE, Granger HY. Autoregulation of superior mesenteric flow in fasted and fed dogs. *Am J Physiol* 1979; **237**: H174–H177.

52. Diabetic Retinopathy Study Research Group. Indications for photocoagulation treatment of diabetic retinopathy: Diabetic Retinopathy Study report no. 14. *Int Ophthalmol Clin* 1987; **27**: 239–53.

53. McLeod D, Marshall J, Kohner EM, Bird AC. The role of axoplasmic transport in the pathogenesis of retinal cotton-wool spots. *Br J Ophthalmol* 1977; **61**: 177–91.

54. Hayreh SS, Servais GE, Virdi PS. Cotton wool spots (inner retinal ischemic spots) in malignant arterial hypertension. *Ophthalmologica* 1989; **198**: 197–215.

55. Kuwabara T, Cogan DG. Retinal vascular patterns (VI): mural cells of the retinal capillaries. *Arch Ophthalmol* 1963; **69**: 492–502.

56. Buzney SM, Franks RW, Varmas SD. Aldose reductase in retinal neural cells. *Invest Ophthalmol Vis Sci* 1977; **16**: 392–6.

57. Sorbinil Retinopathy Trial Research Group. A randomised trial of Sorbinil, an aldose reductase inhibitor, in diabetic retinopathy. *Arch Ophthalmol* 1990; **108**: 1234–44.

58. Kohner EM, Caldwell G, Plehwe WE, Brown R, Rosen E. Ponalrestat in early diabetic retinopathy. *Diabetes* 1990; **39** (Suppl 1): 245 (abstract).

59. Brownlee M, Vlassara H, Cerami A. Nonenzymatic glycosylation and the pathogenesis of diabetic complications. *Ann Intern Med* 1984; **101**: 527–37.

60. Merimee TJ. Diabetic retinopathy: a synthesis of perspectives. *N Engl J Med* 1990; **322**: 978–83.

61. Lubec G, Pollak A. Reduced susceptibility of nonenzymatically glycosylated glomerular basement membrane to proteases: is thickening of diabetic glomerular basement membranes due to reduced proteolytic degradation? *Renal Physiol* 1980; **3**: 4–8.

62. Li W, Shen S, Khatami M, Rocky JH. Stimulation of retinal capillary pericyte protein and collagen synthesis in culture by high glucose concentration. *Diabetes* 1984; **33**: 785–9.

63. De La Rubia G, Oliver FJ, Inoguchi T, King GL. Induction of resistance to endothelin-1's biochemical actions by elevated glucose levels on retinal pericytes. *Diabetes* 1992; **41**: 1533–9.

64. Merimee TJ. A follow-up study of vascular disease in growth-hormone-deficient dwarfs with diabetes. *N Engl J Med* 1978; **298**: 1217–22.

65. Merimee TJ, Zapf J, Froesch ER. Insulin-like growth factors: studies in diabetes with and without retinopathy. *N Engl J Med* 1983; **309**: 527–30.

66. Grant M, Russel B, Fitzgerald C, Merimee TJ. Insulin-like growth factors in vitreous: studies in control and diabetic subjects with neovascularization. *Diabetes* 1986; **35**: 416–20.

67. McCombe M, Lightman S, Eckland DJ, Hamilton AM, Lightman SL. Effect of a long-acting somatostatin analogue (BIM23014) on proliferative diabetic retinopathy: a pilot study. *Eye* 1991; **5**: 569–75.

68. Hyer SL, Sharp PS, Brooks RA, Burrin JM, Kohner EM. Continuous subcutaneous octreotide infusion markedly suppresses IGF-I levels whilst only partially suppressing GH secretion in diabetics with retinopathy. *Acta Endocrinol* 1989; **120**: 187–94.

69. Raymond L, Jacobson B. Isolation and identification of stimulatory and inhibitory cell growth factors in bovine vitreous. *Exp Eye Res* 1982; **34**: 267–86.

70. Kohner EM, Hamilton AM, Saunders SJ, Sutcliffe BA, Bulpitt CJ. The retinal blood flow in diabetes. *Diabetologia* 1975; **11**: 27–33.

71. Patel V, Rassam S, Newsom R, Wiek J, Kohner E. Retinal blood flow in diabetic retinopathy. BMJ 1992; **305**: 678–83.

72. Tooke JE. Microvascular haemodynamics in diabetes mellitus. *Clin Sci* 1986; **70**: 119–25.

73. DAMAD study group. Effect of aspirin alone and aspirin plus dipyridamole in early diabetic retinopathy. *Diabetes* 1989; **38**: 491–8.

74. TIMAD study group. Ticlopidine treatment reduces the progression of non-proliferative diabetic retinopathy. *Arch Ophthalmol* 1990; **108**: 1577–83.

75. Patz A. Retinal neovascularization: early contributions of Professor Michaelson and recent observations. *Br J Ophthalmol* 1984; **68**: 42–6.

76. Atherton A, Hill DW, Keen H, Young S, Edwards EJ. The effect of hyperglycaemia on the retinal circulation of the normal cat. *Diabetologia* 1980; **18**: 233–7.

77. Keen H, Chlouverakis C. Metabolic factors in diabetic retinopathy. In: Graymore CN, ed. *Biochemistry of the retina*. New York, Academic Press, 1965.

78. Tilton RG, Baier LD, Harlow JE, Smith SR, Ostrow E, Williamson JR. Diabetes induced glomerular dysfunction: links to a more reduced cytosolic redox ratio of NADH/NAD$^+$. *Kidney Int* 1992; **41**: 778–88.

79. Patel V, Rassam SMB, Chen HC, Kohner EM. Oxygen reactivity in diabetes mellitus: effect of hypertension and hyperglycaemia. *Clin Sci* 1994; **86**: 689–95.

80. Patel V, Rassam SM, Chen HC et al. Effect of angiotensin-converting enzyme inhibition with perindopril and β-blockade with atenolol on retinal blood flow in hypertensive diabetic subjects. *Metabolism* 1998; **47** (Suppl): 28–33.

81. Drury PL, Bodansky HJ. The relationship of the angiotensin system in type I diabetes to microvascular complications. *Hypertension* 1985; Suppl II: 84–9.

82. Wagener HP, Clay GE, Gipner JF. Classification of retinal lesions in the presence of vascular hypertension. *Trans Am Ophthalmol Soc* 1947; **45**: 57–73. Servier 26.

83. Ferrari-Dileo G, Davis EB, Anderson DR. Angiotensin binding sites in bovine human retinal blood vessels. *Invest Ophthalmol Vis Sci* 1987; **28**: 1747–51.

84. Fernandez WA, Wickler J, Mead A. Neovascularisation produced by angiotensin II. *J Lab Clin Med* 1985; **105**: 141–5.

85. Kohner EM. The renin-angiotensin system and diabetic retinopathy. *Klin Wochenschr* 1992; **69** (Suppl XXIX): 25–7.

86. Kuwabara T, Cogan DG. Retinal vascular patterns (VI): mural cells of the retinal capillaries. *Arch Ophthalmol* 1963; **69**: 492–502.

87. Bates DO, Lodwick D, Williams B. Vascular endothelial growth factor and microvascular permeability. *Microcirculation* 1999; **6**: 1–19.

88. Williams B, Baker AQ, Gallacher B, Lodwick D. Angiotensin II increases vascular permeablity factor (VPF/VEFG) gene expression by human vascular smooth muscle. *Hypertension* 1995; **68**: 160–7.

89. Williams B. Angiotensin II, VEGF and diabetic retinopathy. *Lancet* 1998; **351**: 837–8.

90. Aiello LP, Avery RL, Arrigg PG, et al. Vascular endothelial growth factor in ocular fluid of patients with diabetic retinopathy and other retina; disorders. *N Engl J Med* 1994; **331**: 1480–7.

91. Williams B, Gallacher B, Patel H, Orme C. Glucose-induced protein kinase C activation regulates vascular permeability factor (VPF/VEGF) mRNA expression and peptide production by human vascular smooth muscle cells in vitro. *Diabetes* 1997; **46**: 1497–503.

92. DIRECT study

93. Estacio RO, Savage S, Nagel NJ, Schrier RW. Baseline characteristics of participants in the

appropriate blood pressure control in diabetes trial. *Control Clin Trials* 1996; **17**: 242–57.

94. Estacio RO, Jeffers BW, Gifford N, Schrier RW. Effect of blood pressure control on diabetes microvascular complications in patients with hypertension and type 2 diabetes. *Diabetes Care* 2000; **23** (Suppl 2): B54–B64.

95. Lewis JM, Jovanovic-Peterson L, Ahmadizadeh I, Bevier W, Peterson CM, Williams B. The Santa Barbara County diabetic retinopathy screening feasibility study: significance of diabetes duration and systolic blood pressure. *J Diabetes Complications* 1994; **8**: 51–4.

96. American Diabetes Association Position Statement: Treatment of Hypertension in adults with diabetes. *Diabetes Care* 2002; 134–47 and 199–201.

9

Diabetes and the heart
Adam D Timmis

Introduction

Diabetes is the commonest metabolic disorder encountered in clinical practice. Only about 10% have juvenile onset (type 1) diabetes, the remainder developing type 2 diabetes later in life, often in association with hyperinsulinaemia, obesity, hypertension, and dyslipidaemia. With our ageing, sedentary and increasingly obese population, the number of affected individuals will continue to rise. This will have major implications for cardiological practice since much of the excess morbidity and mortality among diabetic patients is attributable to accelerated atherogenesis. Young diabetics are at particular risk and, by the age of 50, 33% of those requiring insulin have died from coronary heart disease. Indeed, 75% of all deaths in patients with diabetes are from this cause (Table 9.1).[1]

Mechanisms of accelerated atherogenesis

In diabetic individuals, conventional risk factors (smoking, hypertension and dyslipidaemia) increase the risk of coronary heart disease in much the same way as in non-diabetics. Thus, the fact that hypertension and dyslipidaemia are more prevalent in diabetes must itself contribute to the heightened risk of coronary heart disease. The contribution is only partial however, and it is estimated that these conventional risk factors account for less than 25% of the excess risk.[2] In the Multiple Risk Factor Interventional Trial (MRFIT), for example, in which 361,662 men were followed up for 6 years, the mortality risk in both diabetic and non-diabetic individuals increased almost linearly with serum cholesterol.[3] However, at any given cholesterol level diabetics had a 3 to 4-fold excess risk (Fig. 9.1). It is now recognized that much of this excess risk is a consequence of accelerated atherogenesis which, in turn, is attributable to multiple factors.

Acknowledgement: this chapter is an extended version of an earlier publication by the same author and appears by permission of Heart (2001; 85: 463–9)

- 75% of deaths in patients with DM caused by CHD
- By the age of 50, 33% IDDM patients have died of CHD
- Most risk factors for CHD more prevalent in DM
- Conventional risk factors account for <25% of excess risk of CHD in DM
- Aggressive euglycaemic treatment diminishes micro- but not macrovascular complications

Table 9.1
Atherogenesis in diabetes

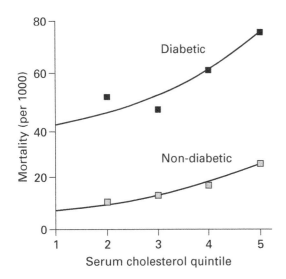

Figure 9.1
CHD Mortality in MRFIT by cholesterol quintile: comparison of diabetic and non-diabetic groups.

Hyperglycaemia

Hyperglycaemia is an important risk factor for microvascular complications of diabetes but its relation with macrovascular disease is less well defined. For example, in the Wisconsin Epidemiologic Study of diabetic Retinopathy, a 1% increase in glycosylated haemoglobin resulted in a 70% increased incidence of retinopathy, but only a 10% increased incidence of coronary heart disease.[4] Insofar as hyperglycaemia is a late event in the long process leading from insulin resistance to the development of diabetes it has not been considered a major player in the pathogenesis of accelerated atherosclerosis.[5] Nevertheless, there has been renewed interest in the atherogenic potential of hyperglycaemia based on recent evidence relating it to mechanisms of increased oxidative stress and lipid peroxidation in diabetes.[6] This damages vascular endothelial cells both physically and function-

ally and initiates a complex chain of events that is now considered central to the early pathogenesis of atherosclerosis. Indeed increased oxidative stress is increasingly regarded as the final common pathway that links all major risk factors for coronary atherosclerosis, including hypertension, smoking and dyslipidaemia. The chronic hyperglycaemia associated with diabetes leads to reversible glycosylation of protein amino groups by enzymatic and non-enzymatic pathways. This has no direct pathological consequences, the glycosylation of haemoglobin providing a useful clinical index of glycaemic control. However, it leads to irreversible oxidation of fructoselysine which produces a variety of advanced glycation end products (AGEs). These react with a specific receptor (RAGE) at the vascular endothelium, the expression of which is increased considerably in diabetes.[7] The AGE-RAGE interaction (Fig. 9.2) increases vascular endothelial production of superoxide anions and other oxidative products with important consequences. These include LDL oxidation, stimulation of monocyte adherence to the blood vessel (one of the earliest events in the atherogenic process), increased vascular permeability (allowing accelerated passage of macromolecules into the vessel wall), increased membrane expression of tissue factor (enhancing the procoagulant state), increased endothelin secretion and inactivation of nitric oxide (promoting vasoconstriction), and increased growth factor secretion (encouraging proliferation of vascular smooth muscle cells). Thus the AGE-RAGE interaction at the vascular endothelium may be a key factor in the accelerated atherogenesis of diabetes. Recent data (Fig. 9.3) indicate that reducing vascular exposure to AGEs by injection of soluble RAGE (which mops up circulating AGEs) suppresses accelerated atherosclerosis in diabetic mice, providing

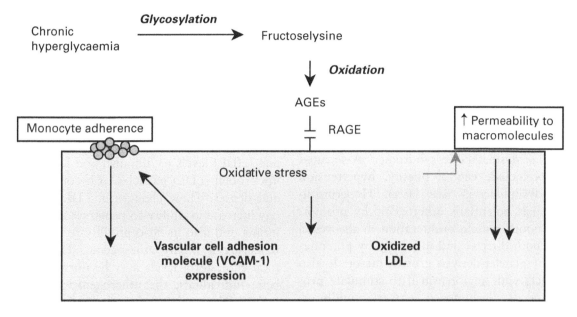

Figure 9.2
Mechanisms of accelerated atherogenesis in diabetes: Advanced Glycation End Products (AGEs).

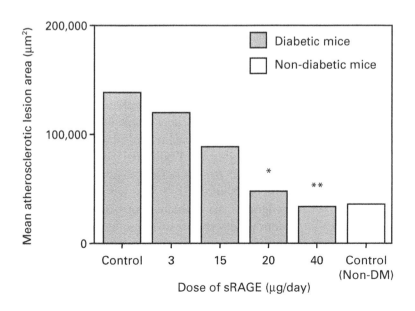

Figure 9.3
sRAGE suppresses accelerated atherosclerosis in diabetic mice (apoE-deficient mice susceptible to atherosclerosis and rendered diabetic using streptozotocin). *Reproduced with permission from Park et al*[8] *Nature Med 1998; 4: 1025–31.*

grounds for optimism about future clinical applications.[8]

Hyperinsulinaemia, insulin resistance and the cardiac dysmetabolic syndrome

Hyperinsulinaemia and insulin resistance are the central metabolic derangements of the cardiovascular dysmetabolic syndrome.[9] Associated factors include central obesity, hypertension and dyslipidaemia (see later). Hyperinsulinaemia is potentially atherogenic by promoting smooth muscle proliferation in the vessel wall, both directly and indirectly by potentiation of platelet-derived growth factor. It also interacts with angiotensin II to stimulate production of plasminogen activator inhibitor. However, insulin also exhibits vasculoprotective effects, notably by stimulation of endothelial nitric oxide production, and net effects on atherogenesis are hard to quantify.[10] The results of epidemiological studies have been contradictory,[11] and although meta-analysis indicates that hyperinsulinaemia may be a weak independent risk factor for accelerated atherogenesis in diabetes, this does not necessarily imply a causal relationship.[12] Insulin resistance appears to correlate better with coronary artery disease and in the Insulin Resistance Atherosclerosis Study was found to have an independent effect on atherogenesis (as reflected by carotid intimal medial wall thickness) following adjustment for smoking, lipid levels, hypertension, diabetes and gender.[13] Speculation has it that insulin resistance might disturb the balance between insulin's vasculoprotective and proliferative effects, favouring atherogenesis by promotion of vascular smooth muscle growth and migration.

Dyslipidaemia

Dyslipidaemia affecting the entire spectrum of lipids and lipoproteins is almost invariable in type 2 diabetes.[14-16] Chylomicrons and atherogenic very low density lipoprotein (VLDL) remnants accumulate, while hypertriglyceridaemia, itself a major risk factor for coronary artery disease,[17] causes high density lipoprotein (HDL) levels to diminish and low density lipoprotein (LDL) particles to become smaller and denser. These changes in LDL morphology increase its ability to penetrate the arterial intima and also its susceptibility to oxidation, rendering it highly atherogenic. Thus, while total cholesterol levels may be normal in diabetic individuals, the atherogenicity of LDL and VLDL is enhanced, and circulating levels of HDL, which protects against atherogenesis by facilitating reverse cholesterol transport, are reduced. The importance of dyslipidaemia in diabetic atherosclerotic disease is reflected in the benefits of lipid lowering therapy reported in randomized trials (see later). Nevertheless, treatment does not reduce risk to the level seen in patients without diabetes and it seems clear, therefore, that dyslipidaemia accounts for only a part of the increased susceptibility to coronary heart disease in diabetes.

Procoagulant factors

Oxidative stress and endothelial dysfunction in diabetes (see earlier) result in deficient production of prostacyclin and plasminogen activator inhibitor. Oxidative stress is also responsible for increased platelet production of thromboxane A2.[18] The net effect of these changes is to enhance vasoconstrictor and thrombotic responses to plaque rupture in diabetes, increasing plaque burden and the risk of myocardial infarction.

Diabetes and cardiovascular risk

Three large epidemiological studies have contributed importantly to current understanding of the natural history of diabetic heart disease.[2,4,19] The Framingham study showed that diabetes increased the relative risk of coronary heart disease by 66% in men and 203% in women followed up for 20 years, after controlling for the effects of age, smoking, blood pressure and cholesterol.[2] The Whitehall study of male civil servants extended these observations by showing that subclinical glucose intolerance, in addition to frank diabetes, also increased coronary risk.[19] The Multiple Risk Factor Interventional Trial (MRFIT) with its very large population of middle-aged men was able to provide more detailed information about the interaction between diabetes and other risk factors in determining coronary risk.[4] This trial confirmed the heightened risk attributable to diabetes, and also the independent effects of serum cholesterol, blood pressure and smoking in men with and without diabetes. MRFIT showed that in men with diabetes, 12-year cardiovascular mortality was much higher at every level of these major risk factors considered singly and in combination, and that with progressively more unfavourable risk factor status the mortality rate rose much more steeply than in men without diabetes (Fig. 9.4).

Risk factor modification for protecting against coronary heart disease in diabetes

Based on their data, the MRFIT investigators recommended "rigorous sustained intervention in people with diabetes to control blood pressure, lower serum cholesterol, and abolish cigarette smoking...". These recommendations remain central to the cardiovascular management of diabetes and their value for primary and secondary prevention has been confirmed in randomized trials. Disappointingly, however, there is not yet clear evidence that the recommendation for more vigorous risk factor modification in diabetes leads to extra protection against coronary heart disease beyond that achieved in non-diabetic individuals, although important protection against microvascular complications (retinopathy, renal disease) does occur. Nevertheless, as our practice evolves from single to multifactorial risk assessment in which an individual's absolute coronary risk can be readily assessed from simple colour coded charts the clinical impact of risk factor modification can be expected to increase, particularly with the recent availability of charts for use in men and women with diabetes.[20]

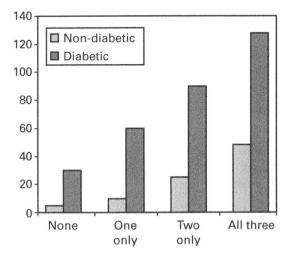

Figure 9.4
MRFIT: Age-adjusted CVD death rates by presence of number of risk factors in men with and without diabetes.

Blood pressure

Hypertension commonly occurs in type 2 diabetes, and contributes importantly to the heightened risk of cardiovascular, renal and retinal disease.[21–24] By the age of 50 more than 40% of patients with type 2 diabetes are hypertensive, the proportion rising to 60% by the age of 75.[21] Subgroup analyses of large trials have suggested that the benefits of treating hypertension apply equally to diabetic and non-diabetic patients, a suggestion emphatically confirmed in the hypertensive cohort of the UK Prospective Diabetes Study (UKPDS).[25] Comparison of patients allocated either to tight blood pressure control (<150/85 mmHg) using captopril or atenolol, or to less-tight control showed that tight control for 8.4 years was associated with significant reduction in the risk of death related to diabetes, and with reductions in all microvascular endpoints (Fig. 9.5). Predictably, reductions in the risk of heart failure and stroke also occurred, but the 21% reduction in the risk of myocardial infarction was not significant. The Hypertension Optimal Treatment (HOT) study also reported reductions in myocardial infarction in patients treated to a target diastolic blood pressure of 80 mmHg compared to targets of 85 or 90 mmHg, but again the changes were not significant.[26] Based largely on these recent trial data, a target blood pressure of <130 mmHg systolic and <80 mmHg diastolic is now recommended for diabetic

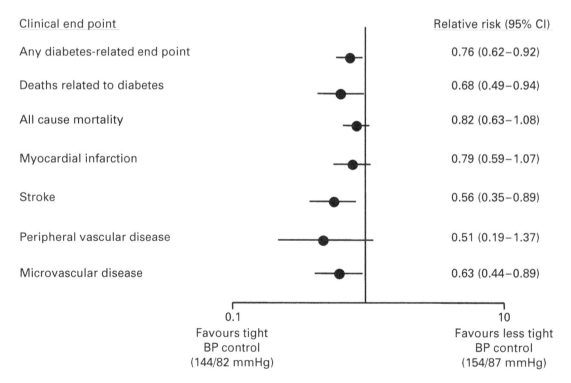

Figure 9.5
UKPDS 38: relative risk reduction with tight BP control.

patients.[27] Lower targets might be appropriate for diabetic patients with microalbuminuria, in whom considerable data support the use of ACE-inhibitors for protecting against deterioration of renal function, a beneficial effect that occurs independently of blood pressure reduction.[28,29] However, UKPDS reported that captopril or atenolol was similarly effective in reducing the incidence of diabetic complications and concluded that for most patients blood pressure reduction itself is more important than the agent used.[30]

Lipid modification with fibrates and statins

Hypertriglyceridaemia with reductions in HDL are the typical abnormalities detected on routine laboratory testing in type 2 diabetes.[14] This provides a logic for fibrate therapy in addition to exercise and weight reduction. The Helsinki study suggested a trend towards reduced coronary events in diabetic patients treated with gemfibrozil for 5 years,[31] but data from other fibrate studies have generally been inconclusive. This contrasts with subgroup analyses of the major statin trials which have shown convincingly that hypercholesterolaemic diabetic patients gain similar relative benefit as non-diabetic patients in the secondary prevention of coronary artery disease, and greater absolute benefit due to their higher event rate (Fig. 9.6).[32–34] Thus, vigorous treatment of all diabetics with known atherosclerotic disease to achieve a total cholesterol of <5.0 mmol/l (LDL <3.0 mmol/l) is recommended, together with correction of hypertriglyceridaemia using additional fibrate therapy, as necessary. In diabetic patients without overt atherosclerotic disease, an

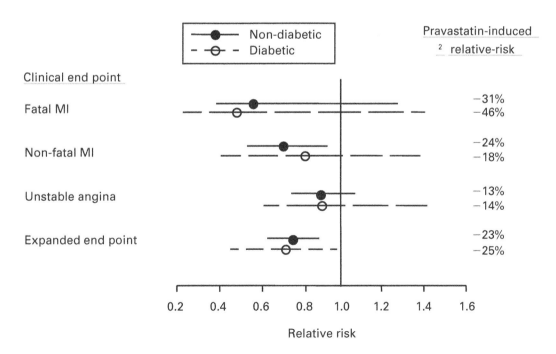

Figure 9.6
CARE trial: pravastatin and cardiovascular events.

absolute risk of 15% of developing coronary heart disease over the next 10 years, as deduced from colour-coded risk prediction charts, is sufficiently high to justify drug treatment.[27]

Smoking

Observational data suggest that the risk of myocardial infarction is reduced by up to 50% within 1 year of quitting smoking, with favourable effects on mortality maintained for up to 10 years. Since the cardiac risk attributable to smoking is magnified considerably in diabetes, as indeed is the risk attributable to all other risk factors, the benefits of quitting are likely to be as great, if not greater in diabetic than non-diabetic patients.[3]

Glycaemic control for protecting against coronary heart disease in diabetes

Strict glycaemic control has long been recommended in diabetes, based on epidemiological surveys that have reported more favourable clinical outcomes for groups with lower plasma glucose and glycosylated haemoglobin concentrations.[4,35,36] However, whether these more favourable outcomes reflected less severe underlying disease rather than the benefits of glycaemic control remained unresolved until publication of UKPDS in which 3867 newly diagnosed patients with type 2 diabetes were randomly assigned to an intensive (sulphonylurea or insulin) or conventional treatment policy.[37] After follow-up for 10 years, glycosylated haemoglobin concentrations in the two groups were 7.0% and 7.9%, respectively, a difference of only 11%. Nevertheless, this trial confirmed the close relationship between glycaemia and the risk of microvascular and macrovascular complications,[38] including coronary heart disease, and also dispelled concerns about the potential adverse cardiovascular effects of sulphonylureas. Importantly, in the group randomized to intense glycaemic control, significant protection against microvascular complications occurred although macrovascular complications were not similarly affected, the 16% reduction in the risk of myocardial infarction being of only borderline statistical significance. In short, therefore, UKPDS has confirmed the importance of strict glycaemic control (glycosylated haemoglobin 7% or lower) for protection against microvascular complications of diabetes. It is tempting to speculate that more substantial protection against macrovascular end-points might have occurred had there been greater differences in glycaemic control (as reflected by glycosylated haemoglobin) between the intensive and conventional treatment groups.

Other strategies for protecting against coronary heart disease in diabetes

Antiplatelet therapy

An overview of randomized trials has shown that the benefits of antiplatelet therapy for secondary prevention of coronary heart disease are similar for groups with and without diabetes.[39] Thus patients with diabetic coronary heart disease should all receive a daily aspirin. Though not strictly evidence-based, aspirin is now recommended for diabetic adults without clinical manifestations of atheromatous disease (primary prevention) since platelet dysfunction is common and the prevalence of subclinical disease high. Evidence for non-aspirin platelet inhibitors in diabetic subgroups is often unavailable, and a convincing case for the glycoprotein IIb/IIIa receptor antagonists in acute coronary syndromes has yet to be made. However, as an adjunct to coronary stenting, glycoprotein IIb/IIIa receptor antagonists have a particularly useful role,[40] reducing the rate of adverse events in patients with diabetes to a level comparable to that of patients without diabetes (see later).

ACE-inhibition

ACE-inhibition protects against the development of atherosclerotic plaque in experimental animals fed lipid-rich diets.[41–43] Potential for similar benefit in humans was reported by the TREND investigators who showed that treatment with quinapril improved coronary endothelial function in patients with coronary disease.[44] This potential has now been confirmed by the Heart Outcomes Prevention Evaluation (HOPE) study (Fig. 9.7) in which significant reductions in the risk of the combined primary outcome (death, myocardial infarction and stroke) occurred in high risk patients randomized to treatment with ramipril.[45] Among these high risk patients were 3577 with diabetes who had a previous cardiac event or at least one other cardio-vascular risk factor, but not heart failure or proteinuria. Within this diabetic subgroup, randomization to ramipril reduced the risk of the combined primary outcome by 25%, with an additional reduction in the risk of overt nephropathy.[46] These important findings are now having a major impact on the management of diabetes, providing indications for ACE-inhibition with ramipril in any diabetic patient with multiple risk factors, established vascular disease, or microalbuminuria.

Screening for coronary heart disease in diabetes

The prevalence of subclinical coronary artery disease in the general population is high, but is almost certainly higher in the diabetic population due to accelerated atherosclerosis.[47,48] Thus, people with diabetes have a long-term rate of myocardial infarction and cardiovascular death comparable to that of nondiabetic patients with a documented history of myocardial infarction.[49] Subclinical disease is commonly non-obstructive due to outward

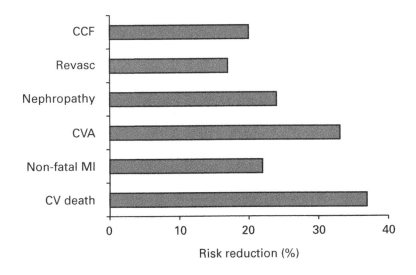

Figure 9.7
HOPE and MICRO-HOPE: effects of ramipril in people with diabetes (n = 3577). *Adapted from HOPE Investigators, Lancet 2000.[46]*

remodelling of the coronary artery.[50] However, obstructive disease may also be clinically silent, particularly in diabetes when autonomic neuropathy may interfere with the perception of cardiac pain such that symptoms take longer to develop after the onset of myocardial ischaemia (prolonged anginal perceptual threshold)[51] or do not occur at all (silent ischaemia).[52]

The relatively high prevalence of subclinical coronary artery disease associated with diabetes has led to debate about the value of screening programmes using non-invasive tests.[53,54] As a universal principal, this can scarcely be justified, the sensitivity of stress testing (electrocardiographic or perfusion imaging) for detecting subclinical disease being low with only a 5–10% incidence of *obstructive* lesions (>50% luminal narrowing at angiography) among asymptomatic diabetic cohorts.[55–57] Moreover, the mere demonstration of obstructive coronary disease does not usually affect ongoing management with strict glycaemic control and risk factor modification. Certainly, there is no evidence to support angioplasty in asymptomatic cases, while the potential prognostic benefits of surgery in the minority with 3 vessel or left main disease need to be balanced against the heightened procedural risk and less favourable longer term outcome in patients with diabetes (see below). Nevertheless, in certain subgroups, screening for coronary artery disease is recommended because it can lead to treatment strategies that favourably affect prognosis. These include diabetic patients needing renal transplantation or major noncardiac vascular surgery in whom coronary revascularization may reduce the procedural risk.[58–60]

Angina and revascularization in diabetes (Table 9.2)

Angina may affect up to 40% of adults with diabetes, although its precise prevalence is hard to deduce from the literature. Symptoms are commonly atypical, perhaps because of abnormalities in the perception of angina caused by autonomic neuropathy,[51,52] and the physician should retain a low threshold for non-invasive investigation (Fig. 9.8). A positive stress test associated with atypical symptoms in the diabetic patient indicates a high probability of underlying coronary disease and the need for specific anti-anginal treatment, often with additional angiographic assessment. The disease is typically diffuse affecting both proximal and distal coronary segments (angiographic observations not always borne out by pathological studies),[61] and this has the potential to intensify ischaemia.[62] There is no evidence of reduced responsiveness to medical therapy in patients with diabetes which should be with nitrates and beta-blockers in the first instance with the addition of calcium channel blockers or potassium channel openers in more resistant cases. However, diffuse disease makes revascularization by angioplasty or bypass surgery more difficult and more

• Appreciation of ischaemic pain blunted: silent ischaemia more common anginal perceptual threshold prolonged silent infarction more common • Abnormalities of pain perception related to autonomic neuropathy • Autonomic neuropathy in DM predicts sudden death

Table 9.2
Angina in diabetes

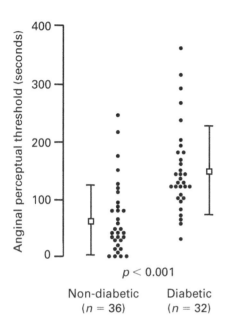

$p < 0.001$

Non-diabetic   Diabetic
($n = 36$)   ($n = 32$)

Figure 9.8
Anginal perceptual thresholds in diabetic and non-diabetic patients with CAD. Reproduced with permission from Ambepityia et al, J Am Coll Cardiol, **15:** 72–7.[51]

- Diffuse and distal disease makes revascularization technically more demanding
- Reduced survival after CABG and PTCA
- Increased restenosis rates after PTCA
- BARI data indicate that for most diabetics CABG is preferable to PTCA
- Recent EPISTENT data point to an important role for stenting and IIb/IIIa receptor blockers in diabetic PTCA

Table 9.3
Revascularization in diabetes

hazardous (Table 9.3). Indeed, diabetes has long been recognized as one of the major independent predictors of long term mortality after surgery.[63] The results of angioplasty also tend to be less good in diabetic compared with non-diabetic patients. Again, diffuse disease makes for technically more difficult angioplasty procedures and, in addition, restenosis rates are consistently higher.[64] In the recent BARI trial of angioplasty versus bypass surgery, subgroup analysis showed that patients without diabetes had comparable results with either revascularization modality. In patients with diabetes, however, the survival curves descended more steeply, particularly those randomized to angioplasty who fared significantly worse than those randomized to bypass surgery (Fig. 9.9). The investigators concluded

that for most diabetics requiring revascularization coronary bypass surgery was preferable to angioplasty.[65] Nevertheless, a predefined subgroup analysis from the EPISTENT trial showed that angioplasty and stenting combined with infusion of abciximab (a glycoprotein IIb/IIIa receptor inhibitor) improves the long-term outcome in diabetic patients substantially, with a 6-month incidence of ischaemic endpoints comparable to that achieved in non-diabetic patients.[40] The data suggest, therefore, that stenting and IIb/IIIa receptor blockade may have an important role in diabetic angioplasty.

Acute myocardial infarction in diabetes (Table 9.4)

Framingham data have shown that the risk of acute myocardial infarction is 50% greater in diabetic men and 150% greater in diabetic women than in nondiabetic individuals.[2] Indeed, acute myocardial infarction accounts for 30% of all diabetic deaths. This propensity to myocardial infarction presumably reflects the increased prevalence of coronary artery disease in diabetes, with associated hypertension predisposing to plaque rupture. More-

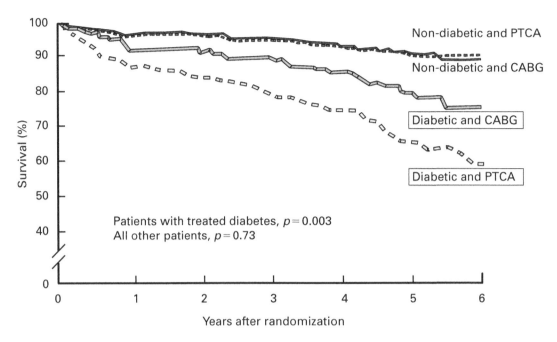

Figure 9.9
BARI: 5-year survival rates. Reproduced with permission of the BARI Investigators. N Engl J Med. *1996;*
***335:** 217–25.[65]*

- Autonomic impairment
  Silent infarction more common
  Loss of circadian and seasonal rhythms
- Multiple risk factors
  Older
  More commonly Asian and female
  Hypertensive
- Increased risk
  ↑ Incidence of AMI
  ↑ Risk of major complications (esp. LVF)
  ↑ Risk of death
- Treatment implications
  Insulin/glucose improves outcome
  Thrombolytic therapy no less effective
  Secondary prevention no less effective

Table 9.4
Diabetic myocardial infarction: summary

over, thrombotic responses to plaque rupture are likely to be exaggerated in diabetes due to haematological abnormalities, particularly increased platelet activation.[18]

It has long been recognized that diabetics are prone to "silent" myocardial infarction and this presumably reflects impaired perception of ischaemic cardiac pain caused by autonomic neuropathy. Thus, in diabetes, acute myocardial infarction is silent or presents with atypical symptoms in 32–42% of cases compared with 6–15% of non-diabetic infarcts.[66] This is disadvantageous because it has the potential to delay access to emergency facilities early after coronary events, increasing the risk of out-of-hospital sudden death and morbid complications of myocardial infarction,

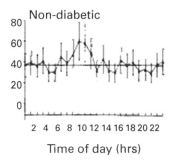

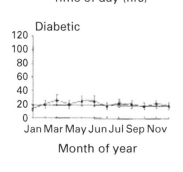

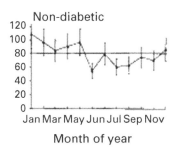

Figure 9.10
*AMI: admission rates by hour of day and month of year (n = 1225). Reproduced with permission from Sayer et al, Heart 1997; **77**: 325–9.[69]*

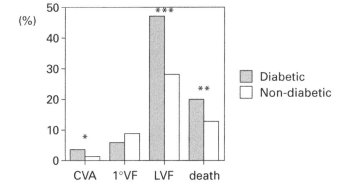

Figure 9.11
Complications of AMI (n = 1829). (Unpublished data from NGH CCU database.)

particularly cardiogenic shock.[67,68] Abnormalities of circadian and seasonal rhythms of acute myocardial infarction, with attenuation of the morning and winter peaks, may also reflect autonomic dysfunction because these rhythms are largely driven by parallel changes in sympathovagal activity (Fig. 9.10).[69] The consequences of this to the patient with diabetes are unclear.

All the major complications of myocardial infarction occur more commonly in diabetes, particularly heart failure which affects nearly 50% of diabetics compared with under 30% of non-diabetics (Fig. 9.11).[70] This difference is not accounted for by infarct size but may reflect the more severe and diffuse disease in diabetes that limits coronary reserve and intensifies ischaemia in noninfarcted segments by a watershed effect.[62] Diabetes-specific myocardial disease may also have a role. Thus, contractile dysfunction remote from the infarct zone is commonly reported in diabetic myocardial infarction.[62] Since heart failure is one of the major determinants of outcome, it is little surprise that both hospital and long-term mortality rates are increased in patients with diabetes.[62,66,70] Thus, in our own coronary care unit, the 30-day and 12-month mortality rates (95% CI) for patients with diabetes are 80.8% (76.9–84.7%) and 73.4% (68.9–77.8%), compared with 87.3% (85.2–89.4%) and 80.9% (78.4–83.4%) for patients without diabetes (Fig. 9.12).

Patients with acute myocardial infarction who have diabetes, or an admission blood glucose concentration = 11.0 mmol/l, should receive insulin and glucose infusion for at least 24 hours based on the findings of the Diabetes Mellitus, Insulin Glucose Infusion in Acute Myocardial Infarction (DIGAMI) investigators who showed that this significantly improves survival (Fig. 9.13).[71] Subcutaneous insulin treatment continued for at least 3 months in this study, a regime that many units find too unwieldy to apply in practice. Certainly treatment during the acute phase of infarction is likely to be particularly beneficial, not only for improving left ventricular function,[72] but also for reducing infarct size and lethal complications, since the shift to anaerobic glucose metabolism that occurs in the myocardium during acute ischaemia is an insulin dependent adjustment that may be deficient in diabetes due to absolute or relative lack of insulin.[73,74]

In other respects the treatment of myocardial infarction in patients with diabetes should be the same as in those without, responses to thrombolytic therapy and the benefits of secondary prevention being similar in the two groups. The Thrombolysis and Angioplasty in Myocardial Infarction (TAMI) investigators, for example, reported that patency rates of the infarct-related artery 90 minutes after thrombolytic therapy were almost identical in patients with and without diabetes (Fig. 9.14).[62] Similarly, diabetes does not appear to affect the benefits of aspirin,[39] nor that of beta blockers (Fig. 9.15)[75] and statins which provide protection against recurrent infarction and death comparable to that seen in patients

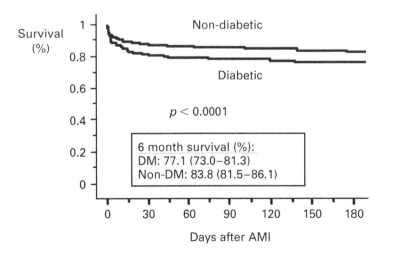

Figure 9.12
Six-month survival after AMI in diabetic and non-diabetic groups (n = 1829). (Data from NGH CCU database.)

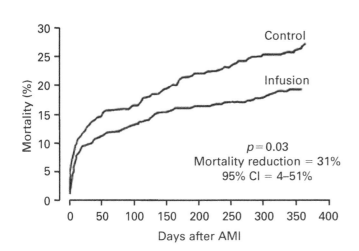

$p = 0.03$
Mortality reduction = 31%
95% CI = 4–51%

Figure 9.13
*DIGAMI study: insulin glucose infusion followed by subcutaneous insulin in AMI (n = 620). Reproduced with permission by Malmberg et al J Am Coll Cardiol 1995; **26**: 57–65.*[71]

	Diabetes (*n* = 148)	No Diabetes (*n* = 923)	P
LV ejection fraction (%)	48.8±12.3	51.3±11.8	ns
Regional LV function (SD/chord)			
infarct zone	−2.7±1.0	−2.5±1.1	0.15
non-infarct zone	−0.13±1.8	0.32±1.7	0.02
Extent of CAD			
0–1 vessel (%)	34	54	
multivessel (%)	66	46	<0.001
Segments per pt with ≥ 25% stenosis	3.4±2.0	2.9±1.8	<0.002
Patency of IRCA 90 mins after t'lysis (%)	71	70	ns

Figure 9.14
TAMI trials: angiographic responses to thrombolytic therapy in AMI (n = 1071).

without diabetes (see Fig. 9.6).[32] ACE inhibitors, in particular, have a special role and should be given to all diabetic patients with acute myocardial infarction, not only because of the heightened risk of left ventricular failure, for which these drugs are of proven benefit, but also because of the protection they afford against microvascular complications (see earlier).

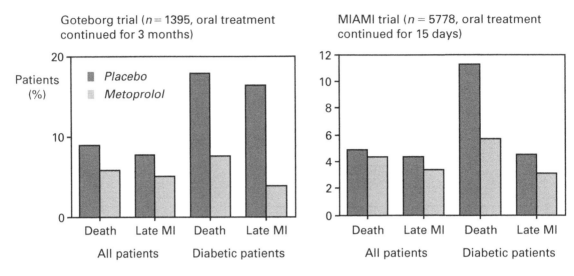

Figure 9.15
Goteborg and MIAMI trials of IV Metoprolol in AMI: comparison of diabetic and non-diabetic patients. Reproduced with permission from Malmberg et al, Eur Heart J *1989;* **10***: 423–8.*[75]

Sudden death in diabetes

Patients with diabetes are at increased risk of sudden death, and this is not always attributable to complications of plaque events.[76,77] There is considerable evidence that autonomic neuropathy plays an important pathophysiological role, through prolongation of QT interval and selective reductions in vagal function (increasing sympathetic activity), both of which may increase susceptibility to lethal arrhythmias.[78–80] In addition, altered perception of ischaemic cardiac pain may deprive diabetic patients of the signal to stop exercising allowing ischaemia to intensify to the point that arrhythmias are triggered (Fig. 9.16).[81] Alterations in pain perception may also prevent the diabetic patient from seeking medical attention in the event of acute coronary syndromes or lead to inappropriate triage decisions in the emergency room such that access to defibrillators is denied and specific

treatment delayed.[82] This emphasizes the importance of retaining low diagnostic thresholds for coronary heart disease in the diabetic patient presenting with atypical symptoms. It also emphasizes the importance of strict glycaemic control in diabetes although whether this indeed protects against neuropathy is unclear.

Heart failure in diabetes (Table 9.5)

Over 20 years ago, the Framingham investigators reported that the annual incidence of heart failure in diabetic men and women was substantially greater across all age groups than in non-diabetic individuals, even after controlling for underlying coronary and rheumatic heart disease (Fig. 9.17).[83] They concluded that diabetes itself might predispose to heart failure independently of concurrent coronary

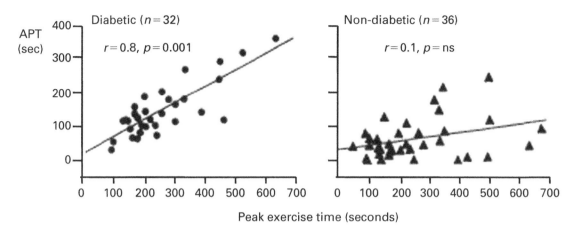

Figure 9.16
*Anginal perceptual threshold and exercise tolerance in diabetic and non-diabetic pts with CAD.
Reproduced with permission from Ranjadayalan et al, J Am Coll Cardiol 1990; 16: 1120–4.[81]*

or rheumatic heart disease. At about the same time post-mortem reports appeared in diabetics with heart failure describing normal coronary arteries and heart valves.[84] Histology, however, may reveal a range of abnormalities including myocyte hypertrophy, interstitial fibrosis, increased PAS-positive material and intramyocardial microangiopathy.[85] These are largely indistinguishable from changes found in hypertensive left ventricular disease and

emphasize the importance of effective anti-hypertensive therapy as reported in UKPDS.[25] In further studies, analysis of systolic time intervals provided evidence of both systolic and diastolic left ventricular dysfunction in diabetic individuals in whom there was no clinical evidence of coronary artery disease.[86] Taken together these epidemiological, pathological and haemodynamic data provide the evidence-base for diabetes-specific myocardial

Pathological evidence
- 1972 – post mortems in diabetics with CCF: myocyte hypertrophy, interstitial fibrosis, increased PAS-positive material and intramyocardial microangiopathy
- Depletion of myocardial catecholamines

Epidemiological evidence
- ↑ Risk of CCF in diabetes, not all explained by CHD
- Diabetics with CAD more likely to be hospitalized with CCF than non-diabetics (SOLVD)

Haemodynamic evidence
- Non-invasive evidence of systolic and diastolic dysfunction

Table 9.5
Evidence for diabetic cardiomyopathy

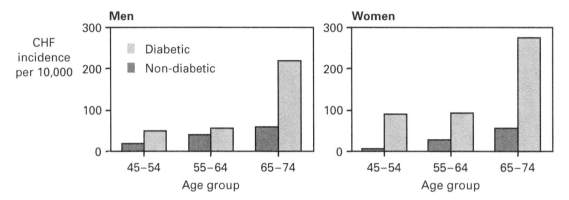

Figure 9.17
*Annual incidence of heart failure in Framingham population in diabetic and non-diabetic individuals (prevalence of antecedent coronary or rheumatic heart disease was almost identical in diabetics and non-diabetics). Reproduced with permission from Kannel et al, Am J Cardiol 1974; **34**: 29–34.*[83]

disease, commonly called "diabetic cardio-myopathy". The pathogenesis is unclear, although possible mechanisms include the synergistic impact of hypertension plus chronic derangement of myocardial metabolism, with increased free fatty acid oxidation and decreased glucose utilization.[87]

While the existence and clinical importance of diabetic cardiomyopathy is fairly well established, it must be emphasized that coronary heart disease is considerably more important as a cause of heart failure in the patient with diabetes. Certainly some of the epidemiological data summarized above may have been distorted by co-existing but asymptomatic coronary heart disease and the pathological data do not rule out the possibility of cardiomyopathy as a coincidental diagnosis or as a response to hypertension. In practical terms, however, the distinction is largely unimpor-

tant, except insofar as it affects revascularization decisions, since treatment strategies are unaffected and are the same as for non-diabetic patients with heart failure. Thus, control of provocative factors, particularly arrhythmias and hypertension, remains essential and conventional treatment should be applied for correcting fluid retention, increasing exercise capacity and improving prognosis. Diuretics may adversely influence metabolic control in diabetes but are mandatory for symptomatic treatment, while the efficacy of ACE-inhibition is undiminished, judging by subgroup analyses of the Studies Of Left Ventricular Dysfunction (SOLVD) prevention and treatment trials.[88,89] Beta-blockers too are recommended although this is based on generalization from randomized trials rather than specific data for patients with diabetes.

References

1. Bierman EL. Atherogenesis in diabetes. *Atheroscler Thromb* 1992; **12**: 647–56.
2. Kannel WB, McGee DL. Diabetes and cardiovascular risk factors: the Framingham Study. *Circulation* 1979; **59**: 8–13.
3. Stamler J, Vaccaro O, Neaton J et al. Diabetes, other risk factors, and 12-yr cardiovascular mortality for men screened in the Multiple Risk Factor Intervention Trial. *Diabetes Care* 1993; **16**: 434–44.
4. Klein R. Hyperglycemia and microvascular and macrovascular disease in diabetes. *Diabetes Care* 1995; **18**: 258–68.
5. Haffner SM, Stern MP, Hazuda HP, Mitchell BD, Patterson JK. Cardiovascular risk factors in confirmed prediabetic individuals: does the clock for coronary heart disease start ticking before the onset of clinical diabetes? *JAMA* 1990; **263**: 2893–8.
6. Chappey O, Dosquet C, Wautier M-P, Wautier JL. Advanced glycation end products, oxidant stress and vascular lesions. *Eur J Clin Invest* 1997; **27**: 97–108.
7. Yan SD, Stern D, Schmidt AM. What's the RAGE? The receptor for advanced glycation end products (RAGE) and the dark side of glucose. *Eur J Clin Invest* 1997; **27**: 179–81.
8. Park L, Raman KG, Lee KJ et al. Suppression of accelerated diabetic atherosclerosis by the soluble receptor for advanced glycation endproducts. *Nat Med* 1998; **4**: 1025–31.
9. Reaven GM. Role of insulin resistance in human disease. *Diabetes* 1988; **37**: 1595–607.
10. Hsueh WA, Law RE. Cardiovascular risk continuum: implications of insulin resistance and diabetes. *Am J Med* 1998; **105**: 4S–14S.
11. Wingard DL, Barret-Connor EL, Ferrara A. Is insulin really a heart disease risk factor? *Diabetes Care* 1995; **18**: 1299–304.
12. Ruige JB, Assendelft WJJ, Dekker JM et al. Insulin and risk of cardiovascular disease: a meta-analysis. *Circulation* 1998; **97**: 996–1001.
13. Howard G, O'Leary DH, Zaccaro D et al. Insulin sensitivity and atherosclerosis. The Insulin Resistance Atherosclerosis Study (IRAS) Investigators. *Circulation* 1996; **93**: 1809–17.
14. Kreisberg RA. Diabetic dyslipidemia. *Am J Cardiol* 1998; **82**: 67U–73U.
15. Haffner SM. Diabetes, hyperlipidemia, and coronary artery disease. *Am J Cardiol* 1999; **83**: 17F–21F.
16. Feher MD, Elkeles RS. Lipid modification and coronary heart disease in type 2 diabetes: different from the general population. *Heart* 1999; **81**: 10–11.
17. Hokanson JE, Austin MA. Plasma triglyceride level is a risk factor for cardiovascular disease independent of high density lipoprotein cholesterol level: a meta-analysis of population-based prospective studies. *J Cardiovasc Risk* 1996; **3**: 213–19.
18. Davi G, Ciabottoni G, Consoli A, Messetti A, Falco A, Santarone S et al. In vivo formation of 8-iso-prostaglandin F2a and platelet activation in diabetes mellitus: effects of improved metabolic control. *Circulation* 1999; **99**: 224–9.
19. Fuller JH, Shipley MJ, Rose G, Jarrett RJ, Keen H. Mortality from coronary heart disease and stroke in relation to degree of glycaemia: the Whitehall study. *BMJ* 1983; **287**: 867–70.
20. Wood D, De Backer G, Faergeman O, Graham I, Mancia G, Neil A, Orth-Gomer K, Pyorala K. *Clinician's Manual on Total Risk Management.* London: Science Press, 2000.
21. Hypertension in Diabetes Study Group, HDS. 1: Prevalence of hypertension in newly presenting type 2 diabetic patients and the association with risk factors for cardiovascular and diabetic complications. *J Hypertens* 1993; **11**: 309–17.
22. Hypertension in Diabetes Study Group, HDS. 2: Increased risk of cardiovascular complications in hypertensive type 2 diabetic patients. *J Hypertens* 1993; **11**: 319–25.
23. United Kingdom Prospective Diabetes Study (UKPDS) Group. Risk factors for coronary

artery disease in non-insulin dependent diabetes (UKPDS 23). *BMJ* 1998; **316**: 823–8.

24. United Kingdom Prospective Diabetes Study (UKPDS) Group. Diabetic retinopathy at diagnosis of type 2 diabetes and associated risk factors (UKPDS 30). *Arch Ophthalmol* 1998; **116**: 297–303.

25. United Kingdom Prospective Diabetes Study (UKPDS) Group. Tight blood pressure control and risk of macrovascular and microvascular complications in type 2 diabetes (UKPDS 38). *BMJ* 1998; **317**: 703–13.

26. Hansson L, Zanchetti A, Carruthers SG et al. Effects of intensive blood pressure lowering and low-dose aspirin in patients with hypertension: principal results of the Hypertension optimal treatment (HOT) randomised trial. *Lancet* 1998; **352**: 1252–68.

27. Wood DA et al. Joint British recommendations on prevention of coronary heart disease in clinical practice. *Heart* 1998; **80** (Suppl 2): 1–26.

28. Lewis EJ, Hunsicker LG, Bain RP, Rohde RD. The effect of angiotensin-converting-enzyme inhibition on diabetic nephropathy. *N Engl J Med* 1993; **329**: 1456–62.

29. Kasiske BL, Kalil RSN, Ma JZ, Liao M, Keane WK. Effect of antihypertensive therapy on the kidneys in patients with diabetes: a metaregression analysis. *Ann Intern Med* 1993; **118**: 129–38.

30. United Kingdom Prospective Diabetes Study (UKPDS) Group. Efficacy of atenolol and captopril in reducing risk of macrovascular and microvascular complications in type 2 diabetes (UKPDS 39). *BMJ* 1998; **317**: 713–20.

31. Koskinen P, Manttari M, Manninen V et al. Coronary heart disease incidence in NIDDM patients in the Helsinki Heart Study. *Diabetes Care* 1992; **15**: 820–5.

32. Pyorala K, Pederson T, Kjekshus J et al, and the Scandinavian Simvastatin Survival Study (4S) Group. Cholesterol lowering with simvastatin improves prognosis of diabetic patients with coronary heart disease: a subgroup analysis of the Scandinavian Simvastatin Survival Study (4S). *Diabetes Care* 1997; **20**: 614–20.

33. Sacks FM, Pfeffer MA, Moye LA et al. The effect of pravastatin on coronary events after myocardial infarction in patients with average cholesterol levels. *N Engl J Med* 1996; **335**: 1001–9.

34. Long-term Intervention with Pravastatin in Ischaemic Disease (LIPID) Study Group. Prevention of cardiovascular events and death with pravastatin in patients with coronary heart disease and a broad range of initial cholesterol levels. *N Engl J Med* 1998; **339**: 1349–57.

35. Moss SE, Klein R, Klein BEK et al. The association of glycemia and cause-specific mortality in a diabetic population. *Arch Intern Med* 1994; **154**: 2473–9.

36. Gaster B, Hirsch IB. The effects of improved glycemic control on complications in type 2 diabetes. *Arch Intern Med* 1998; **158**: 134–40.

37. United Kingdom Prospective Diabetes Study (UKPDS) Group. Intensive blood-glucose control with sulphonylureas or insulin compared with conventional treatment and risk of complications in patients with type 2 diabetes (UKPDS 33). *Lancet* 1998; **352**: 837–53.

38. United Kingdom Prospective Diabetes Study (UKPDS) Group. Association of glycaemia with macrovascular and microvascular complications of type 2 diabetes (UKPDS 35). *BMJ* 2000; **321**: 405–12.

39. Antiplatelet Trialists' Collaboration. Collaborative overview of randomised trials of antiplatelet therapy – 1: prevention of death, myocardial infarction, and stroke by prolonged antiplatelet therapy in various categories of patients. *BMJ* 1994; **308**: 81–106.

40. Marso SP, Lincoff AM, Ellis SG, Bhatt DL, Tanguay JF, Kleiman NS et al. Optimizing the percutaneous interventional outcomes for patients with diabetes mellitus: results of the EPISTENT (Evaluation of platelet IIb/IIIa inhibitor for stenting trial) diabetic substudy. *Circulation* 1999; **100**: 2477–84.

41. Chobanian AV, Haudenschild CC, Nickerson C, Drago R. Anti-atherogenic effect of captopril in the Watanabe heritable hyperlipidaemic rabbit. *Hypertension* 1990; **15**: 327–31.

42. Aberg G, Ferrer P. Effects of captopril on atherosclerosis in Cynomolgus monkeys. *J Cardiovasc Pharmacol* 1990; **15** (Suppl): S65–S72.

43. Rolland PH, Charpiot P, Friggi A et al. Effects of angiotensin-converting enzyme inhibition with perindolol on hemodynamics, arterial structures, and wall rheology in the hindquar-

ters of atherosclerotic mini-pigs. *Am J Cardiol* 1993; **71**: 22E–27E.

44. Mancini GB, Henry GC, Macaya C, O'Neill BJ, Pucillo AL, Carere RG, Wargovich TJ, Mudra H, Luscher TF, Klibaner MI, Haber HE, Uprichard AC, Pepine CJ, Pitt B. Angiotensin-converting enzyme inhibition with quinapril improves endothelial vasomotor dysfunction in patients with coronary artery disease. The TREND (Trial on Reversing ENdothelial Dysfunction) Study. *Circulation* 1996; **94**: 258–65.

45. Yusuf S, Sleight P, Pogue J, Bosch J, Davies R, Dagenais G, for The Heart Outcomes Prevention Evaluation (HOPE) Study Investigators. Effects of an angiotensin-converting-enzyme inhibitor, ramipril, on cardiovascular events in high-risk patients. *N Engl J Med* 2000; **342**: 145–53.

46. Heart Outcomes Prevention Evaluation (HOPE) Study Investigators. Effects of ramipril on cardiovascular and microvascular outcomes in people with diabetes mellitus: result of HOPE study and MICRO-HOPE substudy. *Lancet* 2000; **355**: 253–9.

47. Enos WF, Holmes RH, Beyer J. Coronary disease among United States soldiers killed in action in Korea: preliminary report. *JAMA* 1953; **152**: 1090–3.

48. McGill HC Jr, McMahan A, Zieske AW, Tracy RE, Malcom GT, Herderick EE, Strong JP. Association of coronary heart disease risk factors with microscopic qualities of coronary atherosclerosis in youth. *Circulation* 2000; **102**: 374–9.

49. Haffner SM, Lehto S, Ronnemoa T et al. Mortality from coronary heart disease in subjects with type 2 diabetes and in nondiabetic subjects with and without prior myocardial infarction. *N Engl J Med* 1998; **339**: 229–34.

50. Glagov S, Weisenberg E, Zarins CK et al. Compensatory enlargement of human atherosclerotic coronary arteries. *N Engl J Med* 1987; **316**: 1371–5.

51. Ambepityia G, Kopelman PG, Ingram D, Swash M, Mills PG, Timmis AD. Exertional myocardial ischemia in diabetes: a quantitative analysis of anginal perceptual threshold and the influence of autonomic function. *J Am Coll Cardiol* 1990; **15**: 72–7.

52. Nesto R, Phillips R, Kett K et al. Angina and exertional myocardial ischemia in diabetic and non-diabetic patients: assessment by exercise thallium scintigraphy. *Ann Intern Med* 1988; **108**: 170–5.

53. Sayer JW, Timmis AD. Investigation of coronary artery disease in diabetes; is screening of asymptomatic patients necessary? *Heart* 1997; **78**: 525–6.

54. Nesto RW. Screening for asymptomatic coronary artery disease in diabetes. *Diabetes Care* 1999; **22**: 1393–5.

55. Janand-Delenne B, Savin B, Habib G, Bory M, Vague P, Lassman-Vague V. Silent myocardial ischemia in patients with diabetes: who to screen? *Diabetes Care* 1999; **22**: 1396–400.

56. Milan Study on Atherosclerosis and Diabetes (MiSAD) Group. Prevalence of unrecognised silent myocardial ischemia and its association with atherosclerotic risk factors in non insulin-dependent diabetes mellitus. *Am J Cardiol* 1997; **79**: 134–9.

57. Koistinen MJ. Prevalence of asymptomatic myocardial ischaemia in diabetic subjects. *BMJ* 1990; **301**: 92–5.

58. Manske CL, Wilson RF, Wang Y, Thomas W. Atherosclerotic vascular complications in diabetic transplant candidates. *Am J Kidney Dis* 1997; **29**: 601–7.

59. Nesto RW, Watson FS, Kowalchuk GJ, Zarich SW, Hill T, Lewis SM, Lane SE. Silent myocardial ischemia and infarction in diabetics with peripheral vascular disease: assessment by dipyridamole thallium-201 scintigraphy. *Am Heart J* 1990; **120**: 1073–7.

60. Younis LT, Miller DD, Chaitman BR. Preoperative strategies to assess cardiac risk before noncardiac surgery. *Clin Cardiol* 1995; **18**: 447–54.

61. Waller BF, Palumbo PJ, Roberts WC. Status of the coronary arteries at necropsy in diabetes mellitus with onset after age 30 years. *Am J Med* 1980; **69**: 498–506.

62. Granger CB, Califf RM, Young S, Candela R, Samaha J, Worley S, Kereiakes DJ, Topol EJ, and The Thrombolysis and Angioplasty in Myocardial Infarction (TAMI) Study Group. Outcome of patients with diabetes mellitus and acute myocardial infarction treated with thrombolytic agents. *J Am Coll Cardiol* 1993; **21**: 920–5.

63. Adler DS, Goldman L, O'Neil A et al. Long-term survival of more than 2,000 patients after coronary artery bypass grafting. *Am J Cardiol* 1986; **58**: 195–202.

64. Carrozza JP, Kuntz RE, Fishman RF, Baim DS. Restenosis after arterial injury caused by coronary stenting in patients with diabetes mellitus. *Ann Intern Med* 1993; **118**: 344–9.

65. The Bypass Angioplasty Revascularization Investigation (BARI) Investigators. Comparison of coronary bypass surgery with angioplasty in patients with multivessel disease. *N Engl J Med* 1996; **335**: 217–25.

66. Jacoby RM, Nesto RW. Acute myocardial infarction in the diabetic patient: pathophysiology, clinical course and prognosis. *J Am Coll Cardiol* 1992; **20**: 736–44.

67. Sayer JW, Archbold RA, Wilkinson P, Ray S, Ranjadayalan K, Timmis AD. Prognostic implications of ventricular fibrillation in acute myocardial infarction: new strategies required for further mortality reduction. *Heart* 2000; **84**: 258–61.

68. Uretsky BF, Farquhar D, Berezin A, Hood W. Symptomatic myocardial infarction without chest pain: prevalence and clinical course. *Am J Cardiol* 1977; **40**: 498–503.

69. Sayer JW, Wilkinson P, Ranjadayalan K, Ray S, Marchant B, Timmis AD. Attenuation or absence of circadian and seasonal rhythms of acute myocardial infarction. *Heart* 1997; **77**: 325–9.

70. Stevenson R, Ranjadayalan K, Wilkinson P, Roberts R, Timmis AD. Short and long term prognosis of acute myocardial infarction since introduction of thrombolysis. *BMJ* 1993; **307**: 349–53.

71. Malmberg K, Ryden L, Efendic S et al. for the Diabetes Mellitus, Insulin Glucose Infusion in Acute Myocardial Infarction (DIGAMI) Study Group. Randomized trial of insulin-glucose infusion followed by subcutaneous insulin treatment in diabetic patients with acute myocardial infarction: effects on mortality at 1 year. *J Am Coll Cardiol* 1995; **26**: 57–65.

72. Sasso FC, Carbonara O, Cozzolino D, Rambaldi P, Mansi L, Torella D et al. Effects of insulin-glucose infusion on left ventricular function at rest and during dynamic exercise in healthy subjects and noninsulin dependent dia-betic patients: a radionuclide ventriculographic study. *J Am Coll Cardiol* 2000; **36**: 219–26.

73. Opie LH. Glucose and the metabolism of ischaemic myocardium. *Lancet* 1995; **345**: 1520–1.

74. McGuire DK, Granger CB. Diabetes and ischemic heart disease. *Am Heart J* 1999; **138**: S336–S375.

75. Malmberg K, Herlitz J, Hjalmarson A, Ryden L. Effects of metoprolol on mortality and late infarction in diabetics with suspected acute myocardial infarction. Retrospective data from two large studies. *Eur Heart J* 1989; **10**: 423–8.

76. Watkins P, Mackay J. Cardiac denervation in diabetic neuropathy. *Ann Intern Med* 1980; **92**: 304–7.

77. Ewing D, Campbell I, Clarke B. Assessment of cardiovascular effects in diabetic autonomic neuropathy and prognostic implications. *Ann Intern Med* 1980; **92**: 308–11.

78. Bellavere F, Ferri M, Guarini L et al. Prolonged QT period in diabetic autonomic neuropathy: a possible role in sudden cardiac death? *Br Heart J* 1988; **59**: 379–83.

79. Ewing D, Boland O, Neilson J, Cho C, Clarke B. Autonomic neuropathy, QT interval lengthening, and unexpected deaths in male diabetic patients. *Diabetologia* 1991; **34**: 182–5.

80. Marchant B, Umachandran V, Stevenson R, Kopelman PG, Timmis AD. Silent myocardial ischaemia: the role of subclinical neuropathy in patients with and without diabetes. *J Am Coll Cardiol* 1993; **22**: 1433–7.

81. Ranjadayalan K, Umachandran V, Ambepityia G, Kopelman PG, Mills PG, Timmis AD. Prolonged anginal perceptual threshold in diabetes: effects on exercise capacity and myocardial ischemia. *J Am Coll Cardiol* 1990; **16**: 1120–4.

82. Soler N, Bennet M, Pentecost B, Fitzgerald M, Malins J. Myocardial infarction in diabetics. *Q J Med* 1975; **173**: 125–32.

83. Kannel WB, Hjortland M, Castelli WP. Role of diabetes in congestive heart failure: The Framingham Study. *Am J Cardiol* 1974; **34**: 29–34.

84. Rubler S, Dlugash J, Yucheology Y. New types of cardiomyopathy associated with diabetic glomerulosclerosis. *Am J Cardiol* 1972; **30**: 595–60.

85. Hardin N. The myocardial and vascular pathology of diabetic cardiomyopathy. *Coron Artery Dis* 1996; **17**: 99–108.

86. Zarich S, Nesto R. Diabetic cardiomyopathy. *Am Heart J* 1989; **118**: 1000–5.

87. Solang L, Malmberg K, Ryden L. Diabetes mellitus and congestive heart failure: further knowledge needed. *Eur Heart J* 1998; **20**: 789–95.

88. The Studies Of Left Ventricular Dysfunction (SOLVD) Investigators. Effect of enalapril on survival in patients with reduced left ventricular ejection fractions and congestive heart failure. *N Engl J Med* 1991; **325**: 293–302.

89. The Studies Of Left Ventricular Dysfunction (SOLVD) Investigators. Effect of enalapril on mortality and the development of heart failure in asymptomatic patients with reduced left ventricular ejection fractions. *N Engl J Med* 1992; **327**: 685–91.

10

Diabetic cardiomyopathy

Bryan Williams, Suhkbinder Bassi and David O'Brien

Introduction

Diabetes mellitus is associated with an increased prevalence of congestive heart failure (CHF), which is a major cause of morbidity and mortality.[1] This observation raised the spectre of a specific diabetes-associated cardiac disease that manifests as heart failure, independent of coronary heart disease or valvular disease – a diabetic cardiomyopathy. This concept has been supported by a series of reports describing heart failure in patients with diabetes that is associated with characteristic (although not specific) cardiac structural and functional changes, characteristic histopathological changes in the myocardium and a range of less well characterized biochemical disturbances in cardiac muscle. This has prompted debate as to whether 'diabetic cardiomyopathy' is a specific pathological entity, or a spectrum of changes representing a predictable cardiac structural and functional response to elevated systemic blood pressure, 'silent myocardial ischaemia' and disturbances to the metabolic milieu.[2] The debate surrounding this important clinical complication of diabetes has been fuelled by numerous studies reporting findings in small numbers of patients that are often poorly characterized, particularly with regard to their blood pressure. Thus, apart from a few exceptions, the debate has been hindered by a remarkable lack of firm evidence or systematic detailed study of the heart beyond coronary disease in people

with diabetes. This chapter reviews the current evidence supporting the concept of a specific diabetic cardiomyopathy from an epidemiological, cardiac structural, functional, histological and biochemical perspective.

Epidemiological support for diabetic cardiomyopathy

The most commonly cited evidence in favour of the existence of a diabetic cardiomyopathy is the epidemiological observation of an increased incidence of heart failure among people with diabetes without clinically overt coronary heart disease.[1] Rubler et al.[3] first raised suspicions in 1972 when they reported post-mortem findings in four patients with diabetic nephropathy who had presented with cardiomegaly and CHF, in the absence of atherosclerotic, valvular, congenital, hypertensive or alcoholic heart disease. Herein lies one of the problems with the database in this debate – the small numbers of patients and the unlikelihood that any of the four patients with diabetic nephropathy were 'normotensive'. Soon afterwards, Hamby et al. noted a high incidence of diabetes (22%) among a series of 73 patients with idiopathic cardiomyopathy and normal coronary angiograms.[4] This compared with only 11% of people in an age- and sex-matched cohort of people without cardiomyopathy. More definitive evidence for a direct association between diabetes and the likelihood of developing CHF was provided by the Framingham Heart Study. A follow-up of 5000 people over 18 years revealed that in a cohort of people with diabetes (~10% of the total study group), the annual incidence of heart failure in people with diabetes mellitus was two-fold greater in diabetic men.[5] The age-adjusted risk was even worse in women at over five-fold excess (Fig. 10.1). Increased levels of risk persisted after adjustment for factors relevant to the development of CHF, i.e. age, hypertension and obesity, hypercholesterolaemia and coronary heart disease. This association between diabetes and increased CHF risk, which did not appear to be accounted for by conventional risk factors for CHF, provided strong circumstantial evidence for the existence of a diabetes-specific cardiomyopathy.

Cardiac structural and functional disturbances in diabetes

Left ventricular hypertrophy (LVH) is a major risk factor for morbidity and mortality and the Framingham Heart Study has previously reported that left ventricular wall thickness and mass were disproportionately increased in people with diabetes when compared with people without diabetes.[6] This appeared to be true independent of conventional risk factors for LVH in women but not men. More recently, these observations were extended by a much more comprehensive and definitive study of cardiac structure and function in people with diabetes – the Strong Heart Study.[7] This is a study of cardiovascular risk factors in American Indians. It is important in that almost all previous studies have focused on predominantly white populations with diabetes, whereas diabetes is more common in other ethnic groups. Echocardiography was performed in 1810 people with diabetes and 944 with normal glucose tolerance. When the data were adjusted for all co-variates likely to influence left ventricular wall thickness and mass, both men and women with diabetes had higher left ventricular mass and wall thicknesses. There were also significant functional disturbances in the hearts of people with diabetes, notably, lower left ventricular fractional shortening, mid-wall shortening and stress-corrected mid-wall shortening. These abnor-

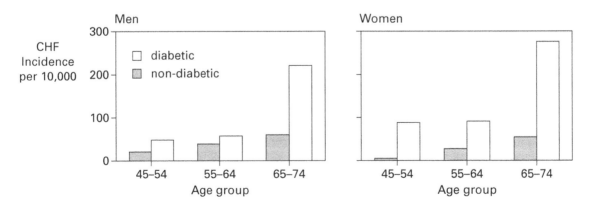

Figure 10.1
Incidence of congestive cardiac failure comparing men and women with and without diabetes. (From reference 5.)

malities in contractility indices are consistent with cardiac disease and have been shown previously to have adverse cardiovascular prognostic significance in hypertensive people without diabetes.[8]

In the Strong Heart Study, diabetes was also associated with a higher cardiac output, lower peripheral resistance and an especially high pulse pressure/stroke volume index, which is indicative of increased arterial stiffness. This index of arterial stiffness was increased by ~12% in men and women with diabetes and was largely accounted for by an increased pulse pressure (mean + 7 mmHg) in people with diabetes. This observation supports the hypothesis presented in Chapter 00 and raises the important question as to whether increased arterial stiffness and its

impact on central arterial pressure may be a major driver of the increased LV mass indices in diabetes.

The data from the Strong Heart Study provide the most comprehensive evidence to date showing disturbances in cardiac structure and function in diabetes that no doubt ante-date the development of clinical heart failure.[7] Previous studies have highlighted characteristic functional disturbances in the diabetic heart. In 1966, Karlefors noted that asymptomatic diabetic men had a lower cardiac output during supine exercise compared with matched controls.[9] Subsequent studies in recently diagnosed type 1 diabetic patients noted lower stroke volumes during exercise than controls, with cardiac output being maintained by a higher heart rate.[10] These abnormalities

Parameter	DM patients (n = 1227)	Glucose-tolerant subjects (n = 478)	p
IVS (cm)	0.95 ± 0.13	0.87 ± 0.11	<0.0001
LVID (cm)	4.85 ± 0.48	4.81 ± 0.42	NS
PWT (cm)	0.87 ± 0.10	0.82 ± 0.09	<0.0001
LV mass (g)	155 ± 40	138 ± 32	<0.0001
LV mass/BSA (g/m^2)	85 ± 21	78 ± 16	<0.0001
LV mass/height (g/m$^{2.7}$)	44.6 ± 11.5	39.2 ± 9.6	<0.0001
LV mass/fat-free mass (g/kg)	3.3 ± 0.8	3.1 ± 0.7	<0.001
Relative wall thickness	0.36 ± 0.05	0.34 ± 0.04	<0.0001
Fractional shortening (%)	35 ± 6	36 ± 5	0.008
Mid-wall shortening (%)	17.3 ± 2.5	18.4 ± 2.1	<0.0001
Stress-corrected mid-wall shortening (% predicted)	103 ± 13	108 ± 11	<0.0001
Cardiac index (l/min/m^2)	2.56 ± 0.57	2.47 ± 0.56	0.01
Peripheral resistance (dyne/s/cm^5)	1716 ± 495	1790 ± 461	0.004
Pulse pressure/stroke volume (mmHg/ml)	0.92 ± 0.41	0.81 ± 0.29	<0.0001

IVS, intraventricular septal thickness; LVID, left ventricular internal dimension; PWT, posterior wall thickness; BSA, body surface area; NS, not significant. Values are mean $\pm$ SD. (Adapted from reference 7.)

Table 10.1
Left ventricular and haemodynamic indices of diabetic and non-diabetic women from the Strong Heart Study

Parameter	DM patients (n = 583)	Glucose-tolerant subjects (n = 466)	p
IVS	0.98 ± 0.14	0.92 ± 0.10	<0.0001
LVID	5.22 ± 0.55	5.19 ± 0.48	NS
PWT	0.90 ± 0.10	0.86 ± 0.08	<0.0001
LV mass (g)	183 ± 44	167 ± 35	<0.0001
LV mass/BSA (g/m^2)	89 ± 22	84 ± 17	0.001
LV mass/height (g/m$^{2.7}$)	42.4 ± 11.0	37.7 ± 8.1	<0.0001
LV mass/fat-free mass (g/kg)	2.85 ± 0.70	2.76 ± 0.59	NS
Relative wall thickness	0.35 ± 0.05	0.33 ± 0.04	<0.0001
Fractional shortening (%)	32 ± 7	33 ± 6	0.001
Mid-wall shortening (%)	16.2 ± 2.9	17.3 ± 2.3	<0.0001
Stress-corrected mid-wall shortening (% predicted)	99 ± 15	104 ± 13	<0.0001
Cardiac index (l/min/m^2)	2.49 ± 0.60	2.43 ± 0.58	NS
Total peripheral resistance (dyne/s/cm^5)	1622 ± 418	1666 ± 512	NS
Pulse pressure/stroke volume (mmHg/ml)	0.77 ± 0.30	0.68 ± 0.27	<0.0001

IVS, intraventricular septal thickness; LVID, left ventricular internal dimension; PWT, posterior wall thickness; BSA, body surface area; NS, not significant. Values are mean ± SD. (Adapted from reference 7.)

Table 10.2
Left ventricular and haemodynamic indices of diabetic and non-diabetic women from the Strong Heart Study

appeared to be reversed after treatment with insulin for 1 year. These findings were obtained in diabetic populations who were free from major coronary vessel disease. Subsequent studies pointed to the fact that microangiopathy may play a role in the development of cardiac dysfunction. Left ventricular dysfunction was found to be commonly associated with clinical microangiopathy.[11-13]

Early in the disease process, systolic time intervals, especially the pre-ejection period/left ventricular ejection time, were frequently found to be abnormal, reflecting decreased contractility and/or a reduced diastolic volume.[11,14,15] Later studies utilizing M-mode echocardiography confirmed the presence of left ventricular dysfunction with a prolongation of the isovolumic relaxation time and

slowing of ventricular filling. This disturbance was shown to be related to the duration of diabetes and was particularly common in the presence of microvascular disease, i.e. proteinuria and/or retinopathy.[11-17]

In subsequent radionucleotide studies of myocardial function in otherwise healthy people with diabetes, there was an impaired cardiac response to exercise, with a less than expected increase in ejection fraction in response to dynamic exercise, despite a normal resting ejection fraction.[18,19] These abnormalities were particularly common in those with microangiopathy or cardiac autonomic neuropathy. Moreover, those with overt hypertension were much more likely to have systolic dysfunction. These findings are consistent with those in the recent Strong Heart Study, which showed decreased contractility indices and reduced left ventricular chamber size, despite an increase in left ventricular mass indices, all of which are consistent with impaired systolic function.[7]

Diastolic function is impaired early in patients with diabetes. This reflects a reduction in left ventricular compliance. Doppler echocardiography studies have demonstrated ventricular asynergy and a subclinical state of diastolic dysfunction, with significantly lower E:A ratios in people with diabetes.[20–22] E and A areas are the components of the total velocity-time integral in the early passive phase of ventricular filling (E) and the late active period of ventricular filling due to atrial contraction (A). A low E:A ratio thus reflects reduced passive ventricular filling in diastole and an increased dependence on atrial contraction – this in turn reflects an increased LV stiffness and reduced left ventricular compliance (Fig. 10.2). These findings are also common in people with LVH due to hypertension without co-existing diabetes and suggest a potentially important role for hypertension in the genesis of early diastolic dysfunction in people with diabetes.

In summary, the current evidence suggests that the earliest manifestations of non-atherosclerotic diabetic heart disease are characterized by the early onset of diastolic dysfunction, with a preserved left ventricular ejection fraction. As the condition progresses, systolic dysfunction develops and becomes clinically dominant. These disturbances are initially detectable and produce symptoms mainly on exertion, but inexorably progress. There are associated changes in left ventricular structure that are characterized by a disproportionate increase in left ventricular wall thickness indices and mass and a reduction in left ventricular chamber size relative to the patient's age, sex, body mass and blood pres-

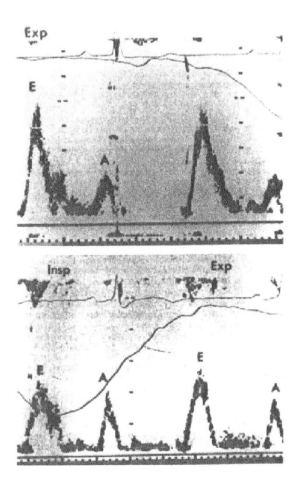

Figure 10.2
The top panel shows a normal transmitral Doppler echocardiogram obtained from an adolescent non-diabetic patient. Note that the early phase of ventricular filling (E-wave) is typically much greater than the late phase of ventricular filling (A-wave). The lower panel shows a similar study in an adolescent patient with diabetes. Note the smaller E-wave and the taller A-wave, consistent with a significantly reduced E:A ratio due to impaired diastolic filling in the patient with diabetes. (From reference 22.)

sure. These changes are more common in diabetic people with evidence of microangiopathy and/or autonomic dysfunction. These changes are also accelerated and greatly magnified in the presence of hypertension. Moreover, they are similar to the changes observed in non-diabetic patients developing LVH due to hypertension. This raises the question as to whether diabetic cardiomyopathy is an exaggerated manifestation of hypertensive heart disease in a population of patients uniquely susceptible to hypertensive cardiac injury.

Cardiac autonomic neuropathy

Autonomic dysfunction is very common in patients with diabetes. Although autonomic disturbances are not a specific feature of diabetic cardiomyopathy, they are relevant to the discussion of cardiomyopathy in that they compound the aforementioned disturbances in cardiac function by promoting a higher resting heart rate and they predispose to sudden cardiac death.

It has been suggested that autonomic dysfunction can be detected in at least 40% of patients by formal autonomic nervous system testing, even though only a few will have symptoms.[23] Autonomic dysfunction is more likely in those with clinical microangiopathy and/or left ventricular diastolic dysfunction.[18,19,24] The latter confirms the likelihood that most diabetic patients with clinical evidence of heart failure are likely to exhibit some evidence of autonomic dysfunction.

Diabetic patients with clinical evidence of autonomic dysfunction are at extremely high risk of sudden death, with a 5-year survival of only 44% compared with 85% in age- and sex-matched diabetic patients without clinical evidence of neuropathy.[19] This excess mortality is not explained by an excess of coronary events. Thus, the development of cardiac autonomic dysfunction is an ominous sign.[25–27]

Initially, early in the course of diabetes, car-diac autonomic neuropathy manifests as an abnormality on the cardiac baroreflex, which is a high gain control system of great importance in the moment-to-moment maintenance of arterial blood pressure, especially during orthostatic stress. With non-invasive techniques such as power spectral analysis of heart rate and blood pressure variability of the baroreceptor-cardiac reflex (a surrogate marker for cardiac autonomic function), studies in normotensive patients with type 1 diabetes have documented early disturbances of the sympathovagal balance in favour of an early decrease in vagal tone and a relative increase in sympathetic activity.[28] Disturbance to sympathetic pathways occurs later. These early subtle disturbances are demonstrable within a couple of years of onset of type 1 diabetes and are associated with an increase in left ventricular mass, reduced day-night heart rate variability, less day-night blood pressure differences, an increased 24 hour blood pressure load, prolonged QTc intervals and reduced baroreceptor cardiac reflex sensitivity.[29,30] It seems likely that the disturbances to baroreceptor function and attenuation of nocturnal blood pressure dipping contribute to the development of hypertension in people with diabetes and may thus be involved in the early pathogenesis of cardiac structural changes. This is important because such patients will often have a 'normal' office blood pressure and the potential role of disturbed blood pressure regulation in the pathogenesis of cardiac structural and functional change will be under-estimated.

Another feature of autonomic dysfunction is QTc prolongation at rest and during exercise on the ECG.[30–33] This is driven by the relative overactivity of the sympathetic nervous system and results in a substantially increased risk of fatal ventricular arrhythmias and sudden cardiac death – the so-called 'dead in bed' syndrome reported in patients with type 1 diabetes.[32] To date, the importance of cardiac autonomic neuropathy with regard to morbidity and mortality in people with diabetes has not been formally evaluated. This is a significant omission where the opportunities for targeted therapeutic intervention designed to augment vagal tone and/or reduce sympathetic overactivity are considered.

Pathology of diabetic cardiomyopathy

The histological characteristics of the heart in patients with long-standing diabetes reveal many features that could potentially explain the functional disturbances noted above. Cardiac histology studies in humans have shown increased deposition of interstitial fibrosis – PAS-positive (periodic acid-Schiff) material comprising interstitial glycoproteins and collagens.[3,4] This is seen around blood vessels and penetrating between muscle cells, thereby disrupting the normal cardiac architecture. This is not necessarily uniform and islands of extensive fibrosis have been reported, which are thought to represent areas of myocytolysis.[34–38] These are surrounded by areas of myocyte hypertrophy. This pattern can be gross, resembling a peculiar nodularity of the myocardial architecture, not unlike the appearance of hepatic cirrhosis at low power[35] (Fig. 10.3). It is likely that the establishment of these changes plays a key role in the functional disturbances in the heart, i.e. diastolic dysfunction due to left ventricular wall stiffening. This is likely to be further compounded by the modification and abnormal cross-linking of interstitial collagens by advanced glycation end-products (AGEs) which form at an enhanced rate in people with diabetes.[39] Such cross-links greatly increase the functional stiffness of the interstitium and are likely to

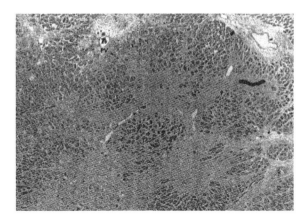

Figure 10.3

Histological section from the heart of a patient with hypertension and diabetes. Note the large areas of replacement fibrosis (R) surrounding islands of myocytes, which are also surrounded by interstitial fibrosis (IS). There is also extensive perivascular fibrosis (PV). (From reference 35.)

compound the effects of the increased interstitial fibrosis on diastolic and systolic function.

A detailed histological study of the hearts from non-diabetic hypertensive patients, normotensive diabetic patients and hypertensive diabetic patients aged 60–70 years at death has reported a spectrum of histological changes in the heart as indicated above, becoming progressively more severe as the diabetic patient develops hypertension.[35] In this report, even the 'normotensive' diabetic patients appeared to have greater heart weights and more histological damage than the non-diabetic patients without hypertension. However, caution is needed in interpreting such data. The definition of hypertension in 1990 was very different to that of today. Moreover, in post-mortem studies, the diagnosis of hypertension is made from the patient records and often hypertension was undiagnosed in life. In support of this conclusion, examination of the renal histology in the diabetic patients designated 'normotensive' in life revealed unequivocal evidence of vascular changes consistent with significant hypertension in a majority. Thus, it seems likely that those patients often designated 'normotensive' in earlier post-mortem studies of the heart were indeed hypertensive and the changes in the diabetic heart labelled as a specific diabetic cardiomyopathy look very much like the histology of severe hypertensive cardiomyopathy (Fig. 10.4).

In addition to changes in myocytes and increased interstitial fibrosis, there are also substantial vascular changes. There is a marked increase in perivascular fibrosis and also accumulation of PAS-positive material within the tunica media of small and medium-sized vessels. There is also hyalinization of ves-

sels without luminal narrowing.[3,35,39–43] These changes are likely to substantially impair the compliance of the coronary circulation (Fig. 10.5).

Microvascular disease has also been documented in the hearts of patients with diabetes.[44–46] These vascular changes in the microcirculation of the heart are very similar to those documented in the retina and glomerular circulations.[44–49] These changes comprise proliferation and thickening of the capillary basement membrane along with the formation of capillary microaneurysms.[45] The latter may either be saccular (Fig. 10.6) or fusiform and are often associated with kinking or irregularities in the diameter of the capillary wall pre- and/or post-aneurysmal dilatation. The functional significance of these aneurysms in the heart is unknown, as is their relationship to microvascular disease in other organs. For example, can we assume that in patients

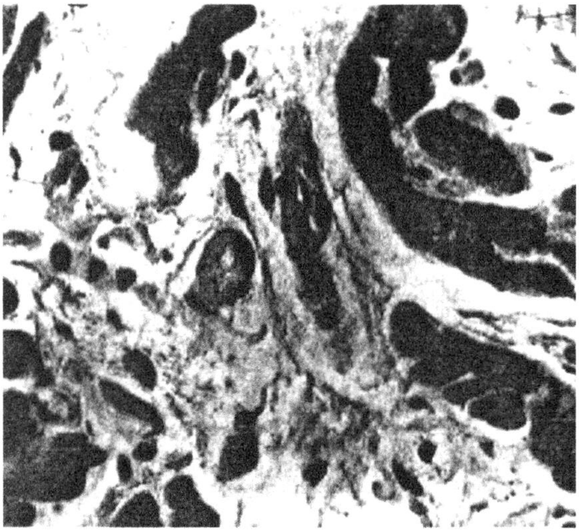

Figure 10.4
The myocardium of a diabetic patient showing atrophied myocytes (left side) compared with more normal myocytes (right side). Note also the extensive interstitial fibrosis in the area of myocyte loss and hyaline thickening of the small arteriolar walls. H&E × 300 magnification. (From reference 43.)

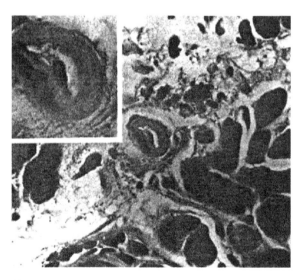

Figure 10.5
Hyalinization without luminal narrowing of a small arteriole (×300) from the heart of a patient with diabetes. Inset the same arteriole (×700). (From reference 43.)

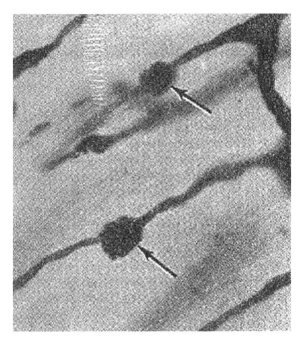

Figure 10.6
Two saccular aneurysms, each of which measures more than three times the vessel diameter of these capillary loops from the heart of a patient with diabetes. Reproduced with permission from Factor et al.[45] © 1980 Massachusetts Medical Society. All rights reserved.

Cellular dysfunction in diabetic cardiomyopathy

A number of cellular abnormalities that may underlie impaired myocyte function in diabetic cardiomyopathy have been identified in animal models of diabetes. These include reduced expression and activity of myocardial cell sodium pumps and the sodium calcium exchanger.[50–53] This leads to intracellular calcium overload and reduced activity of repolarizing potassium currents due to early down-regulation of key cardiac potassium channel genes as a consequence of insulin deficiency.[54–56] This may account for the increased arrhythmogenicity of the diabetic heart and may help to explain the frequently observed changes in QT interval.

Experimental studies from diabetic rodents with cardiomyopathy have revealed significant alterations in the glycerophospholipid composition of cardiac cell membranes.[57,58] This may also be of significance in that the phospholipid composition of cell membranes is of considerable functional importance with regard to cell signalling. Several studies have also highlighted cardiac disturbances of lipid metabolism which have been implicated in the pathogenesis of cardiomyopathy via altered substrate supply and/or utilization.[59–63] Abnormal substrate supply driven by the abnormal metabolic milieu of diabetes results in reduced glucose oxidation and increased fatty acid oxidation in cardiac myocytes which have been strongly associated with impaired contractile function.[62,64] Moreover, cardiomyopathy associated with type 1 diabetes in humans has been associated with carnitine deficiency and/or taurine excess, both important metabolites in the regulation of cardiac fatty acid metabolism and glycolysis.[65,66]

Other reported cellular mechanisms for diabetic cardiomyopathy include altered cell

with proliferative retinopathy, there are likely to be similar microvascular changes in the heart? Or do certain local conditions have to prevail to allow the target organ specific development of microaneurysms? Whatever the answer to these questions, or the functional significance of such aneurysms, their presence reveals a unique pathological feature in the diabetic heart, as such changes have never been reported in the hearts of hypertensive patients without diabetes.

signalling via disturbed expression of key G protein subclasses and activation of protein kinase C.[67-70] Protein kinase C (PKC) is activated in many tissues, including cardiovascular and renal tissues via glucose-dependent pathways.[71,72] There is selective activation of specific PKC isoforms, especially PKC β1, which have been associated with the development of LVH, cardiac fibrosis and impaired left ventricular function.[70] Of potential future therapeutic interest, these changes improved in animals treated with selective PKC inhibitors.[70]

Increased oxidative stress and reduced cardiac antioxidant reserve (presumably due to consumption) have also been strongly implicated in the pathogenesis of human and experimental diabetic cardiomyopathy,[73-75] as has the potential role of pro-inflammatory cytokines, including angiotensin II. Angiotensin II has been implicated in the regulation of diabetic myocyte death and hypertrophy,[76] in addition to cardiac fibrosis, perhaps via the induction of the pro-inflammatory cytokine TGFβ.[77,78] Moreover, correlations between increased tumour necrosis factor-α and interleukin-6 have been established with most types of cardiomyopathy, supporting the hypothesis that diabetic cardiac disease may have a strong inflammatory basis.[79-81]

Conclusions

In summary, the cardiomyopathic heart in patients with diabetes is characterized by an increase in left ventricular wall thickness and mass relative to age-, sex- and weight-matched non-diabetic populations. Histologically there is a spectrum of change typically involving increased deposition of interstitial collagens and glycoproteins, which at its most extreme can take on the appearance of replacement fibrosis, compensating for myocyte loss. There

are extensive vascular changes in vessels of all sizes, typically leading to hyalinization with lumen preservation and microangiopathy. These structural changes are compounded by marked disturbances in cellular function and autonomic dysregulation. Together, these changes culminate in the development of a heart disease characterized by impaired diastolic and systolic function, impaired coronary microcirculatory function, decreased flow reserve and increased arrhythmogenicity (Fig. 10.7). Some of these changes appear to be unique to the diabetic state but many resemble the pathology of hypertensive heart disease. Mindful of the under-estimated significance of disturbed blood pressure regulation in diabetes and the unique vulnerability of diabetics to hypertensive injury (Chapter 00), these observations raise the distinct possibility that diabetic cardiomyopathy is an exaggerated and accelerated form of hypertensive heart disease.

Therapeutic implications

These should be considered in the context of (1) prevention and (2) treatment of the established condition. The latter will involve the conventional management of heart failure, i.e. ACE-inhibition, loop diuretics, β-blockers and spironolactone. Specific studies in patients with diabetes and heart failure have not been conducted, but analysis of diabetic cohorts within trials of patients with heart failure has revealed that patients with diabetes and heart failure fare at least as well as non-diabetic patients with heart failure in response to the aforementioned interventions. With regard to prevention of heart failure, the UKPDS study in patients with type 2 diabetes showed that a 10/5 mmHg reduction in blood pressure resulted in a 56% reduction in the development of clinical heart failure.[82] This supports the hypothesis that blood pressure per se is a key driver of diabetic heart disease. However,

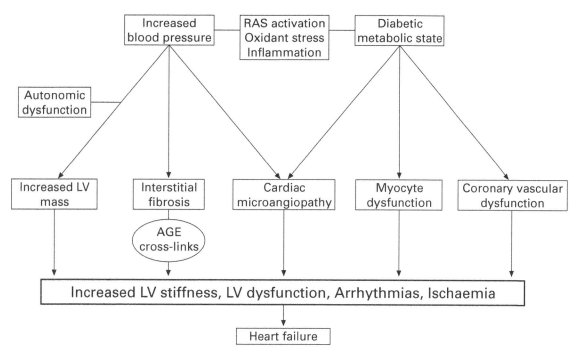

Figure 10.7
The pathogenesis of diabetic cardiomyopathy. Interactions between increased blood pressure and the metabolic disturbances of diabetes, compounded by cardiac renin-angiotensin system (RAS) activation, increased oxidant stress and increased expression of pro-inflammatory cytokines. AGE, advanced glycation end-product; LV, left ventricular.

there may be additional benefits from blockade of angiotensin II. The recent RENAAL trial in patients with type 2 diabetes and advanced nephropathy showed a dramatic 32% reduction in hospitalization for heart failure in patients treated with the angiotensin II antagonist losartan when compared with placebo, both administered in addition to conventional antihypertensive therapy.[83] This benefit was additive to the effect of blood pressure control. These observations suggest that strict blood pressure control and angiotensin II blockade are likely to be a powerful means of attenuating the development of heart failure in people with diabetes. Whether other novel approaches targeted at the basic pathophysiological mechanisms cited above, i.e. selective PKC isoform inhibition, cross-link breakers to inhibit AGEs, or immunomodulation, will add to the armoury awaits further studies.

References

1. Kannel WB, McGee, DL. Diabetes and cardio-vascular disease. The Framingham Study. *JAMA* 1979; **241**: 2035–8.
2. Solang L, Malmberg K, Ryden L. Diabetes and congestive heart failure – further knowledge needed. *Eur Heart J* 1999; **20**: 789–95.
3. Rubler S, Dlugash J, Yucheoglu YZ, et al. New type of cardiomyopathy associated with diabetic glomerulosclerosis. *Am J Cardiol* 1972; 30: 595–602.
4. Hamby RI, Zoneraich S, Sherman L. Diabetic cardiomyopathy. *JAMA* 1974; **229**: 1749–54.
5. Kannel WB, Hjortland M, Castelli WP. Role of diabetes in chronic heart failure: The Framingham Study. *Am J Cardiol* 1974; **34**: 29–34.
6. Factor SM, Minase T, Sonnenblick EM. Clinical and morphological features of human diabetic cardiomyopathy. *Am Heart J* 1980; **99**: 446–58.
7. Devereux RB, Roman MJ, Paranicas BA, et al. Impact of diabetes on cardiac structure and function – the Strong Heart Study. *Circulation* 2000; **101**: 2271–6.
8. De Simone G, Devereux RB, Koren MJ, et al. Midwall left ventricular mechanics: an independent predictor of arterial risk in hypertension. *Circulation* 1996; **93**: 259–65.
9. Karlefors T. Haemodynamic studies in male diabetics. *Acta Med Scand* 1966; **449** (Suppl): 45–73.
10. Carlstrom S, Karlefors T. Haemodynamic studies in newly diagnosed diabetics before and after adequate insulin treatment. *Br Heart J* 1970; **32**: 355–8.
11. Seneviratne B. Diabetic cardiomyopathy – the pre-clinical phase. *BMJ* 1977; **1**: 1444–6.
12. Sanderson JE, Brown DJ, Rivellese A, Kohner E. Diabetic cardiomyopathy? An echocardiographic study of young diabetics. *BMJ* 1978; I: 404–7.
13. D'Elia JA, Weinrauch LA, Healy RA, et al. Myocardial dysfunction without coronary artery disease in diabetic renal failure. *Am J Cardiol* 1979; **43**: 193–9.
14. Shapiro LM, Howat AP, Calter MM. Left ventricular function in diabetes mellitus I: Methodology, prevalence and spectrum of abnormality. *Br Heart J* 1981; **45**: 122–8.
15. Shapiro LM, Leatherdale BA, MacKinnon J, Fletcher RF. Left ventricular function in diabetes mellitus II: Relationship between clinical features and left ventricular function. *Br Heart J* 1981; **45**: 129–32.
16. Shapiro LM. Echocardiographic features of impaired ventricular function in diabetes mellitus. *Br Heart J* 1982; **47**: 439–44.
17. Airaksiner J, Ikaheimo M, Kaila J, et al. Impaired left ventricular filling in young female diabetics. *Acta Scand Med* 1984; **216**: 509–16.
18. Vered A, Battler A, Segal P, et al. Exercise induced left ventricular dysfunction in young men with asymptomatic diabetes mellitus (diabetic cardiomyopathy). *Am J Cardiol* 1984; **54**: 633–7.
19. Kahn JK, Zola B, Juni JE, Vinik AI. Radionuclide assessment of left ventricular diastolic filling in diabetes mellitus with and without cardiac autonomic neuropathy. *J Am Coll Cardiol* 1986; **7**: 1303–9.
20. Labowitz AJ, Pearson AC. Evaluation of left ventricular diastolic function: clinical relevance and recent Doppler echocardiographic insights. *Am Heart J* 1987; **114**: 836–51.
21. Zarich SW, Arbuckle BE, Cohen LR, et al. Diastolic abnormalities in young asymptomatic diabetic patients assessed by pulsed Doppler echocardiography. *J Am Coll Cardiol* 1988; **12**: 114–20.
22. Riggs T, Transue D. Doppler echocardiographic evaluation of left ventricular diastolic function in adolescents with diabetes mellitus. *Am J Cardiol* 1990; **65**: 899–902.
23. Ewing DJ, Martyn CN, Young RJ, Clarke BF. The value of cardiovascular autonomic function tests: a 10 year experience in diabetes. *Diabetes Care* 1985; **8**: 482–91.
24. Monteagudo PT, Moises VA, Kohlmann O, et al. Influence of autonomic neuropathy upon

left ventricular dysfunction in insulin dependent diabetic patients. *Clin Cardiol* 2000; **23:** 371–5.

25. Ewing DJ, Campbell IW, Clarke BF. The natural history of diabetic autonomic neuropathy. *Q J Med* 1980; **49:** 95–108.

26. Ewing DJ, Campbell IW, Clarke BF. Assessment of cardiovascular effects in diabetic autonomic neuropathy and prognostic implications. *Ann Intern Med* 1980; **92:** 308–11.

27. Watkins P, MacKay J. Cardiac denervation in diabetic neuropathy. *Ann Intern Med* 1980; **92:** 304–7.

28. Weston PJ, Bush G, Thurston H. An automatic device for the assessment of cardiovascular autonomic function. *Diabetic Med* 1998; **15:** 700–4.

29. Weston PJ, James MA, McCullough A, et al. Assessment of baroreceptor-cardiac reflex sensitivity using time domain analysis in patients with IDDM. *Diabetologia* 1996; **39:** 1385–91.

30. Weston PJ, Glancy JM, McNally PG, et al. Can abnormalities of ventricular repolarisation identify IDDM patients at risk of sudden death? *Heart* 1997; **78:** 56–60.

31. Weston PJ, Gill GV. Is undetected autonomic dysfunction responsible for sudden death in IDDM? The 'dead in bed' syndrome revisited. *Diabetic Med* 1999; **16:** 626–31.

32. Lawrence IG, Weston PJ, Bennett MA, et al. Is impaired baroreflex sensitivity a predictor or cause of sudden death in IDDM? *Diabetic Med* 1997; **14:** 82–5.

33. Ewing DJ, Boland D, Neilson J, et al. Autonomic neuropathy, QT interval lengthening and unexpected deaths in male diabetic patients. *Diabetologia* 1991; **34:** 182–5.

34. Ledet T. Histological and histochemical changes in the coronary arteries of old diabetic patients. *Diabetologia* 1968; **4:** 268–72.

35. van Hoeven KH, Factor SM. A comparison of the pathological spectrum of hypertensive, diabetic and hypertensive-diabetic heart disease. *Circulation* 1990; **82:** 848–55.

36. Factor SM, Minase T, Sonnenblick EH. Clinical and morphological features of human hypertensive-diabetic cardiomyopathy. *Am Heart J* 1980; **74:** 446–58.

37. Yoarum R, Zirkin H, Stammler G, Rose AG. Human coronary microvessels in diabetes and ischaemia. Morphometric study of autopsy material. *J Pathol* 1992; **166:** 265–70.

38. Sunni S, Bishop SP, Kent SP, Geer JC. Diabetic cardiomyopathy. *Arch Pathol Lab Med* 1986; **110:** 375.

39. Brownlee M, Cerami A, Vlassara H. Advanced glycosylation end products in tissues and the biochemical basis of diabetic complications. *N Engl J Med* 1988; **318:** 1315–21.

40. Blumenthal H, Alex M, Goldberg S. A study of lesions of the intramural coronary by-branches in diabetes mellitus. *Arch Pathol* 1960; **70:** 27–42.

41. Crall F, Roberts W. The extramural and intramural coronary arteries in juvenile diabetes mellitus. *Am J Med* 1978; **64:** 221–30.

42. Zoneraich S, Silverman G, Zoneraich O. Primary myocardial disease, diabetes mellitus and small vessel disease. *Am Heart J* 1980; **5:** 754–5.

43. Sutherland CG, Fisher BM, Frier BM, et al. Endomyocardial biopsy pathology in insulin dependent diabetes patients with abnormal ventricular function. *Histopathology* 1989; **14:** 596–601.

44. Fischer VW, Barner HB, Lewis L. Capillary basal laminar thickness in diabetic human myocardium. *Diabetes* 1979; **28:** 713–19.

45. Factor SM, Okun EM, Minase T. Capillary micro-aneurysms in the human diabetic heart. *N Engl J Med* 1980; **302:** 384–8.

46. McMillan DE. Deterioration of the microcirculation in diabetes. *Diabetes* 1975; **24:** 944–57.

47. Raskin IP. Diabetic regulation and its relationship to microangiopathy. *Metabolism* 1978; **27:** 235–52.

48. Anderson GS. The pathogenesis of diabetic glomerulosclerosis. *J Pathol Bacteriol* 1954; **67:** 241–5.

49. Bloodworth JMB Jr. A re-evaluation of diabetic glomerulosclerosis after the discovery of insulin. *Hum Pathol* 1978; **9:** 429–53.

50. Golfman L, Dixon IM, Takeda N, et al. Cardiac sarcolemmal Na-Ca exchange and Na-K ATPase activities and expression in alloxan-induced diabetes in rats. *Mol Cell Biochem* 1998; **188:** 91–101.

51. Gerbi A, Barbey O, Raccah D, et al. Alteration of Na-K ATPase isoenzymes in diabetic cardiomyopathy: effect of dietary supplementation

with fish oil (n-3 fatty acids) in rats. *Diabetologia* 1997; **40**: 496–505.

52. Schaffer SW, Ballard-Croft C, Boerth S, Allo SN. Mechanisms underlying depressed Na/Ca exchanger activity in the diabetic heart. *Cardiovasc Res* 1997; **34**: 129–36.

53. Ziegelhoffer A, Ravingerova T, Styk J, et al. Mechanisms that may be involved in calcium tolerance of the diabetic heart. *Mol Cell Biochem* 1997; **176**: 191–8.

54. Wong D, Kiyosue T, Arita M, et al. Abnormalities of K^+ and Ca^{2+} currents in ventricular myocytes from rats with chronic diabetes. *Am J Physiol* 1998; **269**: H1288–96.

55. Casis O, Gallego M, Iriarte M, et al. Effects of diabetic cardiomyopathy on regional electrophysiologic characteristics of rat ventricle. *Diabetologia* 2000; **43**: 101–9.

56. Qin D, Huang B, Deng L, et al. Downregulation of $K(+)$ channel gene expression in type I diabetic cardiomyopathy. *Biochem Biophys Res Commun* 2001; **283**: 549–53.

57. Williams SA, Tappia PS, Yu CH, et al. Impairment of the sarcolemmal phospholipase D-phosphatidate phosphohydrolase pathway in diabetic cardiomyopathy. *J Mol Cell Cardiol* 1998; **30**: 109–18.

58. Vecchini A, Del Rosso F, Binaglia L, et al. Molecular defects in sarcolemmal glycerophospholipid subclasses in diabetic cardiomyopathy. *J Mol Cell Cardiol* 2000; **32**: 1061–74.

59. Stanley WC, Lopaschuk GD, McCormack JG. Regulation of energy substrate metabolism in the diabetic heart. *Cardiovasc Res* 1997; **34**: 25–33.

60. Rodrigues B, Cam MC, McNeill JH. Metabolic disturbances in diabetic cardiomyopathy. *Mol Cell Biochem* 1998; **180**: 53–7.

61. Mizushige K, Yao L, Noma T, et al. Alteration in left ventricular diastolic filling and accumulation of myocardial collagen at the insulin-resistant prediabetic stage of a type II diabetic rat. *Circulation* 2000; **101**: 899–907.

62. Belke DD, Larsen TS, Gibbs EM, Severson DL. Altered metabolism causes cardiac dysfunction in perfused hearts from diabetic (db/db) mice. *Am J Physiol Endocrinol Metab* 2000; **279**: E1104–13.

63. van der Vusse GJ, van Bilsen M, Glatz JF. Cardiac fatty acid uptake and transport in health and disease. *Cardiovasc Res* 2000; **45**: 279–93.

64. Matsui H, Okumura K, Mukawa H, et al. Increased oxysterol contents in diabetic rat hearts: their involvement in diabetic cardiomyopathy. *Can J Cardiol* 1997; **13**: 373–9.

65. Malone J, Schocken D, Morrison A, Gilbert-Barness E. Diabetic cardiomyopathy and carnitine deficiency. *J Diabetic Complications* 1999; **13**: 86–90.

66. Militante J, Lombardini J, Schaffer S. The role of taurine in the pathogenesis of the cardiomyopathy of insulin-dependent diabetes mellitus. *Cardiovasc Res* 2000; **46**: 393–402.

67. Yang JM, Cho C, Kong K, et al. Increased expression of G alphaq protein in the heart of streptozotocin-induced diabetic rats. *Exp Mol Med* 1999; **31**: 179–84.

68. Akhter SA, Luttnell LM, Rickman HA, et al. Targetting the receptor Gq interface to inhibit in vivo pressure overload myocardial hypertrophy. *Science* 1998; **280**: 574–7.

69. Adams JW, Sakata Y, Davis MG, et al. Enhanced Galphaq signaling: a common pathway mediates cardiac hypertrophy and apoptotic heart failure. *Proc Natl Acad Sci USA* 1998; **95**: 10140–5.

70. Wakasaki H, Koya D, Schoen F et al. Targeted overexpression of protein kinase C beta2 isoform in the myocardium causes cardiomyopathy. *Proc Natl Acad Sci USA* 1997; **94**: 9320–5.

71. Williams B. Glucose-induced vascular smooth muscle dysfunction: the role of protein kinase C. *J Hypertens* 1995; **13**: 477–86.

72. Koya D, King G. Protein kinase C activation and the development of diabetic complications. *Diabetes* 1998; **47**: 859–66.

73. Kaul N, Hill M, Khaper N, et al. Probucol treatment reverses antioxidant and functional deficit in diabetic cardiomyopathy. *Mol Cell Biochem* 1996; **160–161**: 283–8.

74. Dhalla N, Liu X, Panagia V, Takeda N. Subcellular remodeling and heart dysfunction in chronic diabetes. *Cardiovasc Res* 1998; **40**: 239–47.

75. Singal P, Khaper N, Farahmand F. Oxidative stress in congestive heart failure. *Curr Cardiol Rep* 2000; **2**: 206–11.

76. Fioradaliso F, Li B, Latini R, et al. Myocyte death in streptozotocin-induced diabetes in rats

is angiotensin II dependent. *Lab Invest* 2000; **80:** 513–27.

77. Pfeiffer A, Middleberg-Bisping K, Drewes C, Schatz H. Elevated plasma levels of transforming growth factor-beta I in NIDDM. *Diabetes Care* 1996; **19:** 1113–17.

78. Lijnen PJ, Petrov VV, Fagard RH. Induction of cardiac fibrosis by TGF-beta (1). *Mol Genet Metab* 2000; **71:** 418–35.

79. Mandi Y, Hogye M, Talha E, et al. Cytokine production and antibodies against heat shock protein 60 in cardiomyopathies of different origins. *Pathobiology* 2000; **68:** 150–8.

80. Vadlamani L, Abraham WT. Insights into pathogenesis and treatment of cytokines in cardiomyopathy. *Curr Cardiol Rep* 2000; **2:** 120–8.

81. Mabuchi N, Tsutamoto T, Kinoshita M. Therapeutic use of dopamine and beta-blockers modulate plasma interleukin levels in patients with congestive heart failure. *J Cardiovasc Pharmacol* 2000; **36** (Suppl 2): S87–91.

82. UK Prospective Diabetes Study Group. Tight blood pressure control and risk of microvascular and macrovascular complications in type 2 diabetes. UKPDS 38. *BMJ* 1998; **317:** 703–13.

83. Brenner BM, Copper ME, De Zeeuw D, et al. Effects of losartan on renal and cardiovascular outcomes in patients with type 2 diabetes and nephropathy. *N Engl J Med* 2001; **345:** 861–9.

11

The pathogenesis of diabetic nephropathy

Richard E Gilbert and Mark E Cooper

The pathogenesis of diabetic nephropathy is incompletely understood, but is likely to involve interactions among cells, growth factors, structural proteins and cell receptors for these molecules. Recent advances in cellular and molecular biology have highlighted the complex nature of these molecular interactions (Fig. 11.1), but have also brought significant advances in providing a pathophysiological basis for prevention and therapeutic intervention in diabetic nephropathy.

Matrix accumulation and transforming growth factor-β

The diffuse and nodular glomerulosclerosis described by Kimmelstiel and Wilson in 1936[1] has been followed by an appreciation of the relationship between expansion of the extracellular matrix and declining renal function. Much attention has been focused on the glomerulus, where mesangial expansion and loss of glomerular filtration rate are closely related.[2] However, it is likely that tubulointerstitial pathology similarly contributes to progressive renal impairment in diabetes, where an association between interstitial volume and declining renal function has also been described.[3]

The mechanisms underlying the accumulation of extracellular matrix within the diabetic kidney have begun to be unraveled with information from *in-vitro* studies, experimental

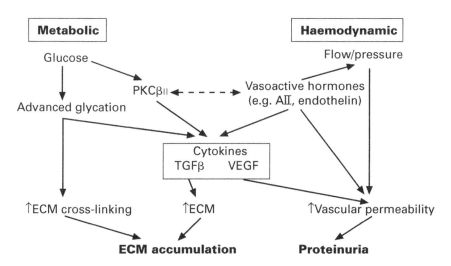

Figure 11.1
Proposed pathways in the pathogenesis of diabetic nephropathy. (From Cooper ME. Pathogenesis, prevention and treatment of diabetic nephropathy. Lancet 1998; 352: 213–19.)

models and clinical trials, suggesting complex interactions among haemodynamic influences, metabolic derangements and vasoactive hormones. In turn, these pathophysiological changes may lead to the stimulation of various locally active cytokines or growth factors. Over the past 5 years considerable experimental evidence has accumulated to support a key role for one such cytokine, transforming growth factor-β (TGF-β) in the pathogenesis of diabetic nephropathy.[4] The mechanisms for this fibrogenic or prosclerotic action of TGF-β are multiple and include both stimulation of extracellular matrix (ECM) synthesis and inhibition of its degradation.[5]

Haemodynamic factors

Diabetic nephropathy is commonly associated with systemic hypertension. In addition to the transmission of such elevated pressures to the glomerulus, micropuncture studies have shown that in experimental diabetes there is an elevation of the intraglomerular pressure, even in the absence of systemic hypertension. Initial studies by Mogensen[6] and Parving et al.[7] demonstrated that in hypertensive type I diabetic patients with nephropathy, aggressive antihypertensive therapy with conventional agents reduced proteinuria and retarded the rate of decline in renal function. At a cellular level, the application of shear stress (the *in-vitro* counterpart of hypertension) to mesangial cells leads to increased production of extracellular matrix proteins in association with increased transcription of the fibrogenic cytokine, TGF-β.[8] These studies suggest that hypertension-induced 'barotrauma' to the glomerulus leads to increased extracellular matrix expression by TGF-β-dependent mechanisms.

Renin-angiotensin system

Angiotensin-converting enzyme (ACE) inhibitors were introduced into the diabetic population in the 1980s and in 1993 were shown in the Collaborative Study Group Trial not only to reduce proteinuria, but also to reduce progression to end-stage renal failure.[9] Similar observations, i.e., renoprotection, have recently been reported for patients with type 2 diabetes and overt nephropathy using angiotension II receptor blockers (ARBs).[10,11] This important clinical trial follows experimental data to suggest that the renin-angiotensin system (RAS) is activated in experimental diabetes[12] and that ACE inhibition reduces glomerular basement membrane thickness in addition to the reduction of proteinuria in this model.[13] In cultured mesangial cells, angiotensin II, the effector molecule of the renin-angiotensin system, stimulates extracellular matrix protein synthesis through induction of TGF-β.[14] Angiotensin II also stimulates TGF-β and matrix protein expression in renal interstitial fibroblasts[15] and in proximal tubular epithelial cells,[16] implicating a RAS-TGF-β axis in the tubular basement membrane thickening and interstitial fibrosis that also develop in diabetic nephropathy. Indeed, in experimental diabetes, blockade of the renin-angiotensin system leads not only to a reduction in glomerular ultrastructural damage[17] and reduced ECM gene transcription in the glomerulus,[18] but also to a reduction in both TGF-β and collagen mRNA in the tubulo-interstitium[19] and vascular wall[20] and enhanced matrix degradation.[21]

Glycaemic control

In vitro, high glucose stimulates extracellular matrix synthesis and TGF-β expression in cultured mesangial[22] and proximal tubular cells.[23] In experimental diabetes, high blood glucose is accompanied by a rapid increase in TGF-β transcription[24] that may relate both to diabetes-associated renal hypertrophy and to the later expansion of extracellular matrix within the glomerulus and tubulo-interstitium. In man, renal expression and urinary excretion of TGF-β is elevated in patients with diabetic nephropathy.[25,26] Furthermore, the magnitude of TGF-β transcription may be directly related to long-term glycaemic control.[27] Several studies, including the landmark Diabetes Control and Complications Trial (DCCT), and the United Kingdom Prospective Diabetes Study (UKPDS) have indicated that intensified glycaemic control may retard the rate of development of both microalbuminuria and overt proteinuria in normoalbuminuric type I diabetic subjects.[28,29] Although large-scale intervention studies in patients with overt nephropathy have not been undertaken, the rate of progression of albuminuria correlates with long-term glycaemic control in both type I and type II diabetes.[30] Indeed, recent studies have emphasised the importance of glycaemic control in reducing the progression of macroproteinuria in patients with type I diabetes.[31] Furthermore, in a recent serial biopsy study, significant reduction in mesangial expansion was noted in diabetic patients whose glycaemic control had been normalised for 10 years by pancreas transplantation.[32] This important study indicates the potential reversibility of the structural changes of diabetic nephropathy.

Glycation

In diabetes, a state of chronic hyperglycaemia, there is an acceleration of the Maillard or browning reaction.[33] This is a spontaneous condensation reaction between reducing sugars and reactive amino groups, particularly those on long-lived proteins such as the collagens. The Maillard consists of a sequence of biochemical changes in which Schiff base intermediates undergo Amadori rearrangement, followed by a series of poorly defined biochemical reactions which ultimately lead to the formation of a range of irreversibly modified advanced glycation end-products (AGEs). These AGEs have been detected immunohistochemically in the kidney in experimental diabetes,[34,35] where they may bind to RAGE (receptor for AGEs) and possibly other proteins. Such AGE-binding sites have been identified in cultured mesangial cells and proximal tubular epithelial cells, where exposing cells to AGEs leads to increased TGF-β expression and extracellular matrix synthesis by a receptor-mediated mechanism.[36] Binding of advanced glycation end products to RAGE on proximal tubular epithelial cells in vitro, also leads to epithelial myofibroblast transdifferentiation which is associated with increased TGFβ expression by these cells.[35] *In vivo*, administration of AGEs leads to glomerulosclerosis and albuminuria[37] and in the diabetic rat, administration of the inhibitor of AGE formation, aminoguanidine, retards the development of these structural and functional changes.[38,39] These experimental studies confirmed deposition of AGEs in both glomeruli and tubules in diabetes and that AGE accumulation could be prevented by aminoguanidine treatment and other more specific inhibitors of advanced glycation.[40] Similar changes have also been described in blood vessels, where aminoguanidine treatment of diabetic rats resulted in reductions in AGE accumulation, ECM expansion and TGF-β expression.[41]

Recently, attention has also been focused on Amadori-modified proteins, early products of non-enzymatic glycation that are also increased in the setting of hyperglycaemia. In culture, mesangial cells exposed to Amadori-modified proteins overexpress type IV collagen mRNA[42] and monoclonal antibodies directed against these proteins (A717) prevent this overexpression. Furthermore, the *in-vivo* administration of the Fab fragments of A717 retards the progression of nephropathy in diabetic (*db/db*) mice.[43] As yet, it is not entirely clear whether this implicates the pathogenetic activity of Amadori-modified proteins or if modification of the proteins prevents their subsequent transformation into AGEs.

In the light of the encouraging experimental findings implicating non-enzymatic glycation in the pathogenesis of diabetic nephropathy, a range of clinical studies are in progress. These studies focus predominantly on the role of aminoguanidine in diabetic patients, with either overt nephropathy or microalbuminuria.[44]

Polyol pathway

A role for the hyperglycaemia-induced acceleration of polyol pathway metabolism in mediating the development of diabetic nephropathy has been suggested by some investigators.[45] In tissues where glucose uptake is independent of insulin, such as the kidney, hyperglycaemia results in increased levels of tissue sorbitol via metabolism of glucose by the NADPH-dependent enzyme aldose reductase. The increased formation and accumulation of sorbitol in these tissues is accompanied by a depletion of free myoinositol, loss of Na^+, K^+-ATPase activity, and increased consumption of the enzyme cofactors NADPH and NAD^+, leading to changes in cellular redox potential. These metabolic derangements have been postulated to result in cellular dysfunction and, ultimately, the morphological lesions that characterise diabetic nephropathy. The aldose reductase inhibitor, epalrestat, was shown to reduce glucose-mediated increase in TGF-β in cultured mesangial cells[46] and several investigators have demonstrated that glomerular hyperfiltration in diabetic rats can be prevented by treatment with aldose reductase inhibitors.[47,48] However, long-term experimen-

tal studies have been conflicting with respect to effects on structural and functional indices of injury in diabetic nephropathy.[49,50] Indeed, although aldose reductase inhibitors have now been available for over 20 years, clinical studies on the role of these agents in the prevention and treatment of diabetic nephropathy have been largely disappointing.

Protein kinase C (PKC)

The adverse effects of hyperglycaemia have been attributed to activation of PKC, a family of serine-threonine kinases that regulates diverse vascular functions, including contractility, blood flow, cellular proliferation and vascular permeability. PKC activity is increased in the retina, aorta, heart and glomeruli of diabetic animals, probably reflecting an increase in *de novo* synthesis of diacylglycerol, a major endogenous activator of PKC. The observation that there is preferential activation of the $β_{II}$ isoform of PKC in diabetes[51] led to the synthesis of an orally effective PKCβ-selective inhibitor, LY333531. This compound is a competitive, reversible inhibitor of $PKCβ_I$ and $PKCβ_{II}$, with a 50-fold lesser effect on other PKC isoenzymes. In studies over 2–8 weeks in diabetic rats, oral administration of LY333531 to diabetic rats resulted in a reduction in the renal overexpression of TGF-β and type IV collagen in addition to a dose-dependent decrease in albuminuria and glomerular hyperfiltration without evidence of toxicity, fall in blood pressure or changes in plasma glucose concentration.[52,53]

Endothelins

Endothelins are a family of three vasoactive peptides cleaved from pro-endothelins by endothelin-converting enzyme (ECE). In the kidneys of both rats and man the predominant endothelin isoform is endothelin-1 (ET-1). Endothelin is synthesised by glomerular endothelial, mesangial and epithelial cells and, in addition, by tubular epithelial and vascular endothelial cells.[54] Nephron-derived endothelins are postulated to function in a paracrine manner in the kidney, with their constitutive expression suggesting a role in vascular tone and extracellular fluid volume homeostasis.[55] Factors which stimulate ET expression are similar to those which have been implicated in renal injury such as TGF-β, angiotensin II, thrombin, interleukin-1, tumour necrosis factor and hypoxia.[56]

Endothelins interact with two receptor types: A (ET$_A$) and B (ET$_B$). Up- and down-regulation of each receptor subtype has been reported with a variety of cytokines and vasoactive hormones.[57] The effects of hyperglycaemia on ET and its receptors are complex. Elevated glucose increases ET-1 secretion by cultured endothelial cells and *in-vitro* studies in mesangial cells suggest a down-regulation of receptor expression,[58] thereby raising the possibility of a dissociation between ET expression and biological action. However, *in vivo*, glomerular ET-1 mRNA in diabetic rats is increased without significant change in either ET$_A$ or ET$_B$ receptor expression.[59] Furthermore, administration of a selective ET$_A$ or combined ET$_A$/ET$_B$ receptor blocker led to a reduction in blood pressure and proteinuria in experimental diabetes[60,61] and in addition was associated with reduced transcription of ECM proteins and TGF-β1.[60]

However, in our more recent studies, blockade of endothelin action, either via the ET-A receptor, or combined blockade of the ET-A and ET-B receptors, did not ameliorate the progression of experimental chronic renal injury. Moreover, addition of such endothelin antagonists to ACE-inhibition did not provide any additional benefit to delay progressive renal injury, over and above that afforded by the ACE-inhibitor alone.[62]

Vascular endothelial growth factor

In addition to the accumulation of extracellular matrix, diabetes is also characterised by increased endothelial permeability to macromolecules. In the kidney, hyperpermeability of glomerular endothelial cells is manifested by proteinuria. Although increased filtration pressure may contribute to the increased transglomerular protein loss, a recently identified permeability-enhancing cytokine, VEGF (vascular endothelial growth factor) has also been implicated in the pathogenesis of proteinuria in diabetic nephropathy.[63] VEGF is among the most potent inducers of vascular permeability identified and has recently been implicated in both capillary exudation[64,65] and ocular neovascularisation.[66,67] Both VEGF and its receptors are expressed in the glomerulus.[68,69]

In-vitro studies have recently shown that the stimuli which increase TGF-β also increase VEGF mRNA. Such stimuli include cell stretch,[70] glucose[71] and angiotensin II.[72] Thus, the ability of RAS blockade to reduce proteinuria[73] and rate of decline of GFR in diabetic nephropathy may be the result of their actions in reducing the overexpression of both VEGF and TGF-β.

In support of this concept, we have recently shown that ACE-inhibitors reduce the expression of VEGF in the retina of diabetic animals and reduce the hyperpermeability associated with diabetes.[10,11,74]

Protein traffic

Diabetic nephropathy is frequently accompanied by heavy proteinuria. Studies by Remuzzi and colleagues suggest that resorption of excessive quantities of protein by the proximal tubule leads to 'activation' of these cells as manifested by increased expression of endothelins and other potentially injurious factors such as monocyte chemotactic protein, MCP-1.[75] The basolateral secretion of these molecules may then lead to an interstitial inflammatory reaction, resulting in extracellular matrix accumulation, fibrosis and loss of renal function. This phenomenon of protein toxicity in the proximal tubule raises the possibility that the beneficial effects of RAS blockade in diabetic renal disease may reflect their potent anti-proteinuric action, in addition to the reduction of AII-mediated effects on glomerular haemodynamics and growth factor activation.[76]

Recent studies provide mechanistic and ultrastructural insights into the non-haemodynamic mechanisms that might be important in mediating this effect of RAS-blockade on protein trafficking across the glomerulus into the urinary space. Changes in podocyte number and morphology have long been implicated in the pathogenesis of proteinuria. We have shown that podocyte foot process effacement (broadening) is increased in experimental models of diabetes and that these ultrastructural abnormalities are attenuated by RAS blockade.[77] Moreover, there has been much recent interest in nephrin; a cytoskeletal protein that localizes to the slit pore of the podocyte in the glomerulus and is thought to be involved in regulating transglomerular protein trafficking.[78] Chronic experimental diabetes and proteinuria are associated with nephrin depletion.[78] Moreover, we have also shown that this depletion of nephrin and the associated proteinuria can be attenuated by RAS blockade in experimental diabetic nephropathy.[79] This observation provides preliminary evidence that modification of glomerular proteins such as nephrin may be involved in the reduction of glomerular hyperpermeability by RAS blockade.

ECM degradation

The increased ECM found in diabetes may reflect reduced degradation in addition to increased synthesis. Several types of enzymes may be involved in the degradation of ECM. In diabetes most studies have focused on the matrix metalloproteinases (MMPs) a group of zinc endopeptidases which are active at neutral pH against a wide variety of ECM proteins including collagens, fibronectin and laminin.[80] *In vitro*, mesangial cell MMP mRNA and the ability of these cells to degrade matrix are reduced by culture in a high glucose medium.[81,82] Gene expression of MMPs has also been examined in glomeruli of long-term diabetic animals, where Nakamura and colleagues have found a reduction in MMP-1 and MMP-3 mRNA, along with an increase in the expression of their inhibitors TIMP-1 and TIMP-2.[83] These findings suggest that both reduced MMP synthesis and activity may contribute to extracellular matrix accumulation in the diabetic kidney.[20,21,83]

HMGCoA reductase inhibition

In addition to their ability to lower cholesterol, HMGCoA reductase inhibitors may influence other aspects of cell function such as proto-oncogene expression,[84] DNA synthesis[85] and growth factor action.[86] These effects may be mediated by a reduction in the isoprenoid, farnesyl, leading to downstream effects on nuclear transcription factors.[87] In cultured mesangial cells, HMGCoA reductase inhibitors have been shown to reduce platelet-derived growth factor expression[88] and cell proliferation.[85] *In vivo*, HMGCoA reductase inhibitor administration to obese Zucker[88] and 5/6 nephrectomy rats[89] reduces glomerular injury. More recently, simvastatin therapy was shown to reduce albuminuria in normotensive microalbuminuric patients with type II diabetes.[90] The mechanisms underlying this beneficial effect are unclear, with only a transient reduction in diabetes-related overexpression of TGF-β reported with lovastatin.[91] These interesting observations suggest that HMGCoA reductase inhibitor may have a renoprotective action in progressive renal injury, although the mechanisms underlying this beneficial effect have not been delineated.

Conclusion

Advances in cellular and molecular biology have highlighted the complex nature of the molecular interactions which may lead to glomerulosclerosis and tubulo-interstitial fibrosis in diabetes. Pathogenetic factors include both glucose-dependent and glucose-independent mechanisms such as the renin-angiotensin and other vasoactive hormone systems. The inter-related pathophysiological changes which develop in diabetes may exert their pathogenetic effects via central cytokine (TGF-β, VEGF and other)-mediated pathways which may in part explain the therapeutic effects of currently available treatments such as blood pressure reduction, good glycaemic control and RAS blockade.[92]

References

1. Kimmelstiel P, Wilson C. Intercapillary lesions in the glomerulus. *Am J Pathology* 1936; **12**: 83–97.
2. Mauer S, Steffes M, Ellis E, Sutherland D, Brown D, Goetz F. Structural–functional relationships in diabetic nephropathy. *J Clin Invest* 1984; **74**: 1143–55.
3. Bader R, Bader E, Grung KE, Markensen-Haen S, Christ H, Bohle A. Structure and function of the kidney in diabetic glomerulosclerosis: correlations between morphological and functional parametes. *Pathol Res Pract* 1980; **167**: 204–16.
4. Border WA, Yamamoto T, Noble NA. Transforming growth factor-β in diabetic nephropathy. *Diabetes/Metab Rev* 1996; **12**: 309–39.
5. Bruijn JA, Roos A, DeGeus B, DeHeer E. Transforming growth factor-beta and the glomerular extracellular matrix in renal pathology. *J Lab Clin Med* 1994; **123**: 34–47.
6. Mogensen CE. Progression of nephropathy in long-term diabetics with proteinuria and effect of initial anti-hypertensive treatment. *Scand J Clin Lab Invest* 1976; **36**: 383–8.
7. Parving H-H, Andersen ER, Smidt U, Hommel E, Mathiesen E. Antihypertensive treatment postpones endstage renal failure in diabetic nephropathy. *Br Med J* 1987; **294**: 1443–7.
8. Yasuda T, Kondo S, Homma T, Harris RC. Regulation of extracellular matrix by mechanical stress in rat glomerular mesangial cells. *J Clin Invest* 1996; **98**: 1991–2000.
9. Lewis EJ, Hunsicker LG, Bain RP, Rohde RD, for the Collaborative Study Group. The effect of angiotensin-converting-enzyme inhibition on diabetic nephropathy. *N Engl J Med* 1993; **329**: 1456–62.
10. Lewis EJ, Hunsicker LG, Clarke WR, et al. Renoprotective effect of the angiotensin receptor antagonist irbesartan in patients with nephropathy due to type 2 diabetes. *N Engl J Med* 2001; **345**: 851–60.
11. Brenner BM, Cooper ME, De Zeeuw D, et al. Effects of losartan on renal and cardiovascular outcomes in patients with type 2 diabetes and nephropathy. *N Engl J Med* 2001; **345**: 861–9.
12. Anderson S, Jung FF, Ingelfinger JR. Renal renin-angiotensin system in diabetes: functional, immunohistochemical, and molecular biological correlations. *Am J Physiol* 1993; **265**: F477–86.
13. Cooper ME, Allen TJ, Macmillan PA, Clarke BE, Jerums G, Doyle AE. Enalapril retards glomerular basement membrane thickening and albuminuria in the diabetic rat. *Diabetologia* 1989; **32**: 326–8.
14. Kagami S, Border WA, Miller DE, Noble NA. Angiotensin II stimulates extracellular matrix protein synthesis through induction of transforming growth factor-beta expression in rat glomerular mesangial cells. *J Clin Invest* 1994; **93**: 2431–7.
15. Ruiz-Ortega M, Egido J. Angiotensin II modulates cell growth-related events and synthesis of matrix proteins in renal interstitial fibroblasts. *Kidney Int* 1997; **52**: 1497–510.
16. Wolf G, Mueller E, Stahl RAK, Ziyadeh FN. Angiotensin II-induced hypertrophy of cultured murine proximal tubular cells is mediated by endogenous transforming growth factor-β. *J Clin Invest* 1993; **92**: 1366–72.
17. Allen TA, Cao Z, Youssef S, Hulthen L, Cooper ME. Role of angiotensin II and bradykinin in experimental diabetic nephropathy. *Diabetes* 1997; **46**: 1612–18.
18. Nakamura T, Takahashi T, Fukui M, et al. Enalapril attenuates increased gene expression of extracellular matrix components in diabetic rats. *J Am Soc Nephrol* 1995; **5**: 1492–7.
19. Gilbert RE, Cox A, Wu LL, et al. Expression of transforming growth factor-β1 and type IV collagen in the renal tubulointerstitium in experimental diabetes: effects of angiotensin converting enzyme inhibition. *Diabetes* 1998; **47**: 414–22.
20. Rumble JR, Gilbert RE, Cox A, Wu L, Cooper ME. Angiotensin II converting enzyme inhibition reduces the expression of transforming growth factor-beta 1 and type IV collagen in

diabetic vasculopathy. *J Hypertension* 1998; **16**: 1603–9.

21. McClennan SV, Kelly DJ, Cox AJ, et al. Decreased matrix degradation in diabetic nephropathy: effect of ACE inhibition on the expression and activities of matrix metalloproteinases. *Diabetilogia* 2002; **45**: 268–75.

22. Ziyadeh FN, Sharma K, Ericksen M, Wolf G. Stimulation of collagen gene expression and protein synthesis in murine mesangial cells by high glucose is mediated by autocrine activation of transforming growth factor-β. *J Clin Invest* 1994; **93**: 536–42.

23. Ziyadeh FN. The extracellular matrix in diabetic nephropathy. *Am J Kidney Dis* 1993; **22**: 736–44.

24. Shankland SJ, Scholey JW, Ly H, Thai K. Expression of transforming growth factor-β1 during diabetic renal hypertrophy. *Kidney Int* 1994; **46**: 430–42.

25. Yamamoto T, Nakamura T, Noble NA, Ruoslahti E, Border WA. Expression of transforming growth factor beta is elevated in human and experimental diabetic nephropathy. *Proc Natl Acad Sci USA* 1993; **90**: 1814–18.

26. Houlihan CA, Akdeniz A, Tsalamandris C, et al. Urinary transforming growth factor beta excretion in patients with type 2 diabetes and elevated albumin excretion rate: effects of angiotensin receptor blockade and sodium restriction. *Diabetes Care* 2002; **25**: 1072–7.

27. Iwano M, Kubo A, Nishino T, et al. Quantification of glomerular TGF-beta-1 mRNA in patients with diabetes mellitus. *Kidney Int* 1996; **49**: 1120–6.

28. Diabetes Control and Complications Trial Research Group. The effect of intensive treatment of diabetes on the development and progression of long-term complications in insulin-dependent diabetes mellitus. *N Engl J Med* 1993; **329**: 977–86.

29. United Kingdom Prospective Diabetes Study group. Intensive blood glucose control with sulphonylureas or insulin compared with conventional treatment and risk of complications in patients with type 2 diabetes: UKPDS 33. *Lancet* 1998; **352**: 837–53.

30. Gilbert RE, Tsalamandris C, Bach L, et al. Glycemic control and the rate of progression of early diabetic kidney disease. *Kidney Int* 1993; **44**: 855–9.

31. Alaveras AE, Thomas SM, Sagriotis A, Viberti GC. Promoters of progression of diabetic nephropathy: the relative roles of blood glucose and blood pressure control. *Nephrol Dial Transplant* 1997; **2**: 71–4.

32. Mauer M. Role of mesangial expansion. Satellite of the XIV International Congress of Nephrology: nephroprotective properties of ACE inhibitors in diabetic and nondiabetic proteinuric nephropathy. Sydney, 1997.

33. Brownlee M. Lilly Lecture 1993. Glycation and diabetic complications. *Diabetes* 1994; **43**: 836–41.

34. Soulis T, Thallas V, Youssef S, et al. Advanced glycation end products and the receptor for advanced glycated end products co-localise in organs susceptible to diabetic microvascular injury: immunohistochemical studies. *Diabetologia* 1997; **40**: 619–28.

35. Oldfield MD, Bach LA, Forbes JM, et al. Advanced glycation end products cause epithelial myofibroblast transdifferentiation via receptor for advanced glycation end products (RAGE). *J Clin Invest* 2001; **108**: 1853–63.

36. Pugliese G, Pricci F, Romeo G, et al. Upregulation of mesangial growth factor and extracellular matrix synthesis by advanced glycation end products via a receptor-mediated mechanism. *Diabetes* 1997; **46**: 1881–7.

37. Vlassara H, Striker LJ, Teichberg S, Fuh H, Li YM, Steffes M. Advanced glycation end products induce glomerular sclerosis and albuminuria in normal rats. *Proc Natl Acad Sci USA* 1994; **91**: 11704–8.

38. Soulis-Liparota T, Cooper M, Papazoglou D, Clarke B, Jerums G. Retardation by aminoguanidine of development of albuminuria, mesangial expansion, and tissue fluorescence in streptozocin-induced diabetic rat. *Diabetes* 1991; **40**: 1328–34.

39. Kelly DJ, Gilbert RE, Cox AL, et al. Aminoguanidine ameliorates overexpression of prosclerotic growth factors and collagen deposition in experimental diabetic nephropathy. *J Am Soc Nephrol* 2001; **12**: 2098–107.

40. Forbes JM, Soulis T, Thallas V, et al. Renoprotective effect of a novel inhibitor of advanced glycation. *Diabetilogia* 2001; **44**: 108–14.

41. Rumble JR, Cooper ME, Soulis T, et al. Vascular hypertrophy in experimental diabetes: role of advanced glycation end products. *J Clin Invest* 1997; **99**: 1016–27.

42. Cohen MP, Hud E, Wu VY, Ziyadeh FN. Albumin modified by Amadori glucose adducts activates mesangial cell type IV collagen gene transcription. *Mol Cell Biochem* 1995; **151**: 61–7.

43. Cohen MP, Sharma K, Jin Y, et al. Prevention of diabetic nephropathy in db/db mice with glycated albumin antagonists. *J Clin Invest* 1995; **95**: 2338–45.

44. Wuerth J-P, Bain R, Mecca T, Park G, Cartwright K, Pimagedine Investigator Group. Baseline data from the Pimagedine Action trials. *Diabetologia* 1997; **40** (Suppl 1): A548.

45. Greene DA, Lattimer SA, Sima AAF. Sorbitol, phosphoinositides, and sodium-potassium-ATPase in the pathogenesis of diabetic complications. *N Engl J Med* 1987; **316**: 599–606.

46. Ishii H, Tada H, Isogai S. An aldose reductase inhibitor prevents glucose-induced increase in transforming growth factor-β and protein kinase C activity in cultured mesangial cells. *Diabetologia* 1998; **41**: 362–4.

47. Tilton RG, Chang K, Pugliese G, et al. Prevention of hemodynamic and vascular albumin filtration changes in diabetic rats by aldose reductase inhibitors. *Diabetes* 1989; **37**: 1258–70.

48. Goldfarb S, Ziyadeh FN, Kern EF, Simmons DA. Effects of polyol-pathway inhibition and dietary myo-inositol on glomerular hemodynamic function in experimental diabetes mellitus in rats. *Diabetes* 1991; **40**: 465–71.

49. McCaleb ML, Sredy J, Millen J, Ackerman DM, Dvornik D. Prevention of urinary albumin excretion in 6 month streptozocin-diabetic rats, with the aldose reductase inhibitor Tolrestat. *J Diabetic Complications* 1988; **2**: 16–18.

50. Beyermears A, Mistry K, Diecke FPJ, Cruz E. Zopolrestat prevention of proteinuria, albuminuria and cataractogenesis in diabetes mellitus. *Pharmacology* 1996; **52**: 292–302.

51. Williams B. Glucose-induced vascular smooth muscle dysfunction: the role of protein kinase C. *J Hypertens* 1995; **13**: 477–86.

52. Ishii H, Jirousek MR, Koya D, et al. Amelioration of vascular dysfunction in diabetic rats by an oral PKC β inhibitor. *Science* 1996; **272**: 728–31.

53. Koya D, Jirousek MR, You-Wei L, Ishii H, Kuboki K, King GL. Characterization of protein kinase C β isoform activation on gene expression of transforming growth factor-β, extracellular matrix components, and prostanoids in the glomeruli of diabetic rats. *J Clin Invest* 1997; **100**: 115–26.

54. Bruzzi I, Benigni A. Endothelin is a key modulator of progressive renal injury: experimental and novel therapeutic strategies. *Clin Exp Physiol Pharmacol* 1996; **23**: 349–53.

55. Kohan DE. Endothelins: renal tubule synthesis and actions. *Clin Exp Physiol Pharmacol* 1996; **23**: 337–44.

56. Egido J. Vasoactive hormones and renal sclerosis. *Kidney Int* 1996; **49**: 578–97.

57. Levin RE. Endothelins. *N Engl J Med* 1995; **333**: 356–63.

58. Koide H, Nakamura T, Ebihara I, Fukui M. Endothelins in diabetic kidneys. *Kidney Int* 1995; **48**: S45–S49.

59. Fukui M, Nakamura T, Ebihara I, et al. Gene expression for endothelin and their receptors in glomeruli of diabetic rats. *J Lab Clin Med* 1993; **122**: 149–56.

60. Nakamura T, Ebihara I, Fukui M, Tomino Y, Koide H. Effect of a specific endothelin receptor A antagonist on mRNA levels for extracellular matrix components and growth factors in diabetic glomeruli. *Diabetes* 1995; **44**: 895–9.

61. Benigni A, Colosio V, Brena C, Bruzzi I, Bertani T, Remuzzi G. Unselective inhibition of endothelin receptors reduces renal dysfunction in experimental diabetes. *Diabetes* 1998; **47**: 450–6.

62. Cao Z, Cooper ME, Wu LL, et al. Blockade of the renin-angiotensin and endothelin systems on progressive renal injury. *Hypertension* 2000; **36**: 561–8.

63. Williams B. A potential role for angiotensin II-induced vascular endothelial growth factor expression in the pathogenesis of diabetic nephropathy. *Mineral and Electrolyte Metab* 1998; **24**: 400–5.

64. Senger DR, Van de Water L, Brown LF, et al. Vascular permeability factor (VPF, VEGF) in tumor biology. *Cancer Metastasis Rev* 1993; **12**: 303–24.

65. Bates DO, Hillman NJ, Williams B, et al. Regulation of microvascular permeability by vascular endothelial growth factors. *J Anatomy* 2002; **200**: 581–97.

66. Ferrara N. Vascular endothelial growth factor. The trigger for neovascularization in the eye. *Lab Invest* 1995; **72**: 615–18.

67. Aiello LP, Avery RL, Arrigg PG, et al. Vascular endothelial growth factor in ocular fluid of patients with diabetic retinopathy and other retinal disorders. *N Engl J Med* 1994; **331**: 1480–7.

68. Simon M, Grone HJ, Johren O, et al. Expression of vascular endothelial growth factor and its receptors in human renal ontogenesis and in adult kidney. *Am J Physiol* 1995; **268**: F240–50.

69. Cooper ME, Vranes D, Youssef S, et al. Increased renal expression of vascular endothelial growth factor (VEGF) and its receptor VEGF-R2 in experimental diabetes. *Diabetes* 1999; **48**: 2229–39.

70. Gruden G, Thomas S, Burt D, et al. Mechanical stretch induces vascular permeability factor in human mesangial cells: mechanisms of signal transduction. *Proc Natl Acad Sci USA* 1997; **94**: 12112–16.

71. Williams B, Gallacher B, Patel H, Orme C. Glucose-induced protein kinase C activation regulates vascular permeability factor mRNA expression and peptide production by human vascular smooth muscle cells in vitro. *Diabetes* 1997; **46**: 1497–503.

72. Williams B, Baker AQ, Gallacher B, Lodwick D. Angiotensin II increases vascular permeability factor gene expression by human vascular smooth muscle cells. *Hypertension* 1995; **25**: 913–7.

73. Laffel LM, McGill JB, Gans DJ. The beneficial effect of angiotensin-converting enzyme inhibition with captopril on diabetic nephropathy in normotensive IDDM patients with microalbuminuria. North American Microalbuminuria Study Group. *Am J Med* 1995; **99**: 497–504.

74. Gilbert RE, Kelly DJ, Cox AJ, et al. Angiotensin converting enzyme inhibition reduces retinal overexpression of vascular endothelial growth factor and hyperpermeability in diabetes. *Diabetilogia* 2000; **43**: 1360–7.

75. Remuzzi G, Ruggenenti P, Benigni A. Understanding the nature of renal disease progression. *Kidney Int* 1997; **51**: 2–15.

76. The GISEN Group (Gruppo Italiano di Studi Epidemiologici in Nefrologia). Randomised placebo-controlled trial of effect of ramipril on decline in glomerular filtration rate and risk of terminal renal failure in proteinuric, nondiabetic nephropathy. *Lancet* 1997; **349**: 1857–63.

77. Mifsud SA, Allen TJ, Bertram JF, et al. Podocyte foot process broadening in experimental diabetic nephropathy: amelioration with renin-angiotensin system blockade. *Diabetilogia* 2001; **44**: 878–82.

78. Forbes JM, Bonnet F, Russo LM, et al. Modulation of nephrin in the diabetic kidney; association with systemic hypertension and increasing albuminuria. *J Hypertension* 2002; **20**: 985–92.

79. Kelly DJ, Aaltonen P, Cox AJ, et al. Expression of the slit-diaphragm protein, nephrin, in experimental diabetic nephropathy: differing effects of antiproteinuric therapies. *Nephrol Dial Transplant* 2002; **17**: 1327–32.

80. Nagase H. Matrix metalloproteinases: a minireview. In: Koide H, Hayashi T, eds. *Extracellular matrix in the kidney*. Basel, Karger, 1994: 85–93.

81. Kitamura M, Kitamura A, Mitarai T, et al. Gene expression of metalloproteinase and its inhibition in mesangial cells exposed to high glucose. *Biochem Biophys Res Commun* 1992; **185**: 1055–61.

82. McLennan SV, Fisher EJ, Yue DK, Turtle JR. High glucose concentration causes a decrease in mesangium degradation. *Diabetes* 1994; **43**: 1041–5.

83. Nakamura T, Fukui M, Ebihara I, Osada S, Tomino Y, Koide H. Abnormal gene expression of matrix metalloproteinases and their inhibitor in glomeruli from diabetic rats. *Renal Physiol Biochem* 1994; **17**: 316–25.

84. Vincent TS, Wulfert E, Merler E. Inhibition of growth factor signaling pathways by lovastatin. *Biochem Biophys Res Commun* 1991; **180**: 1284–9.

85. O'Donnell MP, Kasiske BL, Kim Y, Atluru D, Keane WF. Lovastatin inhibits proliferation of rat mesangial cells. *J Clin Invest* 1993; **91**: 83–7.

86. Grandaliano G, Biswas P, Choudhury GG, Abboud HE. Simvastatin inhibits PDGF-induced DNA synthesis in human glomerular mesangial cells. *Kidney Int* 1993; **44**: 503–8.

87. Goldstein JL, Brown MS. Regulation of the mevalonate pathway. *Nature* 1990; **343**: 425–30.

88. Kasiske BL, O'Donnell MP, Cleary MP, Keane WF. Treatment of hyperlipidaemia reduces glomerular injury in obese Zucker rats. *Kidney Int* 1988; **33**: 667–72.

89. Kasiske BL, O'Donnell MP, Garvis WJ, Keane WF. Pharmacological treatment of hyperlipidaemia reduces glomerular injury in rat 5/6 nephrectomy model of chronic renal failure. *Circ Res* 1988; **62**: 367–74.

90. Tonolo G, Ciccarese M, Brizzi P, et al. Reduction of albumin excretion rate in normotensive microalbuminuric type 2 diabetic patients during long-term simvastatin treatment. *Diabetes Care* 1997; **20**: 1891–5.

91. Han DC, Kim JH, Cha MK, Song KI, Hwang SD, Lee HB. Effect of HMGCoA reductase inhibition on TGF-β1 mRNA expression in diabetic rat glomeruli. *Kidney Int* 1995; **48** (Suppl 51): S61–S65.

92. Cooper ME. Interaction of metabolic and haemodynamic factors in mediating experimental diabetic nephropathy. *Diabetilogia* 2001; **44**: 1957–72.

12

The clinical implications and management of microalbuminuria and proteinuria in type 1 diabetes

Stephen M Thomas and Giancolo F Viberti

Introduction

Diabetic kidney disease (DKD) is now one of the commonest causes of end-stage renal failure (ESRF) requiring renal replacement therapy in Europe and the commonest in the USA.[1] Furthermore, patients with type 1 diabetes have a higher morbidity and mortality than those on renal replacement therapy due to other kidney diseases.[1]

The development of persistent proteinuria in type 1 diabetes heralds the onset of one of the most devastating microvascular complications; in a report in 1983 only 10 per cent of patients with proteinuria had survived >40 years of diabetes, in contrast to a 70 per cent survival rate in those without proteinuria.[2] This depressing statistic was confirmed by Krolewski et al. in 1985 who described a median survival after the onset of proteinuria of 10 years, with 25 per cent of the patients developing ESRF within 6 years and 75 per cent within 15 years.[3]

The ability to measure low urinary albumin concentrations, initially by radioimmunoassay,[4] allowed the first demonstrations of the importance of an elevated urinary albumin concentration – so-called 'microalbuminuria' – for the prediction of the later development of overt proteinuria. Since those early descriptions increasing evidence has accumulated that even at this early stage there is an aggregation of cardiovascular risk factors.

It is to be hoped that the prognosis will be improved in the future by new approaches to treatment of those with DKD. This chapter discusses the importance of microalbuminuria and DKD in type 1 diabetes, and the strategies currently available that may influence these outcomes.

The clinical relevance of microalbuminuria and proteinuria

Diabetic kidney disease

The onset of DKD is signalled, by convention, by the appearance of persistent proteinuria, with a urinary protein excretion of ≥0.5 g/day. The development of persistent proteinuria, or overt DKD, is followed by progressive decline in the glomerular filtration rate (GFR) to ESRF. The fall in GFR appears to be linear with time in all patients, but the rate of decline is variable with up to four-fold differences between individual patients, from 0.6 to 2.4 ml/min/month. Many diverse factors contribute to this variability – the main factor is blood pressure, which is inversely related to the rate of decline of renal function. Other factors impact to a lesser extent, including glycaemic control and, as recent evidence suggests, genetic factors. The amount of proteinuria may also be important pathogenically in renal disease progression rather than

Investigator	Baseline AER (µg/min)	Type of sample	Follow-up (years)	Percentage developing overt nephropathy
Viberti	>30	Overnight	14	88
Parving	>28	24 hours	6	75
Mogensen	>15	Morning	10	86
Mathiesen	>70	24 hours	6	100

Table 12.1
Predictive power of microalbuminuria for overt nephropathy in type I diabetes.

simply representing a consequence of the disease, although this remains unproven. In some cohorts the degree of albuminuria has been related to renal disease progression,[5] but not in all.[6] However, a reduction in albuminuria in response to treatment is predictive of a reduction in the rate of GFR loss in the long-term and treatments with the greatest anti-proteinuric effect reduce both progression to ESRF and mortality.[7,8]

Microalbuminuria, defined as a urinary albumin excretion rate (AER) between 20 and 200 µg/min (30–300 mg/day),[9] can occur within a year of the onset of diabetes, although persistent elevation of the AER is much more common after 5 years.[10] Approximately 80 per cent of patients who develop microalbuminuria progress to DKD within 15 years of the onset of diabetes (Table 12.1),[11] while at levels of ≥100 µg/min the risk of progression to overt renal disease approaches 100 per cent.

It is now clear from biopsy studies that this phase does not merely predict DKD. Micro-albuminuria in type 1 diabetes is associated with definite diabetic glomerular lesions, particularly when there is concomitant retinopathy.[12–16] The glomerular lesions described include glomerular basement membrane thickening, expanded mesangial volume fraction and matrix volume and thickness. It may therefore be time to abandon the nomenclature of 'incipient nephropathy' and to consider persistent microalbuminuria as an early but definite marker of DKD.

Cardiovascular disease

In comparison with the non-diabetic population the relative mortality rate from cardiovascular disease is 37 times higher in those with type 1 diabetes and proteinuria compared with four times higher in those without proteinuria.[17] There are several cardiac sequelae, notably excess coronary artery disease, which is not usually clinically apparent until the late thirties and with a particular excess by the fifth decade of life.[18]

Recent work has shown that left ventricular hypertrophy is also more common in DKD in the microalbuminuria and proteinuria phase. This manifests as an increased left ventricular mass index, a greater prevalence of left ventricular hypertrophy and reduced diastolic function as compared with diabetic subjects with normal AERs.[19,20] This most likely reflects a progressive increase in 24-h blood pressure level in diabetic subjects with DKD (see Chapters 5 and 6). Microalbuminuria is also predictive in the longer term of cardiovascular mortality. In a cohort of patients with type 1 diabetes without overt DKD in Denmark, an elevated urinary albumin excretion at baseline was an independent predictor of atherosclerotic vascular disease[21] and of cardiovascular disease.[22] In a UK cohort followed for 23 years, patients with microalbuminuria at baseline had a higher risk of dying from a cardiovascular cause.[23] Other studies have suggested that even during the phase of microalbuminuria there is often subtle evidence of myocardial dysfunction with a reduced aerobic work capacity[24] and significant, albeit 'silent' coronary artery lesions may be present.[25]

Although not as strong a predictor of cardiovascular mortality as in type 2 diabetes, a clear association exists between renal complications and cardiovascular disease in type 1 diabetic subjects.

Blood pressure

The development of microalbuminuria is accompanied by a rise in blood pressure.[26,27] A larger proportion of type 1 diabetic patients with microalbuminuria have hypertension when compared with age-, sex- and duration-matched patients with a normal AER. The prevalence of hypertension is of course dependent upon the criteria used. In one report it varied from 26 per cent using World Health Organization (WHO) criteria (systolic blood pressure (SBP) ≥160 mmHg, diastolic ≥95 mmHg), to ~50 per cent using criteria from the 5th report of the Joint National Committee on Detection, Evaluation and Treatment of Hypertension (≥130/85).[28]

Even in 'normotensive' patients with microalbuminuria, both sitting and ambulatory 24-h blood pressure levels are higher in patients with microalbuminuria,[29] with evidence that the normal night-time dip, especially in diastolic blood pressure, may be less pronounced.[30,31] The sitting clinic blood pressure rises in the phase of microalbuminuria by an average of 3–4 mmHg per year, as compared with 1 mmHg per year in long-term normoalbuminuric and healthy controls.[32]

In type 1 diabetes the level of blood pressure correlates both with the rate of development of DKD (Viberti, unpublished data) and with the rate of progression of established DKD.[5] Abnormal blood pressure diurnal rhythm may also contribute to a faster progression of DKD.[33]

Glycaemic control and insulin resistance

Poor glycaemic control has been consistently shown to be a factor in the development of microalbuminuria and DKD. Furthermore, DKD makes good blood glucose control more problematic, notwithstanding the treatment modality.[34] In addition, hypoglycaemia may be more troublesome and in those with concomitant heart disease may result in greater morbidity.[34]

Insulin resistance is also a feature of DKD at the microalbuminuria stage,[35] which may contribute to some of the difficulties with glycaemic control. Insulin resistance may even precede the development of microalbuminuria. In a study of 16 patients with type 1 diabetes and normoalbuminuria, seven patients who later developed a urinary albumin excretion rate of >30 mg/24 h had lower glucose disposal at baseline during a euglycaemic hyperinsulinaemic clamp, as compared with those patients who remained normoalbuminuric and six nondiabetic controls.[36] The seven patients whose disease progressed also had a stronger family history of type 2 diabetes.[36] This may have relevance beyond the kidney, as prospective studies have demonstrated a positive relationship between insulin resistance and the future development of cardiovascular disease in the non-diabetic population, although the mechanisms for this association are unclear (see Chapter 3).

Dyslipidaemia

Cross-sectional studies have provided good evidence that disturbances in serum lipids occur early in DKD, with abnormalities being evident (albeit mild) in the phase of micro-albuminuria and more marked as the disease progresses. Jones et al. found significantly higher concentrations of LDL-cholesterol and VLDL-cholesterol with lower concentrations of HDL_2-cholesterol in those with microalbuminuria. Levels of triglycerides, VLDL triglyceride and apolipoprotein B (ApoB) were also higher.[37] Groop et al. described an increase in the IDL sub-fraction in patients with micro- and macroalbuminuria.[38] Several workers have confirmed a reduction in HDL-cholesterol in microalbuminuria while Kahri et al. also described an elevated plasma cholesteryl ester transfer protein, but this did not correlate with HDL concentrations.[39] In addition, there is some evidence that HDL_2-cholesterol (which may be more cardioprotective) is specifically reduced.[37,39,40] Lahdenpera et al. found that patients with a normal AER had larger LDL particles than non-diabetic control subjects. Those with micro- and macroalbuminuria had an increased LDL mass with a tendency towards higher light LDL concentrations and higher dense LDL concentrations as compared with those with a normal AER. However, the differences between the diabetic groups were not significant[41] and it was concluded that the increase in LDL in DKD is primarily due to increased numbers of LDL particles (see Chapter 5).

Lipoprotein(a), which is suggested to pre-dict coronary heart disease, is elevated in patients with microalbuminuria compared with normoalbuminuric diabetic and non-diabetic healthy controls, although the relationship remains uncertain.[42,43]

These abnormalities progress and become quantitatively more important as albuminuria increases.[44] The degree to which the insulin resistance associated with DKD contributes to these lipid abnormalities is also open to question.

Endothelial dysfunction

There is widespread endothelial dysfunction once microalbuminuria is established. In prospective studies subjects with type 1 diabetes and normoalbuminuria who subsequently developed microalbuminuria had higher AER at baseline as compared with subjects who maintained a normal AER.[27] Systemic transcapillary albumin escape rates are higher in patients with microalbuminuria.[45] Circulating levels of von Willebrand factor (vWf), plasminogen activator inhibitor 1 (PAI-1), thrombomodulin, homocysteine and fibrinogen are all increased in microalbuminuria, consistent with endothelial activation.[46–50]

A longitudinal study has shown that vWf levels increase prior to the development of microalbuminuria when the AER is still in the normal stage.[51] These findings reflect a continuum in the disease process and suggest that endothelial dysfunction precedes microalbuminuria in type 1 diabetes. Some investigators have proposed the concept that there may be a 'malignant' microalbuminuria, accompanied by systemic endothelial dysfunction, which has graver consequences than 'benign' microalbuminuria without endothelial dysfunction.[52]

DKD and a familial predisposition to cardiovascular disease

On average, non-diabetic parents of offspring with DKD have raised arterial pressure; this has now been described in several cohorts.[53–57] Other studies have described a higher incidence of cardiovascular disease[58] and of cardiovascular risk factors, including insulin resistance, in the non-diabetic parents of patients with DKD.[59]

Management of DKD in type 1 diabetes

Treatment of blood pressure

The first demonstration of the efficacy of blood pressure treatment in DKD came from Mogensen in 1976 who showed that blood pressure reduction slowed the rate of GFR decline and stabilised albuminuria in patients with type 1 diabetes.[60] Parving et al. confirmed this effect in a 6-year prospective cross-over study.[61] In that study, effective blood pressure treatment reduced the rate of fall of GFR, from 0.94 ml/min/month to 0.29 ml/min/month during the first 3 years and to ~0.10 ml/min/month for the following 6 years. The authors suggested that blood pressure treatment could delay the progression to ESRF from 7–10 years to >20 years.[62] These studies used the conventional anti-hypertensives of the day, β-blockers, vasodilators and diuretics, and are remarkable in that a significant beneficial effect of blood pressure treatment was seen in the small numbers studied, demonstrating the importance and efficacy of blood pressure control. Later studies demonstrated equally conclusively that blood pressure treatment was associated with a lower cumulative mortality, from >50 per cent to 18 per cent at 10 years.[63,64]

Information on blood pressure treatment in different ethnic groups is sparse in type 1 diabetes. In a prospective study of black patients with type 2 diabetes in the USA, hypertension ($\geq$140/90 or mean arterial pressure (MAP) $\geq$106 mmHg) was associated with a fall of GFR in those with a diabetes duration >1 year, whereas GFR remained stable after >10 years of diabetes in normotensive patients.[65]

It is therefore now beyond dispute that effective blood pressure control is of critical importance in the management of DKD. The questions now centre around what are the optimum treatment strategies and blood pressure targets.

We performed an observational study of mean 8 years' follow-up of 58 patients with type 1 diabetes and DKD. At a MAP >106 mmHg the rate of GFR fall was 7.6 ml/min/year as compared with 4.4 ml/min/year at a MAP between 91 and 106, with no further significant fall in the rate of progression at lower MAPs.[6] This study supports the concept of a blood pressure threshold above which progression accelerates, although no attempt to accurately define the threshold was made. Regression analyses based upon observational studies have suggested that a MAP <105 mmHg may be an appropriate goal to retard the progression of DKD.[66] Lower targets may be necessary to prevent progression from microalbuminuria to overt DKD. In a prospective study of the risk factors of progression to microalbuminuria, those who maintained normal AERs throughout the study consistently had MAP $\leq$90 mmHg (~125/75). Regression analyses also suggest that this level is protective.[66]

The latest recommendations from the US Joint National Committee for the Prevention, Detection, Evaluation and Treatment of Blood Pressure (JNC VI) suggest a blood pressure target in diabetes mellitus of 130/85, with no specific target for those with kidney disease.[67] The current World Health Organization/International Society of Hypertension (WHO/ISH) guidelines have made similar recommendations. More recently, the American Diabetes Association issued a position statement on the management of diabetic nephropathy which recommended a target blood pressure in all adults with diabetes of <130/80 mmHg.[68] To date none of these targets have been validated in clinical trials in type I diabetes.

It is clear that the priority in anti-hypertensive treatment should be the attainment of good blood pressure control, although the concept of what level of blood pressure this implies may continue to change.

What agents should be used?

Studies in animals suggest that angiotensin-converting enzyme (ACE) inhibitors ameliorate diabetes-induced rises in glomerular capillary pressure.[69] In addition, *in vitro* studies suggest that angiotensin II also acts at the cellular level, especially in the context of a diabetes-induced haemodynamic insult.[70,71]

The largest clinical study of DKD in type I diabetes to date was published in 1993;[72] 409 patients with type 1 diabetes, persistent proteinuria and a serum creatinine concentration <221 µmol/l were randomised to receive either captopril or placebo. Other anti-hypertensive treatment was added as required to ensure good blood pressure control (<140/90 mmHg). Treatment with captopril (ACE inhibitor) halved the risk of a doubling of the serum creatinine over a median follow-up period of 3 years with a 50 per cent risk reduction in a combined end-point of death or renal replacement therapy. Blood pressure was slightly lower in the captopril-treated group, but as this was considered non-significant the effect of captopril on slowing down the progression of DKD was thought to be independent of blood pressure control. This remains controversial.

Other studies, albeit smaller, promote the claims of calcium antagonists, especially non-dihydropyridine calcium antagonists and β-blockers.[73,74]

A meta-analysis of studies of type 1 diabetes with microalbuminuria or 'overt' proteinuria, treated for 4 weeks with anti-hypertensive agents, found that ACE inhibitor treatment reduced proteinuria more than treatment with β-blockers, diuretics or calcium antagonists ('conventional therapy') despite a similar average reduction in blood pressure. In a linear regression analysis it was calculated that ACE inhibitor treatment would reduce proteinuria by 30 per cent even if there were zero blood pressure change. Nifedipine treatment was associated with a rise in proteinuria, while conventional treatment in the analysis had no anti-proteinuric effect without a blood pressure-lowering effect. Lowering of MAP by 20 mmHg by any therapy resulted in around a 60 per cent lowering in 24-h urine albumin or protein.[75]

Two large placebo-controlled studies have compared captopril and placebo in normotensive patients with type 1 diabetes and micro-albuminuria, with a combined total of 225 patients studied. In all, 25 of 114 placebo-treated patients (21.9 per cent) and 8 of 111 captopril-treated patients (7.2 per cent) progressed to persistent clinical albuminuria over 24 months. There was a significant 69 per cent (95 per cent CI: 31.7–86.1 per cent) reduction in the risk of progression by captopril which persisted after adjustment for differences in time-averaged MAP. AER increased by an average of 14.2 per cent per year in the placebo-treated group compared with a reduction of 9.6 per cent (−18.6 to 0.4 per cent) per year in the captopril-treated group (Fig. 12.1).[76] Furthermore, a recent meta-analysis of clin-

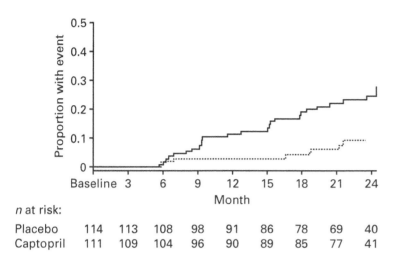

Figure 12.1
Probability of progression to clinical albuminuria after treatment with captopril (broken line) or placebo (solid line) in IDDM patients with microalbuminuria. Risk reduction: Unadjusted = 69.2% (95% CI: 31.7–86.1%), p = 0.004. Adjusted for current MAP = 62.9% (16.1 to 83.6%), p = 0.017

n at risk:	Baseline	3	6	9	12	15	18	21	24
Placebo	114	113	108	98	91	86	78	69	40
Captopril	111	109	104	96	90	89	85	77	41

ical trials of ACE inhibitors in patients with type 1 diabetes and microalbuminuria found that ACE inhibitors reduced progression to macroalbuminuria by 79 per cent, with regression to normoalbuminuria occurring 2.64-fold more often in patients on ACE inhibitors. In addition, the anti-proteinuric effect of ACE inhibitors seemed to be greater in those with the highest AER, an 81 per cent reduction at an AER of 200 µg/min compared with 26 per cent at 20 µg/min (ACE inhibitor triallist group), unpublished data).

Other studies have raised the question of whether dihydropyridine calcium antagonists should be used as first-line agents,[77] although these studies have predominantly investigated type 2 diabetes (see Chapter 17).

Advances in molecular genetics have raised the issue that individual responses to treatment with ACE inhibitors may be in part dependent upon the ACE genotype. A 287-bp deletion in the ACE gene gives rise to a deletion (D) allele and an insertion (I) allele with the suggestion of faster progression and per-

haps less response to ACE inhibition in those homozygous for the D allele, which is associated with higher plasma ACE levels.[77,78] In the future, it is conceivable that treatment may be tailored according to genotype, although these associations need confirmation in larger scale studies.

In conclusion, the clear message is the importance of blood pressure control, which will often require more than one agent. Current data support the use of ACE inhibitors as first-line therapy, although some authorities also advocate combination therapy with a calcium antagonist.[79] The recent position statement from the American Diabetes Association on diabetic nephropathy acknowledges the importance of renin-angiotensin system blockade, alongside blood pressure control for protection against the progression of nephropathy.[68] This review statement also acknowledges that at present, "grade A level" evidence favours the use of ACE-inhibition in hypertensive and non-hypertensive patients with type 1 diabetes and microalbuminuria or

Glycaemic control and the progression of diabetic kidney disease

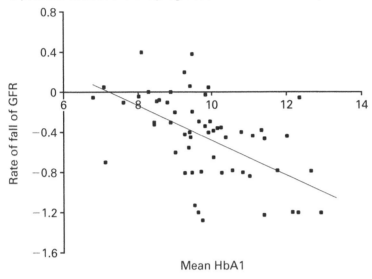

Figure 12.2
The relationship between the time averaged HbA1 and the rate of fall of GFR in 54 patients with type 1 diabetes.

clinical albuminuria as first line therapy. In type 2 diabetes, the weight of evidence is more in favour of angiotensin receptor blockers (ARB) but if one class is not tolerated, the other should be substituted. i.e. in type 1 diabetes, if an ACE-inhibitor is not tolerated, then an ARB would be a suitable alternative for renoprotection. Diabetes and DKD (especially as it progresses) are usually associated with salt and water retention which can blunt the efficacy of any anti-hypertensive strategy. Advice on salt restriction is important (see Chapter 16) and the use of diuretics along with other antihypertensive medications is often essential to achieve optimal blood pressure control.

Glycaemic control

There is no longer any doubt that improved glycaemic control is effective in the primary prevention of DKD, i.e. in preventing the tran-

sition from normoalbuminuria to microalbuminuria. In the Diabetes Control and Complications Trial (DCCT), intensive insulin therapy resulted in a 39 per cent reduction in the risk of developing microalbuminuria.[80] However, at later stages of the disease, i.e. once microalbuminuria is established, the relationship is less clear-cut.

In the Microalbuminuria Collaborative Study Group trial of 70 patients, no beneficial effect on urinary albumin excretion was demonstrated in the intensively treated group compared to the conventionally treated group over a median 5-year period of follow-up, with six patients in each group progressing to overt proteinuria.[81] In the Diabetes Control and Complications Trial, 73 patients had microalbuminuria at baseline; eight patients in both the intensively treated and conventionally treated groups developed clinical proteinuria.[82]

Conversely, in a study of 36 patients with

	HbA1%	Rate of fall of GFR (ml/min/year)	MAP (mmHg)	n
I	(<8.6)	1.1	99 ± 8	10
II	(8.6–10.3)	4.4*	97 ± 8	33
III	(>10.3)	8.1**#	99 ± 11	15
* II vs I $P = 0.0091$ ** III vs I $P = <0.0001$ # III vs II $P = 0.008$				

Table 12.2
Relationship between tertiles of HbA1% and rate of fall of GFR.

type 1 diabetes and microalbuminuria at the Steno Memorial hospital, five patients in a conventionally treated group developed 'overt nephropathy' while none progressed in an intensively treated group using insulin infusion pumps. MAP rose in the conventionally treated group by an average of 2.7 mmHg and by 0.1 mmHg in the intensively treated group.[83]

One study addressed the effect of glycaemic control on renal structure. Improved glycaemic control for ~3 years in patients with microalbuminuria stabilised renal histology. In patients receiving conventional rather than intensified insulin therapy there were greater increases in basement membrane thickness, matrix/mesengial volume and matrix star volume. There was, however, no reduction in AER in this study.[84]

At the stage of macroalbuminuria there is similar controversy regarding the benefits of glycaemic control on the progression of DKD.

A cohort of 58 patients (55 Caucasian, 3 Afro-Caribbean) were followed at Guy's hospital for a median of 7 years.[6] The rate of fall of GFR inversely correlated with both the baseline and mean, time-averaged, HbA1, i.e.

the higher the baseline HbA1 the faster the rate of fall of GFR (Fig. 12.2). In stepwise weighted multivariate regression analysis HbA1 and diastolic blood pressure were independently related to the rate of decline of GFR. An important feature of this study was that the mean MAP during follow-up was 97 mmHg. A tertile analysis of the distribution of mean HbA1 showed that for each tertile, those with the lower HbA1 had a slower rate of decline of GFR as compared with the higher tertile, with no evidence of a threshold effect (Table 12.2).

Other observational studies where blood pressure has been well controlled have also described similar associations.[85,86] However, these observational studies do not prove that intervention and improvement of glycaemic control would affect progression of DKD.

There have been few controlled intervention studies in overt nephropathy and their sample sizes were small. A study in 1986 randomized 12 patients with intermittent proteinuria to either continuous subcutaneous insulin infusion (CSII) or to conventional insulin therapy.[87,88] Over a 2-year follow-up period the improved glycaemic control in the CSII group did not produce a significant difference in the rate of fall of GFR. Tamborlane et al. found no improvement in renal function after 2 years of good metabolic control in 17 patients. One uncontrolled prospective study showed that improved glycaemic control for 36 months had an impact on the rate of fall of GFR only when combined with anti-hypertensive treatment and a low protein diet.[89]

Data on the effect of solitary pancreas transplantation on renal histology have also been published.[90] An initial analysis after 5 years failed to show any improvement in diabetic glomerular changes. However, by 10 years glomerular basement membrane thickness decreased, as did the mesangial fractional volume and the mesangial matrix fractional volume. The mesangial cell fractional volume increased from baseline to 5 years and then decreased to the baseline value by 10 years.

There is a similar paucity of data on the effect of improved glycaemic control on mortality. In the DCCT study the number of deaths due to cardiovascular disease was lower in the intensively treated group.[91] However, given the small numbers in the study this did not achieve statistical significance. In a study of secondary prevention in all forms of diabetes, the 'Digami' study, 620 patients with all kinds of diabetes and a myocardial infarction received either an insulin-glucose infusion for at least 24 h, followed by subcutaneous insulin four times daily for at least 3 months, or standard treatment.[92] A total of 306 patients receiving intensive insulin treatment and 314 controls were followed for a mean of 3.4 years. During the initial year of follow-up those in the insulin group had a relative reduction in mortality of 30 per cent compared with the control group.

The definitive study to determine the benefits of intensification of glycaemic control on renal and cardiovascular progression has not been done, and may remain the case. In the context of an overall treatment strategy, particularly with good blood pressure control, it would seem reasonable to aim for as good glycaemic control as is practicable without significant hypoglycaemia.

Lipid lowering

Not only is DKD associated with dyslipidaemia, but this may contribute to both renal and cardiovascular morbidity. Watts et al. investigated 53 patients with normal AER at baseline and found that increasing albuminuria was associated with baseline serum total LDL and non-HDL-cholesterol, with baseline serum ApoB concentration being an independent predictor of progression of DKD.[93] In a sub-analysis of 439 patients with DKD who had taken part in a multi-centre diabetic retinopathy trial, elevated serum cholesterol was an independent predictor of both the rate of decline in renal function and of cardiovascular mortality.[94] Similarly, another prospective study with smaller numbers found low serum cholesterol to be a strong predictor of a better renal prognosis.[95]

In prospective studies of type 1 diabetes and microalbuminuria, serum cholesterol was significantly associated with changes in AER. Nevertheless there have been no adequate intervention studies of the effect of lipid-lowering treatment on the rate of progression of DKD in type 1 diabetes.

Dietary treatment

In a self-controlled study of 19 patients with type 1 diabetes and DKD a reduction in protein intake from 1.1 to ~0.7 g/kg body weight per day resulted in a slowing of the rate of GFR fall from 0.6 to 0.1 ml/min/month.[96] Not all patients responded, however, and blood pressure changes may have accounted for some of the effect seen.

Reduction of dietary protein by approximately 50 per cent has also been shown to reduce the fractional clearance of albumin in patients with microalbuminuria. There is also evidence that a change from animal to vegetable proteins may be beneficial.[97]

The St Vincent Declaration guidelines recommend that it is probably reasonable to limit the protein intake in patients with microalbuminuria to approximately 0.8–1 g/kg body weight per day. It is further recommended that a reduction in animal protein intake should be considered in patients with clinical nephropathy to a level of between 0.6 and 0.7 g/kg body weight per day.

Smoking

There is evidence that smoking may be related to both the development and progression of microalbuminuria and DKD.[27,98] Although this evidence is not conclusive and the relationship is weak, the strong association with cardiovascular disease means that smoking should be particularly discouraged in patients with DKD.

Summary

The detection of microalbuminuria and proteinuria has enormous implications for both morbidity and mortality in patients with type 1 diabetes. New treatment strategies offer hope that the disease processes can be modified or stabilised, justifying appropriate screening and management protocols.[79,99]

References

1. United States Renal Data Service. The USRDS 1998 Annual Data Report. 1998; 2, Incidence and Prevalence of End-Stage Renal Disease: 23–37.
2. Andersen AR, Christiansen JS, Anderson JK, Kreiner S, Deckert T. Diabetic nephropathy in type 1 (insulin dependent) diabetes: an epidemiological study. *Diabetologia* 1983; **25:** 496–501.
3. Krolewski AS, Warram JH, Christlieb AR, Busick EJ, Kahn CR. The changing natural history of nephropathy in type 1 diabetes. *Am J Med* 1985; **78:** 785–94.
4. Keen H, Chlouverakis C. An immunoassay method for urinary albumin at low concentration. *Lancet* **2:** 913–14.
5. Rossing P, Hommel E, Smidt UM, Parving HH. Impact of arterial blood pressure and albuminuria on the progression of diabetic nephropathy in IDDM patients. *Diabetes* 1993; **42:** 715–19.
6. Alaveras AE, Thomas SM, Sagriotis A, Viberti GC. Promoters of progression of diabetic nephropathy: the relative roles of blood glucose and blood pressure control. *Nephro Dial Transplant* 1997; **12**(Suppl 2): 71–4.
7. Rossing P, Hommel E, Smidt UM, Parving HH. Reduction in albuminuria predicts a beneficial effect on diminishing the progression of human diabetic nephropathy during antihypertensive treatment. *Diabetologia* 1994; **37:** 511–16.
8. Rossing P, Hommel E, Smidt UM, Parving HH. Reduction in albuminuria predicts diminished progression in diabetic nephropathy. *Kidney Int* 1994; Suppl 45: S145–9.
9. Mogensen CE. Microalbuminuria as a predictor of clinical diabetic nephropathy. *Kidney Int* 1987; **31:** 673–89.
10. Marshall SM, Alberti KG. Comparison of the prevalence and associated features of abnormal albumin excretion in insulin-dependent and non-insulin-dependent diabetes. *Q J Med* 1989; **70:** 61–71.
11. Almdal T, Norgaard K, Feldt-Rasmussen B, Deckert T. The predictive value of microalbuminuria in IDDM. A five-year follow-up study. *Diabetes Care* 1994; **17:** 120–5.
12. Chavers BM, Mauer SM, Ramsay RC, Steffes MW. Relationship between retinal and glomerular lesions in IDDM patients. *Diabetes* 1994; **43:** 441–6.
13. Fioretto P, Mauer M. Glomerular changes in normo- and microalbuminuric patients with long-standing insulin-dependent diabetes mellitus. *Adv Nephrol* 1997; **26:** 247–63.
14. Fioretto P, Steffes MW, Sutherland DE, Mauer M. Sequential renal biopsies in insulin-dependent diabetic patients: structural factors associated with clinical progression. *Kidney Int* 1995; **48:** 1929–35.
15. Fioretto P, Steffes MW, Mauer M. Glomerular structure in nonproteinuric IDDM patients with various levels of albuminuria. *Diabetes* 1994; **43:** 1358–64.
16. Walker JD, Close CF, Jones SL, et al. Glomerular structure in type-1 (insulin-dependent) diabetic patients with normo- and micro-albuminuria. *Kidney Int* 1992; **41:** 741–8.
17. Borch-Johnsen K, Kreiner S. Proteinuria: value as predictor of cardiovascular mortality in insulin dependent diabetes mellitus. *BMJ* 1987; **294:** 1651–4.
18. Krolewski AS, Kosinski EJ, Warram JH, et al. Magnitude and determinants of coronary artery disease in juvenile-onset, insulin-dependent diabetes mellitus. *Am J Cardiol* 1987; **59:** 750–5.
19. Sato A, Tarnow L, Parving HH. Increased left ventricular mass in normotensive type 1 diabetic patients with diabetic nephropathy. *Diabetes Care* 1998; **21:** 1534–9.
20. Sato A, Tarnow L, Parving HH. Prevalence of left ventricular hypertrophy in Type 1 diabetic patients with diabetic nephropathy. *Diabetologia* 1999; **42:** 76–80.
21. Deckert T, Yokoyama H, Mathiesen E, et al. Cohort study of predictive value of urinary

albumin excretion for atherosclerotic vascular disease in patients with insulin dependent diabetes. *BMJ* 1996; **312:** 871–4.

22. Rossing P, Hougaard P, Borch-Johnsen K, Parving HH. Predictors of mortality in insulin dependent diabetes: 10 year observational follow up study. *BMJ* 1996; **313:** 779–84.

23. Messent JW, Elliot TG, Hill RD, Jarrett RJ, Keen H, Viberti GC. Prognostic significance of microalbuminuria in insulin-dependent diabetes mellitus: a twenty-three year follow-up study. *Kidney Int* 1992; **41:** 836–9.

24. Jensen T, Richter EA, Feldt-Rasmussen B, Kelbaek H, Deckert T. Impaired aerobic work capacity in insulin dependent diabetics with increased urinary albumin excretion. *Br Med J (Clin Res Ed)* 1998; **296:** 1352–4.

25. Earle KA, Mishra M, Morocutti A, et al. Microalbuminuria as a marker of silent myocardial ischaemia in IDDM patients. *Diabetologia* 1996; **39:** 854–6.

26. Feldt-Rasmussen B, Borch-Johnsen K, Mathiesen ER. Hypertension in diabetes as related to nephropathy. Early blood pressure changes. *Hypertension* 1985; **7:** 18–20.

27. Microalbuminuria Collaborative Study Group United Kingdom. Risk factors for development of microalbuminuria in insulin dependent diabetic patients: a cohort study. Microalbuminuria Collaborative Study Group, United Kingdom. *BMJ* 1993; **306:** 1235–9.

28. Tarnow L, Rossing P, Gall MA, Nielsen FS, Parving HH. Prevalence of arterial hypertension in diabetic patients before and after the JNC-V. *Diabetes Care* 1994; **17:** 1247–51.

29. Hansen KW, Christensen CK, Andersen PH, Pedersen MM, Christiansen JS, Mogensen CE. Ambulatory blood pressure in microalbuminuric type 1 diabetic patients. *Kidney Int* 1992; **41:** 847–54.

30. Hansen KW, Mau Pedersen M, Marshall SM, Christiansen JS, Mogensen CE. Circadian variation of blood pressure in patients with diabetic nephropathy. *Diabetologia* 1992; **35:** 1074–9.

31. Voros P, Lengyel Z, Nagy V, Nemeth C, Rosivall L, Kammerer L. Diurnal blood pressure variation and albuminuria in normotensive patients with insulin-dependent diabetes mellitus. *Nephrol Dial Transplant* 1998; **13:** 2257–60.

32. Mogensen CE. Systemic blood pressure and glomerular leakage with particular reference to diabetes and hypertension. *J Intern Med* 1994; **235:** 297–316.

33. Farmer CK, Goldsmith DJ, Quin JD, et al. Progression of diabetic nephropathy – is diurnal blood pressure rhythm as important as absolute blood pressure level? *Nephrol Dial Transplant* 1998; **13:** 635–9.

34. Bending JJ, Pickup JC, Viberti GC, Keen H. Glycaemic control in diabetic nephropathy. *BMJ* 1984; **288:** 1187–91.

35. Yip J, Mattock MB, Morocutti A, Sethi M, Trevisan R, Viberti GC. Insulin resistance in insulin-dependent diabetic patients with microalbuminuria. *Lancet* 1993; **342:** 883–7.

36. Ekstrand AV, Groop PH, Gronhagen-Riska C. Insulin resistance precedes microalbuminuria in patients with insulin-dependent diabetes mellitus. *Nephrol Dial Transplant* 1998; **13:** 3079–983.

37. Jones SL, Close CF, Mattock MB, Jarrett RJ, Keen H, Viberti GC. Plasma lipid and coagulation factor concentrations in insulin dependent diabetics with microalbuminuria. *BMJ* 1989; **298:** 487–90.

38. Groop PH, Elliott T, Ekstrand A, et al. Multiple lipoprotein abnormalities in type I diabetic patients with renal disease. *Diabetes* 1996; **45:** 974–9.

39. Kahri J, Groop PH, Elliott T, Viberti GC, Taskinen MR. Plasma cholesteryl ester transfer protein and its relationship to plasma lipoproteins and apolipoprotein A-I-containing lipoproteins in IDDM patients with microalbuminuria and clinical nephropathy. *Diabetes Care* 1994; **17:** 412–19.

40. Winocour PH, Durrington PN, Bhatnagar D, Ishola M. Influence of early diabetic nephropathy on very low density (VLDL), intermediate density lipoprotein (IDL), and low lipoprotein (LDL) composition. *Atherosclerosis* 1991; **89:** 49–57.

41. Lahdenpera S, Groop PH, Tilly-Kiesi M, et al. LDL subclasses in IDDM patients: relation to diabetic nephropathy. *Diabetologia* 1994; **37:** 681–8.

42. Earle KA, Mattock M, Morocutti A, Aravanitis D, Viberti GC. Lipoprotein(a) and atherosclerotic disease in insulin-dependent diabetic

patients with declining glomerular filtration rate. *Diabetic Med* 1996; **13**: 1071–2.

43. Groop PH, Viberti GC, Elliott TG, et al. Lipoprotein(a) in type 1 diabetic patients with renal disease. *Diabetic Med* 1994; **11**: 961–7.

44. Haaber AB, Kofoed-Enevoldsen A, Jensen T. The prevalence of hypercholesterolaemia and its relationship with albuminuria in insulin-dependent diabetic patients: an epidemiological study. *Diabetic Med* 1992; **9**: 557–61.

45. Feldt-Rasmussen B. Increased transcapillary escape of albumin in Type 1 (insulin-dependent) diabetic patients with microalbuminuria. *Diabetologia* 1986; **29**: 282–6.

46. Greaves M, Malia RG, Goodfellow K, et al. Fibrinogen and von Willebrand factor in IDDM: relationships to lipid vascular risk factors, blood pressure, glycaemic control and urinary albumin excretion rate: the EURODIAB IDDM Complications Study. *Diabetologia* 1997; **40**: 698–705.

47. Gruden G, Pagano G, Romagnoli R, Frezet D, Olivetti C, Cavallo-Perin P. Thrombomodulin levels in insulin-dependent diabetic patients with microalbuminuria. *Diabetic Med* 1995; **12**: 258–60.

48. Gruden G, Cavallo-Perin P, Bazzan M, Stella S, Vuolo A, Pagano G. PAI-1 and factor VII activity are higher in IDDM patients with microalbuminuria. *Diabetes* 1994; **43**: 426–9.

49. Gruden G, Cavallo-Perin P, Romagnoli R, Olivetti C, Frezet D, Pagano G. Prothrombin fragment 1 + 2 and antithrombin III-thrombin complex in microalbuminuric type 2 diabetic patients. *Diabetic Med* 1994; **11**: 485–8.

50. Hofmann MA, Kohl B, Zumback MS, et al. Hyperhomocyst(e)inemia and endothelial dysfunction in IDDM. *Diabetes Care* 1998; **21**: 841–8.

51. Stehouwer CD, Fischer HR, van Kuijk AW, Polak BC, Donker AJ. Endothelial dysfunction precedes development of microalbuminuria in IDDM. *Diabetes* 1995; **44**: 561–4.

52. Stehouwer CD, Yudkin JS, Fioretto P, Nosadini R. How heterogenous is microalbuminuria in diabetes mellitus? The case for 'benign' and 'malignant' microalbuminuria. *Nephrol Dial Transplant* 1998; **13**: 2751–4.

53. Barzilay J, Warram JH, Bak M, Laffel LM, Canessa M, Krolewski AS. Predisposition to hypertension: risk factor for nephropathy and hypertension in IDDM. *Kidney Int* 1992; **41**: 723–30.

54. Earle K, Viberti GC. Familial, hemodynamic and metabolic factors in the predisposition to diabetic kidney disease. *Kidney Int* 1994; **45**: 434–7.

55. Krolewski AS, Canessa M, Warram JH, et al. Predisposition to hypertension and susceptibility to renal disease in insulin-dependent diabetes mellitus. *N Engl J Med* 1988; **318**: 140–5.

56. Viberti GC, Keen H, Wiseman MJ. Raised arterial pressure in parents of proteinuric insulin dependent diabetics. *BMJ* 1987; **295**: 515–17.

57. Fagerudd JA, Tarnow L, Jacobsen P, et al. Predisposition to essential hypertension and development of diabetic nephropathy in IDDM patients. *Diabetes* 1998; **47**: 439–44.

58. Earle KA, Walker J, Hill C, Viberti GC. Familial clustering of cardiovascular disease in patients with insulin-dependent diabetes and nephropathy. *N Engl J Med* 1992; **326**: 673–7.

59. De Cosmo S, Bacci S, Piras GP, et al. High prevalence of risk factors for cardiovascular disease in parents of IDDM patients with albuminuria. *Diabetologia* 1997; **40**: 1191–6.

60. Mogensen CE. Progression of nephropathy in long-term diabetics with proteinuria and effect of initial anti-hypertensive treatment. *Scand J Clin Lab Invest* 1976; **36**: 383–8.

61. Parving HH, Andersen AR, Smidt UM, Hommel E, Mathiesen ER, Svendsen PA. Effect of antihypertensive treatment on kidney function in diabetic nephropathy. *BMJ* 1987; **294**: 1443–7.

62. Parving HH, Smidt UM, Hommel E, et al. Effective antihypertensive treatment postpones renal insufficiency in diabetic nephropathy. *Am J Kidney Dis* 1993; **22**: 188–95.

63. Parving HH. Impact of blood pressure and antihypertensive treatment on overt nephropathy, retinopathy, and endothelial permeability mellitus. *Diabetes Care* 1991; **14**: 260–9.

64. Parving HH. The impact of hypertension and antihypertensive treatment on the course and prognosis of diabetic nephropathy. *J Hypertens* 1990; 8(Suppl): S187–91.

65. Chaiken RL, Palmisano J, Norton ME, et al. Interaction of hypertension and diabetes on renal function in black NIDDM subjects. *Kidney Int* 1995; **47**: 1697–702.

66. Mogensen CE, Hansen KW, Pedersen MM, Christensen CK. Renal factors influencing blood pressure threshold and choice of treatment for hypertension in IDDM. *Diabetes Care* 1991; **14**(Suppl 4): 13–26.

67. Joint National Committee on Prevention, Evaluation and Treatment of high blood pressure. The sixth report of the Joint National Committee on prevention, detection, evaluation, and treatment of high blood pressure. *Arch Intern Med* 1997; **157**: 2413–46.

68. American Diabetes Association Position Statement – Diabetic Nephropathy. *Diabetes Care*, 2002; **25**: S85–S89.

69. Zatz R, Rentz Dunn B, Mayer TW, Anderson S, Rennke HG, Brenner BM. Prevention of diabetic glomerulopathy by pharmacological amelioration of glomerular capillary hypertension. *J Clin Invest* 1986; **77**: 1925–30.

70. Gruden G, Thomas SM, Burt D, et al. Interaction of angiotensin II and stretch in the production of vascular endothelial growth factor by human mesangial cells (Abstract). *FASEB J* 1998; **12**: 599.

71. Gruden G, Thomas SM, Burt D, et al. Angiotensin II and mechanical stretch independently induces Vascular Permeability Factor (VPF) in human mesangial cells (Abstract). *Diabetes* 1997; **46**(Suppl 1): 121A.

72. Lewis EJ, Hunsicker LG, Bain RP, Rohde RD. The effect of angiotensin-converting-enzyme inhibition on diabetic nephropathy. The Collaborative Study Group. *N Engl J Med* 1993; **329**: 1456–62.

73. Bakris GL, Stein JH. Diabetic nephropathy. *Dis Mon* 1993; **39**: 573–611.

74. Elving LD, Wetzels JF, van Lier HJ, de Nobel E, Berden JH. Captopril and atenolol are equally effective in retarding progression of diabetic nephropathy. Results of a 2-year prospective, randomized study. *Diabetologia* 1994; **37**: 604–9.

75. Weidmann P, Schneider M, Bohlen L. Therapeutic efficacy of different antihypertensive drugs in human diabetic nephropathy: an updated meta-analysis. *Nephrol Dial Transplant* 1995; **10**(Suppl 9): 39–45.

76. Microalbuminuria Captopril Study Group. Captopril reduces the risk of nephropathy in IDDM patients with microalbuminuria. *Diabetologia* 1996; **39**: 587–93.

77. Estacio RO, Jeffers BW, Hiatt WR, Biggerstaff SL, Gifford N, Schrier RW. The effect of nisoldipine as compared with enalapril on cardiovascular outcomes in patients with non-insulin-dependent diabetes and hypertension. *N Engl J Med* 1998; **338**: 645–52.

78. Jacobsen P, Rossing K, Rossing P, et al. Angiotensin converting enzyme gene polymorphism and ACE inhibition in diabetic nephropathy. \Kidney Int 1998; **53**: 1002–6.

79. Cooper ME. Pathogenesis, prevention, and treatment of diabetic nephropathy. *Lancet* 1998; **352**: 213–19.

80. Diabetes Control and Complications Trial Research Group. The effect of intensive treatment of diabetes on the development and progression of long-term complications in insulin-dependent diabetes mellitus. *N Engl J Med* 1993; **329**: 977–86.

81. Microalbuminuria Collaborative Study Group United Kingdom. Intensive therapy and progression to clinical albuminuria in patients with insulin dependent diabetes mellitus and microalbuminuria. *BMJ* 1995; **311**: 973–7.

82. Diabetes Control and Complications Trial (DCCT) Research Group. Effect of intensive therapy on the development and progression of diabetic nephropathy in the Diabetes Control and Complications Trial. *Kidney Int* 1995; **47**: 1703–20.

83. Feldt-Rasmussen B, Mathiesen ER, Deckert T. Effect of two years of strict metabolic control on progression of incipient nephropathy in insulin-dependent diabetes. *Lancet* 1986; **2**: 1300–4.

84. Bangstad HJ, Osterby R, Dahl-Jorgensen K, Berg KJ, Hartmann A, Hanssen KF. Improvement of blood glucose control in IDDM patients retards the progression of morphological changes in early diabetic nephropathy. *Diabetologia* 1994; **37**: 483–90.

85. Nyberg G, Blohme I, Norden G. Impact of metabolic control in progression of clinical diabetic nephropathy. *Diabetologia* 1987; **30**: 3082–6.

86. Mulec H, Blohme G, Grande B, Bjorck S. The

effect of metabolic control on rate of decline in renal function in insulin-dependent diabetes mellitus with overt diabetic nephropathy. *Nephrol Dial Transplant* 1998; **13**: 651–5.

87. Bending JJ, Viberti GC, Watkins PJ, Keen H. Intermittent clinical proteinuria and renal function in diabetes: evolution and the effect of glycaemic control. *BMJ* 1986; **292**: 83–6.

88. Viberti GC, Bilous RW, Mackintosh D, Bending JJ, Keen H. Long term correction of hyperglycaemia and progression of renal failure in insulin dependent diabetes. *BMJ* 1983; **286**: 598–602.

89. Manto A, Cotroneo P, Marra G, et al. Effect of intensive treatment on diabetic nephropathy in patients with type I diabetes. *Kidney Int* 1995; **47**: 231–5.

90. Fioretto P, Steffes MW, Sutherland DE, Goetz FC, Mauer M. Reversal of lesions of diabetic nephropathy after pancreas transplantation. *N Engl J Med* 1998; **339**: 69–75.

91. Diabetes Control and Complications Trial Research Group. Effect of intensive diabetes treatment on the development and progression of long-term complications in adolescents with insulin-dependent diabetes mellitus: Diabetes Control and Complications Trial. *J Pediatr* 1994; **125**: 177–88.

92. Malmberg K. Prospective randomised study of intensive insulin treatment on long term survival after acute myocardial infarction in patients with diabetes mellitus. DIGAMI (Diabetes Mellitus, Insulin Glucose Infusion in Acute Myocardial Infarction) Study Group. *BMJ* 1997; **314**: 1512–15.

93. Watts GF, Powrie JK, O'Brien SF, Shaw KM. Apolipoprotein B independently predicts progression of very-low-level albuminuria in insulin-dependent diabetes mellitus. *Metabolism* 1996; **5**: 1101–7.

94. Krolewski AS, Warram JH, Christlieb AR. Hypercholesterolemia – a determinant of renal function loss and deaths in IDDM patients with nephropathy. *Kidney Int* 1994; Suppl 45: S125–31.

95. Mulec H, Johnsen SA, Wiklund O, Bjorck S. Cholesterol: a renal risk factor in diabetic nephropathy? *Am J Kidney Dis* 1993; **22**: 196–201.

96. Walker JD, Bending JJ, Dodds RA, et al. Restriction of dietary protein and progression of renal failure in diabetic nephropathy. *Lancet* 1989; **2**: 1411–15.

97. Barnes DJ, Pinto J, Viberti GC. The patient with diabetes mellitus. In: Cameron S, Davison AM, Grunfeld J, Kerr D, Ritz E, Winearls C, eds. *Oxford textbook of clinical nephrology*, 2nd edn. Oxford Medical Publications, Oxford, 1998: 723–77.

98. Sawicki PT, Muhlhauser I, Bender R, Pethke W, Heinemann L, Berger M. Effects of smoking on blood pressure and proteinuria in patients with diabetic nephropathy. *J Intern Med* 1996; **239**: 345–52.

99. Mogensen CE, Keane WF, Bennett PH, et al. Prevention of diabetic renal disease with special reference to microalbuminuria. *Lancet* 1995; **346**: 1080–4.

13

The clinical implications and management of microalbuminuria and proteinuria in type II diabetic subjects

Mark E Cooper

Introduction

In the 1930s Kimmelsteil and Wilson characterised the pathological features of diabetic nephropathy. They described the classical lesions of nodular glomerulosclerosis associated with proteinuria and hypertension.[1] In that report of seven cases, the average age was 59 years and the average duration of diabetes was 4 years, consistent with these patients having type II diabetes. Diabetic nephropathy is now the major cause of end-stage renal failure in the Western world. Renal disease remains a major cause of morbidity and mortality in the population with type I diabetes and is becoming an increasingly important clinical problem in type II diabetes. Indeed, as the prevalence of type II diabetes is at least five-fold higher than type I diabetes, this form now contributes at least 50 per cent of diabetic patients in end-stage renal failure programmes.

Natural history of nephropathy in type II diabetes

Although there are some minor differences in the natural history of diabetic nephropathy in type I and type II diabetes there are many similarities.[2] In particular, the classification of nephropathy by Mogensen into a number of distinct phases can, in general, be used for both forms of diabetes.[3] The initial changes, which include glomerular hyperfiltration, have been shown to occur in type II diabetes although not as prominently as reported in type I.[4] This is followed by a silent phase which is associated with subtle morphological changes including glomerular basement membrane thickening, glomerular hypertrophy, mesangial expansion and modest expansion of the tubulo-interstitium. This is followed by a phase known as microalbuminuria or incipient diabetic nephropathy.[5] This is characterised by a modest increase in excretion of albumin into the urine. On renal biopsy, there is evidence of significant glomerular injury,[6] although in type II diabetic patients the pattern is more heterogenous, suggesting a more complex pathogenesis than in type I diabetes.[7] Microalbuminuria is commonly associated with other diabetic complications as well as with cardiovascular disease.[8] Multiple explanations have been provided for the relationship between microalbuminuria and cardiovascular disease. These include common pathogenetic pathways or risk factors such as endothelial dysfunction,[9] hypertension, abnormalities in lipid metabolism, insulin resistance,[10] smoking and metabolic pathways linked to glucose or glucose-derived proteins such as advanced glycated lipoproteins.

Treatment – glycaemic control

There is a range of theoretical reasons for optimising glycaemic control in diabetic patients, as a number of pathogenetic pathways for diabetic nephropathy are glucose-dependent.[11] As in type I diabetes, it has been shown in type II diabetes that hyperglycaemia is a major determinant of progression of diabetic nephropathy.[12] In a Japanese study of type II diabetic subjects, intensified glycaemic control was also shown to reduce the rate of development of diabetic nephropathy.[13] Although the effects of intervention with intensive glycaemic control have not been studied as thoroughly in type II diabetes as in type I, this 6-year study in 110 relatively young (mean age approximately 50 years), non-obese type II diabetic patients from Kumamoto, Japan, indicated a beneficial effect of intensive insulin therapy.[13] Intensive insulin therapy reduced the risk of microalbuminuria by 62 per cent and albuminuria by 100 per cent in the primary prevention cohort. In the secondary intervention cohort, defined by the presence of retinopathy, improved glycaemic control reduced the risk of microalbuminuria by 52 per cent and albuminuria by 100 per cent. In this Japanese study, an assessment was also made of the relationship between mean HbA_{1c} and rates of worsening of diabetic nephropathy. This showed that diabetic nephropathy did not worsen if mean HBA_{1c} was kept below 6.5 per cent (normal range 4.8–6.4 per cent). Above this glycaemic threshold, any improvement in glycaemic control was associated with slower progression of nephropathy. The above evidence in Japanese type II diabetic subjects provides strong support for the concept that improved glycaemic control attenuates early diabetic nephropathy, as reflected by microalbuminuria. However,

evidence to support the importance of metabolic control in obese Caucasian patients with type II diabetes has only recently been obtained. For instance, no benefits with regard to the development of diabetic nephropathy were observed with intensive insulin therapy after 7 years in the University Group Diabetes Program. The United Kingdom Prospective Diabetes study (UKPDS) helped clarify the role of glycaemic control in preventing the development of microalbuminuria defined as urinary protein excretion rate of >50 mg/l. This study showed that intensified control of blood glucose with sulfonylureas or insulin reduced the risk of developing microalbuminuria by approximately 30% after 15 years of follow-up (Fig. 13.1).[14] Nevertheless, this implies that even after considerable effort to optimize glycaemic control in type 2 diabetes, many patients are still at risk of developing nephropathy. The recent American Diabetes Association position statement on the prevention and management of nephropathy in type 2 diabetes recommend aiming for a glycosylated haemoglobin of <7%.[15]

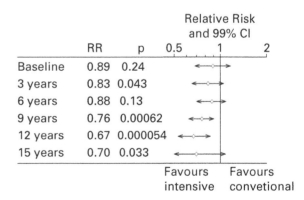

	RR	p	Relative Risk and 99% CI		
			0.5	1	2
Baseline	0.89	0.24			
3 years	0.83	0.043			
6 years	0.88	0.13			
9 years	0.76	0.00062			
12 years	0.67	0.000054			
15 years	0.70	0.033			
			Favours intensive	Favours convetional	

Figure 13.1
The relative risk (1/2 99% confidence intervals) of developing microalbuminuria (urine protein excretion of >50 mg/l) in UKPDS, comparing intensified versus conventional glycaemic control (difference in glycated HbAlc of ,1%). Adapted from reference 14.

Treatment – antihypertensive therapy

Proteinuria

In type I diabetic subjects, the initial studies by Mogensen and Parving et al. clearly demonstrated the importance of antihypertensive agents in overt diabetic nephropathy.[16,17] The possibility of an additional renoprotective effect of angiotensin-converting (ACE) inhibitors was suggested by the Collaborative Study Group, who showed that captopril reduced proteinuria and was associated with less end-stage renal failure in a population of predominantly hypertensive type I diabetic subjects with macroproteinuria. However, the role of ACE inhibitors has not been as clearly defined in type II diabetes. Over the last few years, several studies with duration ⩾12 months have also indicated a role for antihypertensive agents in macroproteinuric type II diabetic subjects (Table 13.1).

The impact of ACE inhibitors, calcium channel blockers (CCBs) and conventional antihypertensive agents on renal function has been evaluated in both normotensive and hypertensive type II diabetic subjects with persistent proteinuria and variable degrees of renal impairment.[18] In hypertensive type II diabetic subjects with persistent proteinuria studied for periods of up to 6 months, ACE inhibitors[19,20] and certain CCBs[20–22] reduced albuminuria. Comparable responses were also obtained with the beta-blocker atenolol, but not with the thiazide diuretic, chlorthalidone, despite similar reduction in blood pressure.[23]

A number of recent studies have confirmed that ACE inhibitors are superior to other antihypertensive agents, including the dihydropyridine calcium channel blockers (in particular nifedipine)[24,25] as well as the vasodilator, hydralazine,[26] in reducing albuminuria in hypertensive type II diabetic subjects with macroproteinuria. However, Parving's group has reported a disparity in effects on albuminuria and renal function.[27] Whereas lisinopril was more effective than atenolol in reducing albuminuria, both agents were similar in efficacy in terms of rate of decline in GFR.

The Heart Outcomes Prevention Evaluation study (HOPE) reported that the ACE-inhibitor ramipril reduced the risk of developing overt nephropathy by 24% (placebo: 8.4% versus ramipril: 6.5%, RR 0.74, CI: 0.6–0.97, $p < 0.027$) in 'normotensive' patients (BP <140/90 mmHg ± antihypertensive therapy) with type 2 diabetes and normoalbuminuria or microalbuminuria at baseline.[28] These data were derived from a large cohort of patients with type 2 diabetes and at least one additional cardiovascular risk factor and mean age of 65 years. The study duration was 5 years and 56% of the patients were defined as hypertensive and the mean blood pressures of the total study population at baseline were; placebo 142.3/79 mmHg, ramipril: 147.7/80 mmHg. The authors have attributed the outcome of the study to the benefits of ramipril therapy, concluding that the final differences in blood pressure between the ramipril and placebo (~ −2/1 mmHg) were insufficient to account for the benefits observed in the ramipril treated patients.

There have been significant differences in the effect on albuminuria obtained with various CCBs, which has been attributed by Bakris and co-workers to the particular class of CCB.[29,30] Bakris et al. have reported an antiproteinuric effect with the CCB, verapamil, as well as with ACE inhibition.[29] In contrast, nifedipine, a dihydropyridine CCB, given for 6 weeks to 14 hypertensive type II diabetic patients with baseline renal impairment, precipitated an increase in albuminuria and a deterioration in renal function, despite

Agent	Duration	n	AER (%)*	GFR	BP	Reference no.
Lisinopril	18 months	10	↓ (−42)	→	↓	28
Diltiazem		10	↓ (−45)	→	↓	
Frusemide and atenolol		10	↓	↓	↓	
Lisinopril	36 months	17	↓ (−55)	↓	↓	26
Atenolol		19	↓ (−15)	↓	↓	
Enalapril	12 months	18	↓ (−87)	→	↓	24
Nifedipine		12	→	→	↓	
Enalapril	52 weeks	7	↓ (−71)	→	↓	23
Nifedipine		10	→		↓	
Captopril	18 months	24	↓ (−27)	→	↓	25
Hydralazine		18	→		↓	
Lisinopril (L)	12 months	8	↓ (−59)	↓	↓	27
Verapamil (V)		8	↓ (−50)	↓	↓	
L + V		8	↓ (−78)	↓	↓	
G + H		6	→	↓	↓	
Verapamil (V)	>4 years	18	↓ (−60)	↓	↓	31
Atenolol		16	↓ (−20)	↓↓	↓	
Lisinopril (L)	5 years	18	↓ (−25)	↓	↓	32
Atenolol		16	→	↓↓	↓	
V or Diltiazem		16	↓ (−18)	↓	↓	

AER, albumin excretion rate; GFR, glomerular filtration rate; BP, blood pressure;
G + H, guanfacine + hydrochlorothiazide.
*In some of these studies proteinuria rather than AER was measured.

Table 13.1
The effect of antihypertensive agents on albuminuria, renal function and blood pressure in hypertensive type II diabetic subjects with established nephropathy.

equivalent blood pressure reduction to diltiazem.[22] In contrast, it has been shown by several groups that the dihydropyridine class of CCB is not as efficacious at reducing albuminuria.[24,25,31] A study in African American type II diabetic subjects with hypertension and macroproteinuria, isradipine was associated with an increase in proteinuria, whereas captopril reduced proteinuria.[32]

Slataper et al. have reported that in a randomised parallel group study comparing diltiazem, lisinopril and conventional therapy (atenolol and frusemide) in hypertensive type II diabetic subjects with nephrotic range proteinuria and renal insufficiency, after 18 months of therapy the rate of decline of glomerular filtration rate was attenuated with either diltiazem or lisinopril when compared with the conventional therapy group, despite comparable blood pressure reduction.[30] The beneficial changes in glomerular filtration rate were paralleled by changes in albuminuria with significant reduction in the diltiazem and lisinopril groups, but no change in the conventionally treated group.

Pursuing this theme, Bakris et al. have reported the findings of two studies in hypertensive type II diabetic subjects with macroproteinuria followed for over 4 years.[33,34] In both studies, the beta-blocker atenolol was associated with a more rapid decline in GFR and less efficacy in terms of reduction in albuminuria than the non-dihydropyridine CCBs, verapamil and diltiazem,[33,34] or the ACE inhibitor, lisinopril.[33]

The aforementioned studies had used a reduction in proteinuria as a surrogate end point for nephroprotection in patients with type 2 diabetes. What was clearly needed were longer-term studies that evaluated the effectiveness of therapeutic intervention at delaying the progression of nephropathy towards end stage renal disease (ESRD) in patients with type 2 diabetes. Two studies have recently reported that addressed this key question; the Irbesartan Diabetic Nephropathy Trial (IDNT)[35] and the Reduction of Endpoints in NIDDM with Angiotensin II Antagonist Losartan (RENAAL)[36] studies. Both studies evaluated the effectiveness of angiotensin receptor blocker (ARB)-based therapy on a similar primary composite end-point, comprising a doubling of baseline creatinine, progression to ESRD, or death in people with type 2 diabetes and nephropathy (proteinuria). A comparison of the studies is shown in Tables 13.2–13.4. These studies were important because they systematically evaluated the effectiveness of renin angiotensin system (RAS) blockade in delaying the progression of nephropathy in type 2 diabetes for the first time. Although it seemed likely that the pathogenesis of nephropathy was similar for both

type 1 and type 2 diabetes, it was important to establish in patients with type 2 diabetes whether or not blockade of the RAS would provide nephro-protection, over and above that attributable to blood pressure reduction. Moreover, the studies evaluated an alternative strategy to ACE-inhibition for blockade of the RAS, notably the ARBs.

The IDNT study:[35] This study randomly assigned 1715 hypertensive patients with type diabetes and nephropathy to treatment with irbesartan (300 mg daily), or amlodipine 10 mg daily or placebo 10 mg daily for a mean duration of follow-up of 2.6 years. The target blood pressure was 135/85 mmHg or less, thus most patients received additional antihypertensive therapies (excluding ACE-inhibitors, calcium channel blockers and other angiotensin II antagonists) in an endeavour to achieve these goals. The inclusion of a treatment arm in which patients were randomised to receive amlodipine-based therapy was important for two reasons; first, it ensured better control for blood pressure differences that have previously plagued the interpretation of trials in which the active drug always seemed to achieve better blood pressure control than placebo-based therapy (even though all patients receive additional antihypertensive therapy as required to control blood pressure). Second, it allowed a direct examination of the effectiveness of a CCB-based therapy at nephroprotection. The patients had a mean age of ~59 years and about 2/3 were men. These were patients with advanced nephropathy, excreting almost 3 g of urinary protein per 24 hours at baseline. The base-line blood pressure was ~159/87 across the groups and the patients on average required at least 3 additional drugs to control their blood pressure. The mean blood pressures during the study, on treatment, were 140/77 in the irbesartan group, 141/77 in the amlodipine group and

	RENAAL	IDNT
Design:	Multi-centered, multi-national, triple-blind, randomized, placebo-controlled – Usual Care (placebo) vs losartan 50, 100 mg QD	Multi-centered, multi-national, double-blind, randomized, placebo-controlled – Usual Care (placebo) vs amlodipine vs irbesartan 75, 150, 300 mg QD
Primary Endpoints:	Doubling of serum creatinine, end-stage renal disease or death	Doubling of serum creatinine, end-stage renal disease or death
Secondary Endpoints:	Cardiovascular events, progression of renal disease, and changes in proteinuria	Fatal or non-fatal cardiovascular events

Tables 13.2

	RENAAL	IDNT
Target BP:	< 140/90 mmHg	< 135/85 mmHg
Patients:	1,513 97% Hypertensive and 3% Normotensive 751 Losartan + conventional therapy 762 Placebo + conventional therapy	1,715 Hypertensive 579 irbesartan + usual care 567 amlodipine + usual care 569 Placebo + usual care
Duration:	Average 3.4 Years	Average 2.6 Years

Tables 13.3

RENAAL	IDNT
Age: 60 ± 7.5 years sCr: 1.9 ± 0.5 mg/dl Baseline BP: 152/82 ± 19/10 mmHg HbA1C: 8.5 ± 1.6% UA/Cr 1867 ± 2701 mg/g (~3.9 g/24 hr)	Age: 59 ± 8 years sCr: 1.7 ± 0.6 mg/dl Baseline BP: 156/85 ± 18/11 mmHg HbA1C: 8.1 ± 1.7% UPE: 4.2 ± 4.1 g/24 hr

Tables 13.4

Tables 13.2–13.4
Comparison of characteristics of the IDNT and RENAAL studies.[35,36]
sCr = baseline serum creatinine. UA/Cr = urinary albumin/urinary creatinine ratio. UPE = urinary protein excretion

144/80 in the placebo group. Thus once again, the placebo group had on average a higher systolic blood pressure by 3–4 mmHg. Moreover, the goal blood pressure was not achieved. The primary composite end-point was a combination of doubling of serum creatinine, progression to end-stage renal failure or death from any cause. Irbesartan-based therapy was associated with a 20% reduction in the primary end-point when compared to placebo, largely driven by a 33% reduction in the rate of doubling of serum creatinine. Amlodipine-based therapy was little different from placebo-based therapy. There was no difference in the rates of death between the groups. This suggests that despite equivalent blood pressure control between the irbesartan and amlodipine groups, irbesartan-based therapy was associated with greater protection against progression of renal disease in patients with type 2 diabetes and advanced diabetic nephropathy.

The absolute rates of change in creatinine clearance were significantly reduced in the irbessartan group; placebo;-6.5 ± 0.37 ml/min/$1.73\,m^2$/year, irbesartan; -5.5 ± 0.36, amlodipine; -6.8 ± 0.37. Proteinuria was reduced by an average of 33% in the irbesartan group compared to 6% and 10% in the amlodipine and placebo groups respectively.

The RENAAL study:[36] This study also focussed on patients with type 2 diabetes and advanced nephropathy. Many of the characteristics of the patients studied were similar to those studied in IDNT cited above (Tables 13.2–13.4). This study randomized 1513 patients with type 2 diabetes and nephropathy to either placebo or losartan-based therapy, in addition to other antihypertensive patients as required (excluding ACE-inhibitors or other ARBs). The patients were followed for a mean of 3.4 years and the composite primary outcome was similar to that cited for IDNT, i.e.

doubling of serum creatinine, progression to ESRD or death. The mean blood pressures at base-line were similar in both arms of the study 152/82 mmHg in the losartan group and 153/82 mmHg in the placebo group. Over 90% of the patients were receiving antihypertensive therapy. At the end of the study, the blood pressures were on average 142/74 in the placebo group and 140/74 in the losartan group. Thus there was a difference of ~2 mmHg systolic between the groups at the end of the study with greater differences earlier in the study. Like irbesartan in the IDNT study, losartan in the RENAAL study significantly reduced the frequency of the primary end-point (-16% versus placebo, $p < 0.024$). This was primarily driven by a reduction in the rate of doubling of serum creatinine (-25%), and reduction in the rate of progression to end-stage renal failure (-28%) (Table 13.5). Most (71%) patients received losartan at the higher dose used in the study, i.e. 100 mg daily. Importantly, over 70% of patients receiving losartan or placebo, also received calcium antagonists and on average patients required at least three additional drugs to control their blood pressure. Of interest, there was also a highly significant reduction in the losartan treated patients in one of the components of the secondary end-point, notably first hopitalization for heart failure (-32%, $p < 0.005$).

What do the IDNT and RENAAL studies tell us? These studies demonstrate that the rate of progression of established nephropathy in patients with type 2 can be delayed by effective antihypertensive therapy and blockade of the angiotensin receptor either with irbesartan 300 mg daily or losartan 100 mg daily, in addition to conventional antihypertensive therapy. The rate of loss of GFR in such patients will be stablized at ~ -5 mls/min/year, which compares very favourably with the usual rate of

End Point	IDNT						RENAAL				
	Ibesartan (n = 579) N (%)	Amiodipine (n = 567) N (%)	Placebo (n = 569) N (%)	Risk reduction Irbesartan vs. Placebo	95% CI	P-value	Losartan (n = 751)	Placebo (n = 762)	Risk reduction	85% CI	P-value
DsCr ESRD Death	189 (32.6)	233 (41.1)	222 (39.0)	19%	1–33	0.03	327 (43.5)	359 (47.1)	16%	2–28	0.02
DsCr	98 (16.9)	144 (25.4)	135 (23.7)	29%	8–46	0.009	162 (21.6)	198 (26.0)	25%	8–39	0.006
ESRD	82	104 (18.3)	101	17%	−11–38	0.19	147 (19.6)	194 (25.5)	28%	11–42	0.002
Death	87 (15.0)	83 (14.6)	93 (16.3)	6	−27–30	0.69	158 (21.0)	155 (20.3)	−2%	−27–19	0.88
Secondary CVD	138 (23.8)	128 (22.6)	144 ()25.3)	9	−14–28	0.40	247 (32.9)	268 (35.2)	10%	−8–24	0.26

Table 13.5
The primary and secondary end-points and outcomes for the IDNT and RENAAL studies. DsCr = doubling of baseline serum creatinine. ESRD = End Stage Renal Disease. CVD = Cardiovascular disease end-points. CI = confidence intervals. Data from references 35 and 36.

loss of GFR in untreated hypertensive patients with overt diabetic nephropathy, i.e. 10–12 ml/min/year.

No such data exists with ACE-inhibitor therapy in this patient population. The recently completed Appropriate Blood Pressure Control in Diabetes (ABCD) study did not confirm superiority of ACE inhibitor-based therapy (Enalapril) over CCB-based therapy (nisoldipine) in terms of rate of change of creatinine clearance over 5 years.[37,38] Nevertheless, the characteristics of the reno-protective effect observed with ARBs in patients with type 2 diabetes and nephropathy, in terms of proteinuria reduction and the magnitude of the effect on the primary endpoint, are similar to those observed with ACE-inhibitor therapy in type 1 diabetes. This suggests that the mechanisms for benefit are most likely dependent on eliminating the actions of Ang II, either by blunting its production with ACE-inhibition, or blockade of its action with ARBs. Whether AIIAs would be as effective in type 1 diabetic nephropathy, or ACE-inhibition in type 2 diabetic nephropathy is not known but seems likely. Nevertheless, it seems unlikely that such "head-to-head" trials between ACE-inhibition and ARBs in patients with nephropathy will ever be performed to specifically answer this question.

The IDNT study also suggests that once the patient with type 2 diabetes has developed nephropathy (proteinuria), CCBs (i.e. amlodipine) without co-existing blockade of the RAS, is less effective at protecting against progression of renal disease than treatment regimes that do include RAS blockade. Importantly however, the RENAAL study confirmed that CCBs can be very effective when used in combination with ARBs to achieve blood pressure goals and that this does not negate the reno-protective effect of the ARB alone.

Most patients with incipient or overt nephropathy require at least three different antihypertensive drugs to control blood pressure to target. This will invariably include a diuretic. Loop diuretics (e.g. frusemide) are preferred once a patient has developed renal impairment and high dose loop diuretics (e.g. fruesemide 250 mg+ daily) are often required once the serum creatinine exceeds 200 µmol/l. In this setting, hypokalaemia due to high dose diuretic therapy is hardly ever encountered, particularly as they will be used in combination with RAS blockade.

In the past, there has been caution, perhaps over-caution, in the use of drugs that block the RAS in patients with established renal impairment, because of perceived risks of substantial declines in renal function and hyperkalaemia. Both IDNT and RENAAL studied patients with advanced nephropathy and confirmed that hyperkalaemia was a very uncommon cause for the need to discontinue therapy (<2%), even in patients with advanced renal impairment, probably because of co-existing prescription of higher dose loop diuretics. Nevertheless, blood potassium should be monitored closely in patients with established renal impairment.

It is interesting to note that despite the best efforts of the study investigators, it was not possible to lower systolic blood pressure to below 140 mmHg. This has been a consistent feature of many studies in patients with type 2 diabetes.

Microalbuminuria and hypertension (Table 13.6)

The use of antihypertensive therapy in type II diabetic subjects with hypertension and microalbuminuria has been evaluated by an increasing number of investigators over the last decade.[18] Gambardella and co-workers[39] showed that indapamide 2.5 mg daily did not

Patients	Agent	Duration of study	n	Δ in AER (%)	Δ in GFR	Δ in BP	Reference no.
Micro HT	Indapamide	36 months	10	↓ (−64)	→	↓	39
Micro HT	Captopril M or HCTZ	36 months	9 12	↓ (−65) →	→ →	↓ ↓	40
Micro HT	Enalapril (E) Nifedipine (N)	12 months	16 15	↓ (−70) →	→ →	↓ ↓	24
Micro HT	E + N Nifedipine	48 months	11 13	↓ (−42) ↑ (+29)	→ →	↓ ↓	48
Micro HT	Lisinopril Nifedipine	12 months	15 6 15 8	↓ (−37) →	→ →	↓ ↓	43
Micro HT	Cilazipril Amlodipine	3 years	9 9	↓ (−27) ↓ (−31)	↓ ↓	↓ ↓	42
Micro HT	R ± Felodipine A ± HCTZ	12 months	46 45	→ ↑	→ ↓	↓ ↓	41
Micro HT	Placebo Irbesartan	24 months	590	+9 −46		↓ ↓	44
Micro HT	Amlodipine Valsartan	24 weeks	332	→ ↓		↓ ↓	45

Micro, microalbuminuria; HT, hypertensive; AER, albumin excretion rate; GFR, glomerular filtration rate; BP, blood pressure; HCTZ, hydrochlorothiazide; M, metoprolol; A, atenolol.

Table 13.6
The effect of antihypertensive agents on albuminuria, renal function and blood pressure in type II diabetic subjects with hypertension and microalbuminuria.

alter albuminuria or glomerular filtration rate over a 24-month period in hypertensive normoalbuminuric patients despite a significant reduction in blood pressure. A double-blind study by Lacourciere et al. compared captopril with conventional therapy (metoprolol and hydrochlorothiazide) in normoalbuminuric and microalbuminuric hypertensive type II diabetic subjects over a 3-year period.[40] Both regimens reduced blood pressure without

altering albuminuria in the normoalbuminuric type II diabetic subjects. However, their findings in hypertensive type II diabetic patients with microalbuminuria indicated that despite a comparable reduction in blood pressure, only the ACE inhibitor induced a persistent decline in albuminuria during the 36 months of therapy.

Schnack et al. have reported that ramipril with or without felodipine stabilised albuminuria. In contrast, atenolol with or without diuretic treatment was associated with an increase in urinary albumin excretion.[41] Furthermore, the ramipril-treated group had stable renal function, whereas the group receiving beta-blockers had a decline in GFR. A reduction in albuminuria by ACE inhibition has also been observed by a number of other investigators.[24,42,43]

In the Melbourne Diabetic Nephropathy Study, nifedipine was shown to produce a similar response to perindopril in decreasing albuminuria over 12 months in the type II diabetic subjects with microalbuminuria.[46] It has been reported by Chan et al. that the ACE inhibitor, enalapril, was more effective than nifedipine in reducing albuminuria in a group of hypertensive microalbuminuric subjects.[24] Recently, several new studies have been reported which have compared calcium channel blockade with ACE inhibition in hypertensive microalbuminuric type II diabetic subjects.[42,43] In a study over 3 years, in a relatively small number of subjects, amlodipine was as effective as the ACE inhibitor, cilazapril, in reducing albuminuria, with both treatment groups having similar declines in renal function.[42] However, in a much larger multicentre study of >300 subjects, the ACE inhibitor, lisinopril, reduced albuminuria over 12 months, whereas nifedipine failed to significantly influence urinary albumin excretion.[43]

Recently, two studies have reported the first data on the use of ARBs in patients with type 2 diabetes, hypertension and microalbuminuria.

Effect of Irbesartan in type 2 diabetic patients with incipient nephropathy (microalbuminuria) (IRMA2). This multinational study enrolled 590 patients with type 2 diabetes, hypertension and microalbuminuria.[44] The patients were randomized to receive either placebo or irbesartan 150 mg daily or 300 mg

daily, in addition to any other antihypertensive medications (excluding ACE-inhibitors or other ARBs). The baseline blood pressures in all three groups was very similar ~153/90 mmHg and the baseline urinary albumin excretion rate was 50–60 µg/min. The patients all had a normal baseline GFR (~110 ml/min/1.73m²). At the end of 2 years follow-up, nephropathy (overt proteinuria) developed in 30 patients in the placebo group, compared to only 19 in the group receiving irbesartan 150 mg/day and 10 receiving irbesartan 300 mg/day. This was a highly significant reduction in the likelihood of progression to nephropathy by 70% in the group receiving irbesartan 300 mg/day (Fig. 13.2). There was a significant 3 mmHg difference in the average trough systolic blood pressure between the placebo and the irbesartan 300 mg/day group, suggesting that the effect was mediated via angiotensin II receptor blockade and blood pressure reduction. Mindful of the fact that urinary albumin excretion would be expected

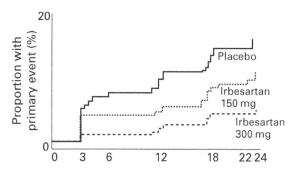

Figure 13.2
Percent of patients with type 2 diabetes progressing from microalbuminuria to overt nephropathy (proteinuria) according to treatment allocation in the IRMA-2 study.[44]

to rise year-on-year in patients with established microalbuminuria, there was an impressive reduction in albuminuria in the patients receiving irbesartan (−38% in the group receiving irbesartan 300 mg/day vs placebo) and this appeared to be drug-dose dependent in that irbesartan 300 mg/day produced a greater reduction in albuminuria than 150 mg irbesartan daily. This important study suggests that improved blood pressure control, targeting to a pressure below 140/80 mmHg, and blockade of the angiotensin II receptor with higher dose irbesartan will help delay the progression of incipient to overt type 2 diabetic nephropathy. In fact the rate of decline of GFR in patients with microalbuminuria, treated in this way will be stabilized to ~ −2 ml/min/yr. This is greater than the normal age-related decline in GFR of −1 ml/min/yr but does represent an impressive stabilization of the clinical course of the disease process.

Microalbuminuria Reduction with Valsartan (MARVAL) Trial: This recently reported study in patients with type 2 diabetes and microalbuminuria complements the IRMA-2 study. The MARVAL study[45] compared the ARB valsartan with the CCB amlodipine in 332 patients with type 2 diabetes and microalbuminuria. The mean baseline blood pressures were similar in both groups (~147/85) and 65% were considered to be hypertensive (≥140/90 mmHg) at baseline. The patients were randomized to amlodipine or valsartan and the dose was uptitrated and other antihypertensive therapies were added when necessary to achieve a goal blood pressure of <135/85 mmHg. The average fall in blood pressure was ~11.5/6 mmHg and was similar in both treatment groups. Despite this, after 24 weeks of study, there were marked differences in the anti-proteinuric effects of ARB versus CCB-based therapies. Whilst valsartan-based therapy reduced urinary albumin excretion by ~40%, there was little change in the group randomized to amlodipine and these differences were highly significant (p<0.001). Moreover, more patients were restored to a normal albumin excretion rate after 24 weeks with valsartan based therapy (49%) was greater than that with amlodipine-based therapy (23%), p<0.001.

These two studies along with the HOPE study[28] that blockade of RAS, either with ACE-inhibition or an ARB, in combination with blood pressure reduction, delays the progression of microalbuminuria to proteinuria in people with type 2 diabetes. This appears to be true irrespective of whether the patient is "normotensive" (blood pressure <140/90 mmHg) or hypertensive (blood pressure ≥140/90 mmHg) at baseline. This has led to the recommendation that RAS blockade should form part of the treatment of all patients with type 2 diabetes and microalbuminuria.[15]

Microalbuminuria and normotension (Table 13.7)

The possibility that early therapy will postpone or retard progression of renal injury in diabetes has led to the use of antihypertensive agents in normotensive subjects. In the Melbourne Diabetic Nephropathy study[46] there was no change in albuminuria after treatment for 12 months with either nifedipine or perindopril in normotensive microalbuminuric patients, despite a small but significant reduction in blood pressure of ~4 mmHg. Nonetheless, on stopping therapy at 12 months, a dramatic increase in albuminuria was detected in the type II but not in the type I diabetic subjects, which was independent of mode of treatment.[47] The inability of either agent to reduce albuminuria in the normotensive cohort coupled with the rapid rise after stopping therapy

Patients	Agent	Duration of study	n	Δ in AER (%)	Δ in GFR	Δ in BP	Reference no.
Micro NT	Nifedipine	12 months	13	→	→	→	46
	Perindopril		11	→	→	→	
Micro NT	Enalapril	48 months	12	↓ (−47)	→	↓	48
	Placebo		12	→	→	→	
Micro NT	Enalapril	5 years	49	→	→	→	50
	Placebo		45	↑ (+152)	↓	→	
Micro NT	Enalapril	5 years	52	↓ (−64)	→	→	49
	Placebo		51	↑ (+60)	→	→	

Micro, microalbuminuria; NT, normotensive; AER, albumin excretion rate; GFR, glomerular filtration rate; BP, blood pressure.

Table 13.7
The effect of antihypertensive agents on albuminuria, renal function and blood pressure in type II diabetic subjects with microalbuminuria and 'normal' blood pressure.

needs to be considered in the setting of the natural history of microalbuminuria. Albuminuria would be anticipated to rise by an average of 20–50 per cent if left untreated for 12 months in microalbuminuric type II diabetic subjects. This phenomenon of a rapid rise in albuminuria was not as clearly apparent in the type I diabetic patients and may indicate a difference in the underlying aetiology and pathogenesis of albuminuria in type II as compared with type I diabetes. It is possible that there are differences in the sensitivity to structural damage incurred from blood pressure between type I and type II diabetes. To further explore this issue, a placebo-controlled study by the Melbourne Diabetic Nephropathy Study Group is now in progress and it is anticipated that after 5 years of treatment, it will be possible to determine if there are significant advantages of certain antihypertensive regimens in the microalbuminuric type II diabetic population. It should be appreciated that

the Melbourne Diabetic Nephropathy Study is being performed in a predominantly Europid population and may not reflect the recent reports of placebo-controlled studies from Japan, India and Israel.[48–50]

The first long-term placebo-controlled double-blind randomised study to evaluate the effect of an antihypertensive agent in normotensive microalbuminuric subjects was reported by Ravid et al.[50] During the first year of treatment albuminuria decreased in the enalapril-treated group from an initial mean of 143 mg/24 hours to a mean of 122 mg/24 hours. In the placebo-treated patients, a gradual increase in albuminuria occurred from a baseline of 123–310 mg/24 hours over the 5 years. In contrast, there was no significant increase in albuminuria in the enalapril-treated group over the 5-year study period. Overt nephropathy, defined as a urinary albumin excretion >300 mg/24 hours occurred in only 6/49 (12.2 per cent) of the enalapril group compared with 19/45 (42.2 per cent) of the placebo-treated group. Although the assessment of renal function (assessed as 100/serum creatinine) was rather crude in the enalapril-treated group, there was no change in this parameter, whereas in the placebo group there was a 13 per cent decrease in the reciprocal of serum creatinine. This study suggests that there is both an antiproteinuric effect of an ACE inhibitor in normotensive type II diabetic patients with microalbuminuria and a preservation of renal function. A follow-up report after treatment for 7 years has confirmed a renoprotective effect of ACE inhibition in this cohort.[51]

Sano et al. have observed in a 4-year study that enalapril treatment reduced albuminuria, whereas placebo treatment was associated with no change in albuminuria in a group of normotensive, microalbuminuric type II diabetic patients.[48] Recently, Ahmad et al. have reported similar effects on albuminuria after 5 years of ACE inhibitor therapy in a group of Indian normotensive type II diabetic subjects with microalbuminuria.[49] Enalapril treatment was associated with a reduction in albuminuria, whereas in the placebo group there was a progressive rise in urinary albumin excretion. Of particular interest was the finding that these effects were observed in the absence of a discernible difference in blood pressure between the two groups. Whether these effects of ACE inhibitors in normotensive patients will also be observed with other antihypertensive agents such as CCBs is the subject of a new placebo-controlled study by the Melbourne Diabetic Nephropathy Study Group.[52]

Combination therapy

The aforementioned studies have all emphasized that combinations of antihypertensive therapies will be required to achieve recommended goals in patients with type 2 diabetes

and incipient or overt nephropathy.

It has been proposed that the combination of a calcium antagonist with a converting enzyme inhibitor should result in a greater reduction in urinary protein excretion and slowed morphological progression of nephropathy.[53] Bakris et al. have compared the renal haemodynamic and antiproteinuric effects of a calcium antagonist (verapamil) and an ACE inhibitor (lisinopril) alone and in combination in three groups of type II diabetic subjects with documented nephrotic range proteinuria, hypertension and renal insufficiency.[29] Patients treated with the combination of a calcium antagonist and an ACE inhibitor manifested the greatest reduction in albuminuria. In addition, the decline in GFR was the lowest in this group.

Sano et al. have shown that the addition of enalapril to nifedipine conferred an additional effect in decreasing albuminuria in a group of microalbuminuric type II diabetic subjects.[48] A recent report by Bakris et al. has suggested that the combination of verapamil and trandolapril, administered in a fixed dose combination, is more effective at reducing proteinuria than either drug alone, despite similar effects on blood pressure.[54] Similar findings have now been reported by Fogari et al., who have shown that benazepril plus amlodipine tended to be more effective than benazepril alone in reducing albuminuria in microalbuminuric, hypertensive type II diabetic patients.[55]

The RENAAL study also confirmed that the addition of a CCV to ARB-based therapy did not diminish the antiproteinuric effect of the ARB and was essential to optimise blood pressure control in most of the patients studied.[36]

The studies described above focus on the combination of ACE inhibitor and calcium antagonist. However, other combinations also need to be considered. For example, diuretics have been shown to potentiate the hypotensive actions of agents which inhibit the renin-angiotensin system and will usually be required as additional therapy in the diabetic patient with a suboptimal response in terms of blood pressure or albuminuria.[56] Other approaches to consider include dietary salt restriction, which has been shown experimentally to reduce diabetic renal injury.[57]

As indicated above, inhibition of the RAS with either ACE-inhibition or ARBs has been shown to be particularly effective at reducing proteinuria in patients with type 1 or type 2 diabetes with nephropathy. This has led to the suggestion that these agents might be combined to provide more effective interuption of the RAS cascade and thus further reduce proteinuria. The combination of the ACE-inhibitor lisinopril (20 mg daily) with the ARB candesartan (16 mg daily) produced greater blood pressure reduction and a greater antiproteinuric effect than either agent alone.[58] In a more recent study, candesartan 8m daily was added to existing therapy in 18 patients with type 2 diabetes, hypertension and overt nephropathy (proteinuria > 1 g/day). All of the patients were receiving an ACE-inhibitor e.g. enalapril or lisinopril 20 mg daily, usually in combination with other antihypertensive drugs i.e. diuretics and/or CCBs. The addition of candesartan, producing dual blockade of the RAS, further reduced albuminuria by 25% and 24 hour systolic blood pressure by an average of 10 mmHg.[59] What these studies highlight is the fact that the ACE-inhibitors or ARBs are probably under-dosed when given as monotherapy when a key objective of therapy is to reduce proteinuria. What is unclear from both of these studies is what would have happened if the dose of either the ACE-inhibitor or the ARB had been doubled as a monotherapy. Further studies are required to define the optimal dose of ACE-inhibition or ARB needed to achieve a maximal antiproteinuric effect and to determine whether there is additional gain from the combination of ACE-inhibition and ARBs at such doses.

References

1. Kimmelsteil P, Wilson C. Intercapillary lesions in the glomeruli in the kidney. *Am J Pathol* 1936; **12**: 83–97.
2. Parving HH. Initiation and progression of diabetic nephropathy. *N Engl J Med* 1996; **335**: 1682–3.
3. Mogensen CE. How to protect the kidney in diabetic patients: with special reference to IDDM. *Diabetes* 1997; **46** (Suppl 2): S104–S111.
4. Vedel P, Obel J, Nielsen FS, et al. Glomerular hyperfiltration in microalbuminuric NIDDM patients. *Diabetologia* 1996; **39**: 1584–9.
5. Mogensen CE, Keane WF, Bennett PH, et al. Prevention of diabetic renal disease with special reference to microalbuminuria. *Lancet* 1995; **346**: 1080–4.
6. Chavers BM, Bilous RW, Ellis EN, Steffes MW, Mauer SM. Glomerular lesions and urinary albumin excretion in type I diabetes without overt proteinuria. *N Engl J Med* 1989; **320**: 966–70.
7. Fioretto P, Mauer M, Brocco E, et al. Patterns of renal injury in NIDDM patients with microalbuminuria. *Diabetologia* 1996; **39**: 1569–76.
8. Mogensen CE. Microalbuminuria predicts clinical proteinuria and early mortality in maturity-onset diabetes. *N Engl J Med* 1984; **310**: 356–60.
9. Stehouwer CD, Nauta JJ, Zeldenrust GC, Hackeng WH, Donker AJ, den Ottolander GJ. Urinary albumin excretion, cardiovascular disease, and endothelial dysfunction in non-insulin-dependent diabetes mellitus. *Lancet* 1992; **340**: 319–23.
10. Yip J, Mattock MB, Morucutti A, Sethi M, Trevisan R, Viberti G. Insulin resistance in insulin-dependent diabetic patients with microalbuminuria. *Lancet* 1993; **342**: 883–7.
11. Cooper ME, Jerums G, Gilbert RE. Diabetic vascular complications. *Clin Exp Pharmacol Physiol* 1997; **24**: 770–5.
12. Gilbert RE, Tsalamandris C, Bach L, et al. Glycemic control and the rate of progression of early diabetic kidney disease: a nine year longitudinal study. *Kidney Int* 1993; **44**: 855–9.
13. Ohkubo Y, Kishikawa H, Araki E, et al. Intensive insulin therapy prevents the progression of diabetic microvascular complications in Japanese patients with non-insulin-dependent diabetes mellitus: a randomized prospective 6-year study. *Diabetes Res Clin Pract* 1995; **28**: 103–17.
14. UK Prospective Diabetes Study (UKPDS) Group. Intensive blood-glucose control with sulphonylureas or insulin compared with conventional treatment and risk of complications in patients with type 2 diabetes (UKPDS 33). *Lancet* 1998; **352**: 837–53.
15. American Diabetes Association Position Statement: Diabetic Nephropathy. *Diabetes Care* 2002; **25** (Suppl 1): S85–9.
16. Mogensen CE. Long-term antihypertensive treatment inhibiting progression of diabetic nephropathy. *BMJ* 1982; **285**: 685–8.
17. Parving H-H, Andersen AR, Smidt UM, Svendsen PA. Early aggressive antihypertensive treatment reduces rate of decline in kidney function in diabetic nephropathy. *Lancet* 1983; **i**: 1175–9.
18. Cooper ME, McNally PG. Antihypertensive treatment in NIDDM, with special reference to abnormal albuminuria. In: Mogensen CE, ed. *The kidney and hypertension in diabetes mellitus*, 4th edn. Norwell, Massachusetts, Kluwer Academic Publishers, 1998: 427–40.
19. Stornello M, Valvo E, Vasques E, Leone S, Scapellato L. Systemic and renal effects of chronic angiotensin converting enzyme inhibition with captopril in hypertensive diabetic patients. *J Hypertens* 1989; **7** (Suppl 7): S65–S67.
20. Bakris GL. Effects of diltiazem or lisinopril on massive proteinuria associated with diabetes mellitus. *Ann Intern Med* 1990; **112**: 701–2.
21. Stornello M, Valvo EV, Scapellato L. Hemodynamic, renal, and humoral effects of the cal-

cium entry blocker nicardipine and converting enzyme inhibitor captopril in hypertensive Type II diabetic patients with nephropathy. *J Cardiovasc Pharmacol* 1989; **14**: 851–5.

22. Demarie BK, Bakris GL. Effects of different calcium antagonists on proteinuria associated with diabetes mellitus. *Ann Intern Med* 1990; **113**: 987–8.

23. Stornello M, Valvo EV, Scapellato L. Comparative effects of enalapril, atenolol and chlorthalidone on blood pressure and kidney function of diabetic patients affected by arterial hypertension and persistent proteinuria. *Nephron* 1991; **58**: 52–7.

24. Chan JC, Cockram CS, Nicholls MG, Cheung CK, Swaminathan R. Comparison of enalapril and nifedipine in treating non-insulin dependent diabetes associated with hypertension: one year analysis. *BMJ* 1992; **305**: 981–5.

25. Ferder L, Daccordi H, Martello M, Panzalis M, Inserra F. Angiotensin converting enzyme inhibitors versus calcium antagonists in the treatment of diabetic hypertensive patients. *Hypertension* 1992; **19**: II237–42.

26. Liou HH, Huang TP, Campese VM. Effect of long-term therapy with captopril on proteinuria and renal function in patients with non-insulin-dependent diabetes and with non-diabetic renal diseases. *Nephron* 1995; **69**: 41–8.

27. Nielsen FS, Rossing P, Gall MA, Skott P, Smidt UM, Parving HH. Long-term effect of lisinopril and atenolol on kidney function in hypertensive NIDDM subjects with diabetic nephropathy. *Diabetes* 1997; **46**: 1182–8.

28. The Heart Outcomes Prevention Evaluation Study Investigators. Effects of ramipril on cardiovascular and microvascular outcomes in people with diabetes mellitus: results of the HOPE study and MICRO-HOPE substudy. *Lancet* 2000; **355**: 253–9.

29. Bakris GL, Barnhill BW, Sadler R. Treatment of arterial hypertension in diabetic humans: importance of therapeutic selection. *Kidney Int* 1992; **41**: 912–19.

30. Slataper R, Vicknair N, Sadler R, Bakris GL. Comparative effects of different antihypertensive treatments on progression of diabetic renal disease. *Arch Intern Med* 1993; **153**: 973–80.

31. Fogari R, Zoppi A, Pasotti C, et al. Comparative effects of ramipril and nitrendipine on albuminuria in hypertensive patients with non insulin dependent diabetes mellitus and impaired renal function. *J Hum Hypertens* 1995; **9**: 13–15.

32. Guasch A, Parham M, Zayas CF, Campbell O, Nzerue C, Macon E. Contrasting effects of calcium channel blockade versus converting enzyme inhibition on proteinuria in African Americans with non-insulin-dependent diabetes mellitus and nephropathy. *J Am Soc Nephrology* 1997; **8**: 793–8.

33. Bakris GL, Mangrum A, Copley JB, Vicknair N, Sadler R. Effect of calcium channel or beta-blockade on the progression of diabetic nephropathy in African Americans. *Hypertension* 1997; **29**: 744–50.

34. Bakris GL, Copley JB, Vicknair N, Sadler R, Leurgans S. Calcium channel blockers versus other antihypertensive therapies on progression of NIDDM associated nephropathy. *Kidney Int* 1996; **50**: 1641–50.

35. Lewis EJ, Hunsicker LG, Clarke WR et al. Renoprotective effect of the angiotensin receptor antagonist irbesartan in patients with nephropathy due to type 2 diabetes. *N Engl J Med.* 2001; **345**: 851–60.

36. Brenner BM, Cooper ME, De Zeeuw D et al. Effects of losartan on renal and cardiovascular outcomes in patients with type 2 diabetes and nephropathy. *N Engl J Med* 2001; **345**: 861–9.

37. Estacio RO, Jeffers BW, Gifford N, Schrier RW. Effect of blood pressure control on diabetic microvascular complications in patients with hypertension and type 2 diabetes. *Diabetes Care* 2000: **23** (Suppl 2): B54–B64.

38. Schrier RW, Estacio RO, Esler A, Mehler P. Effects of aggressive blood pressure control in normotensive type diabetic patients on albuminuria, retinopathy and strokes. *Kidney Int* 2002; **61**: 1086–97.

39. Gambardella S, Frontoni S, Lala A, et al. Regression of microalbuminuria in type II diabetic, hypertensive patients after long-term indapamide treatment. *Am Heart J* 1991; **122**: 1232–8.

40. Lacourciere Y, Nadeau A, Poirier L, Tancrede G. Captopril or conventional therapy in

hypertensive type II diabetics. Three-year analysis. *Hypertension* 1993; **21**: 786–94.

41. Schnack C, Hoffmann W, Hopmeier P, Schernthaner G. Renal and metabolic effects of 1-year treatment with ramipril or atenolol in NIDDM patients with microalbuminuria. *Diabetologia* 1996; **39**: 1611–16.

42. Velussi M, Brocco E, Frogato F, et al. Effects of cilazapril and amlodipine on kidney function in hypertensive NIDDM patients. *Diabetes* 1996; **45**: 216–22.

43. Agardh CD, Garcia Puig J, Charbonnel B, Angelkort B, Barnett AH. Greater reduction of urinary albumin excretion in hypertensive type II diabetic patients with incipient nephropathy by lisinopril than by nifedipine. *J Hum Hypertens* 1996; **10**: 185–92.

44. Parving H-H, Lehnert H, Brochner-Mortensen J et al. The effect of irbesartan on the development of diabetic nephropathy in patients with type 2 diabetes. *N Engl J Med* 2001; **345**: 870–8.

45. Viberti G, Wheeldon NM; MicroAlbuminuria Reduction With VALsartan (MARVAL) Study Investigators. Microalbuminuria reduction with valsartan in patients with type 2 diabetes mellitus: a blood pressure-independent effect. *Circulation* 2002; **106**: 643–5.

46. Melbourne Diabetic Nephropathy Study Group. Comparison between perindopril and nifedipine in hypertensive and normotensive diabetic patients with microalbuminuria. *BMJ* 1991; **302**: 210–16.

47. Jerums G, Allen TJ, Tsalamandris C, Cooper ME, Melbourne Diabetic Nephropathy Study G. Angiotensin converting enzyme inhibition and calcium channel blockade in incipient diabetic nophropathy. *Kidney Int* 1992; **41**: 904–11.

48. Sano T, Kawamura T, Matsumae H, et al. Effects of long-term enalapril treatment on persistent micro-albuminuria in well-controlled hypertensive and normotensive NIDDM patients. *Diabetes Care* 1994; **17**: 420–4.

49. Ahmad J, Siddiqui MA, Ahmad H. Effective postponement of diabetic nephropathy with enalapril in normotensive type 2 diabetic patients with microalbuminuria. *Diabetes Care* 1997; **20**: 1576–81.

50. Ravid M, Savin H, Jutrin I, Bental T, Katz B, Lishner M. Long-term stabilizing effect of angiotensin-converting enzyme inhibition on plasma creatinine and on proteinuria in normotensive type II diabetic patients. *Ann Intern Med* 1993; **118**: 577–81.

51. Ravid M, Lang R, Rachmani R, Lishner M. Long-term renoprotective effect of angiotensin-converting enzyme inhibition in non-insulin-dependent diabetes mellitus. A 7-year follow-up study. *Arch Intern Med* 1996; **156**: 286–9.

52. Jerums G. Angiotensin converting enzyme inhibition and calcium channel blockade in diabetic patients with microalbuminuria. *Nephrology* 1997; **3** (Suppl 1): S41.

53. Bakris G. Combination therapy for hypertension and renal disease in diabetics as compared to non-diabetics. In: Mogensen CE, ed. *The kidney and hypertension in diabetes mellitus*, 3rd edn. Norwell, Massachusetts, Kluwer Academic, 1997: 561–8.

54. Bakris GL, Weir MR, Dequattro V, McMahon FG. Effects of an ACE inhibitor calcium antagonist combination on proteinuria in diabetic nephropathy. *Kidney Int* 1998; **54**: 1283–9.

55. Fogari R, Zoppi A, Mugellini A, Lusardi P, Destro M, Corradi L. Effect of benazepril plus amlodipine vs benazepril alone on urinary albumin excretion in hypertensive patients with type II diabetes and microalbuminuria. *Clin Drug Invest* 1997; **13**: 50–5.

56. Parving HH, Rossing P. The use of antihypertensive agents in prevention and treatment of diabetic nephropathy. *Curr Opin Nephrol Hypertens* 1994; **3**: 292–300.

57. Allen TJ, Waldron MJ, Casley D, Jerums G, Cooper ME. Salt restriction reduces hyperfiltration, renal enlargement and albuminuria in experimental diabetes. *Diabetes* 1997; **46**: 119–24.

58. Mogensen CE, Neldam S, Tikkanen I, et al. Randomised controlled trial of dual blockade of renin angiotensin system in patients with hypertension, microalbuminria, and non insulin dependent diabetes: the candesartan and lisinopril microalbuminuria (CALM) study. *BMJ* 2000; **321**: 1440–4.

59. Rossing K, Christensen PK, Jensen BR, Parving H-H. Dual blockade of the renin-angiotensin system in diabetic nephropathy: a randomised double blind cross-over study. *Diabetes Care* 2002; **25**: 95–100.

14

Renovascular disease in diabetes: clinical implications for the management of hypertension

Bryan Williams and David O'Brien

Introduction

Diabetes mellitus is a state of accelerated and often widespread macrovascular disease. Atherosclerotic renovascular disease is more common in patients with clinical evidence of vascular disease, particularly peripheral vascular disease. Consequently there is a need to consider the possibility of renal artery stenosis (RAS) in a diabetic patient with hypertension. This diagnosis has particular significance in the hypertensive diabetic patient for a number of reasons: 1) Diabetic patients are frequently treated with ACE-inhibition or angiotensin receptor antagonists which can precipitate a decline in renal function in patients with RAS. 2) RAS is a potentially remediable cause of hypertension and/or heart failure. This is an important consideration mindful of the devastating effects of uncontrolled hypertension in people with diabetes and the common occurrence of heart failure. 3) RAS can contribute to a progressive decline in renal function which can be erroneously attributed to diabetic nephropathy if the RAS remains undetected.

This chapter reviews the prevalence of RAS in patients with diabetes, the clinical presentation of RAS and the indications for surgical intervention or intervention via angioplasty and stenting. Finally, the overall implications of RAS with regard to the management of hypertension will be considered.

The prevalence of RAS in diabetes mellitus

Because of the increased prevalence of atherosclerotic disease in diabetes, it has been assumed that atherosclerotic renovascular disease is also more common. Surprisingly there is very little data with regard to the true prevalence of RAS in people with diabetes. This no doubt reflects one of the great conundrums, how is RAS best detected? Various imaging techniques have been adopted to try and identify structural stenoses within renal arteries. These include renal ultrasonography, colour Doppler studies of blood flow across renal arteries, magnetic resonance angiography and the "gold standard" approach i.e. renal angiography. The problems with these approaches is that whilst they may provide evidence of unilateral or bilateral RAS, they provide no direct information with regard to the functional significance of the RAS. More direct assessment of the functional significance of RAS has been attempted in some studies using isotope renograms post-captopril provocation and the measurement of captopril-stimulated plasma renin activity, to determine the activity of the renin-angiotensin axis as discussed below.

Prevalence of RAS at autopsy in people with diabetes mellitus

A retrospective audit of autopsy data from 5194 unselected consecutive cases found RAS (defined as a reduction in renal artery lumen diameter of >50%) to be present in 10.1% of people with a history of both hypertension and diabetes, compared to only 6.1% of people with a prior history of hypertension alone.[1] RAS was found in 4.4% of diabetic people without hypertension and only 1% of non-diabetic people without hypertension. Thus, the overall frequency of anatomical RAS was low in this very large study, although there did appear to be an excess of RAS in people with diabetes, irrespective of whether they were hypertensive or not. Moreover, bilateral RAS was more common in diabetes. However, the vast majority of the lesions in all groups were unilateral. The authors concluded that RAS should be seriously considered in diabetic patients with hypertension, although this conclusion is not justified by the data. The problem with autopsy data is that it provides no information about the functional significance of the vascular stenosis. Since many of the people in the autopsy study with RAS were previously normotensive, it is unlikely that many of the anatomical stenoses were functionally important. It is also important to note that these autopsy studies and the various imaging techniques discussed below are primarily directed towards the detection of main renal artery or major branch stenoses, they are less likely to detect smaller branch stenoses which may also have important haemodynamic consequences.

Prevalence of RAS in clinical studies in people with diabetes mellitus

In living diabetic patients, the prevalence of renal artery stenosis has only been evaluated in a few small studies.[2-7] Some of these studies have suggested a higher prevalence of RAS in diabetics with hypertension when compared to normotensive controls but other studies have reported no difference. A small cross-sectional study using digital subtraction angiography in 24 hypertensive type 2 diabetic patients, under the age of 70 years, revealed a stenosis in five patients (~20%). However, when more detailed functional studies were performed on these patients, including radioisotope renal scans and bilateral renal vein sampling of plasma renin activity, the authors concluded that in most patients the stenosis was functionally insignificant and unlikely to be the cause of the hypertension.[2] A retrospective analysis of renal arteriograms in 28 diabetic patients identified RAS in 10 (36%).[3] In another study, renal investigations were performed in a sub-group of 20 diabetic patients with refractory hypertension. Five were shown to have RAS (25%), two having bilateral disease. In all five, there was a good clinical response in terms of blood pressure control after surgical intervention or angioplasty.[4] However, whether this response has persisted long-term has not been reported. Nevertheless, refractory hypertension appeared to provide a clue to the presence of RAS. Pursuing this theme, a Swedish study reported a prevalence of RAS of 30% in diabetic patients with refractory hypertension requiring three or more drugs.[5] In another clinical study of 60 hypertensive type 2 diabetic patients requiring three or more antihypertensive agents, 22% were found to have RAS angiographically.[6] In a more recent study using magnetic resonance angiography, RAS was detected in 17% of 117 hypertensive type 2 diabetics, with 20 having unilateral disease and only one with bilateral disease. Interestingly, the plasma renin response to a single dose of oral captopril was negative in all patients with RAS. However, the fall in blood pressure in response to captopril was significantly greater in those with RAS. The authors concluded that RAS is common in people with type 2 diabetes and was more likely to be unilateral.[7] They conceded, however, that the functional significance of RAS detected by magnetic resonance angiography was unclear. This limited database suggests that when compared to the non-diabetic hypertensive population, RAS may be more common in hypertensive type 2 diabetic patients, particularly those with refractory hypertension. However, in general, RAS does not appear to be a common cause for hypertension in diabetic patients and even when present, it is not always, or indeed often, functionally significant.

Clinical clues to the presence of RAS in diabetic patients with hypertension

There have been several recent studies that have evaluated possible clinical clues to the presence of RAS in patients with hypertension although the specific impact of diabetes has not always been assessed (Table 10.1). In a cross-sectional study of patients presenting with symptoms of peripheral vascular disease, the severity of peripheral vascular disease correlated closely with the presence of RAS.[8] Importantly, diabetes *per se* was not identified as an added risk factor for RAS. A similar association was identified in another study with 34% of patients with peripheral vascular

disease and hypertension having co-existent RAS.[9] However, in this latter study, the specific influence of diabetes was not examined. Another study of patients undergoing cardiac angiography confirmed the relationship between RAS and coronary disease and reported that this relationship was not influenced by the presence or absence of diabetes. The only study specifically to characterize the impact of various risk factors on the likelihood of detecting RAS in people with hypertension and type 2 diabetes used magnetic resonance angiography to detect RAS in 17% of 117 patients studied.[7] These patients all had type 2 diabetes and hypertension. Importantly, this was a prospective study and none of the patients were preselected for study on the basis of refractory hypertension or the presence of renal impairment. They found that the presence of a femoral bruit on clinical examination was most predictive of RAS. They also found that prior treatment with statin therapy (presumably indicative of hypercholesterolaemia) was also significantly associated with the presence of RAS. Perhaps surprisingly, other clinical features of atherosclerotic vascular disease, i.e. smoking status, sex, age, ethnicity, duration of diabetes, blood pressure, retinopathy, neuropathy, serum creatinine and markers of glycaemic control were not predictive of RAS patients with type 2 diabetes and hypertension.[7] Together, these observations suggest that in a diabetic patient with hypertension, the presence of clinically evident vascular disease, particularly symptomatic peripheral vascular disease, and the presence of a femoral bruit are the best predictors of RAS. Clearly the presence of renal impairment associated with hypertension is most often due to diabetic nephropathy but may also be due to RAS. Moreover, the presence of refractory hypertension increases the likelihood of detecting RAS. These observations also suggest that

Severe or refractory hypertension
Sudden onset of hypertension in middle age
Male sex more commonly affected
More common in smokers
Clinical symptoms of peripheral vascular disease
Clinical evidence of peripheral vascular disease (femoral artery bruit)
Clinical evidence of a renal artery bruit (absence does not exclude RAS)
Renal impairment more likely but not invariably present
Deterioration in renal function after treatment with ACE-inhibitors or angiotensin II receptor antagonists. (Note – there may be no change in serum creatinine in patients with unilateral RAS.)

Table 14.1
Clinical pointers to atherosclerotic renovascular disease

diabetes *per se* does not directly influence the prevalence of RAS and that the increased prevalence of RAS in hypertensive patients with diabetes is primarily attributable to the impact of diabetes on the development of atherosclerotic vascular disease, particularly peripheral vascular disease.

One caveat worthy of note is that these observations primarily apply to older and predominantly type 2 diabetic patients. There are many rarer causes of RAS that are not specific to diabetes that may also manifest in patients with diabetes. Most important is fibromuscular dysplasia of the renal artery which usually presents in younger people (most often female) and thus may be a cause of hypertension in a young type 1 diabetic patient with refractory hypertension. It is important to detect this lesion as it is much more amenable to angioplasty than atherosclerotic RAS, with excellent longer term results in terms of renal artery patency and blood pressure control.

Clinical detection of RAS

At present there are no specific recommendations from any of the national societies with regard to the most appropriate clinical screening methods for RAS in people with diabetes and hypertension. Since there is no convincing evidence that diabetes independent of the existence of peripheral vascular disease is associated with a dramatically increased prevalence of RAS, the presence of diabetes *per se* is not a justification for the routine screening of patients for RAS. There are however clinical features which are associated with an increased prevalence of RAS which should increase clinical suspicion (Table 14.1). Atherosclerotic RAS is more common in older people (>50 yrs), in people with a history of smoking, in those with clinical evidence of generalized vascular disease, particularly peripheral vascular disease, and especially those with a femoral bruit. RAS is also more likely in those with hypertension refractory to treatment. Another clue is the sudden onset of severe hypertension in middle age in a patient in whom blood pressure records have revealed no previous history of hypertension. In some cases "malignant or accelerated" hypertension may be the first presentation of RAS and any patient presenting with malignant hypertension must be actively investigated to exclude RAS as a potentially remediable cause.

In patients with RAS, clinical examination

may reveal the presence of a femoral or renal bruit but their absence does not preclude the diagnosis of RAS. Patients with renal impairment associated with severe or refractory hypertension may also have RAS but renal function *per se* is not a good discriminator. Clearly such patients are more likely to have diabetic nephropathy. Moreover, in patients with significant unilateral RAS, renal function as determined by serum creatinine may appear to be normal. It should be noted that serum creatinine is a poor discriminator of early renal impairment, particularly in women and people with low muscle mass.

Where a strong clinical suspicion exists, it would be prudent to investigate the patient prior to commencing therapy with agents that inhibit the renin-angiotensin system (i.e. ACE inhibitors or angiotensin II receptor antagonists). Renal ultrasonography may reveal asymmetry in renal size, the smaller kidney indicative of potential RAS on that side, with compensatory renal hypertrophy sometimes

present on the contralateral side. Colour Doppler studies of renal artery blood flow are a very useful addition to renal ultrasonography and can help define whether there are abnormalities in the flow characteristics across a renal artery, indicative of stenosis. However, both of these techniques are strongly dependent on operator expertise. Moreover, such non-invasive imaging can be difficult if not impossible in obese patients, a characteristic not uncommon in people with type 2 diabetes. More detailed structural studies can be made via magnetic resonance angiography (MRA) or spiral computerized tomography.[11] These techniques are expensive but accurate in defining a stenosis of >50%. In this regard the sensitivity and specificity of MRA for the detection of RAS has been shown to be 84% and 91% respectively.[12]

The aforementioned studies may define an anatomical lesion (Fig. 14.1) but they provide little information about its functional significance. Gadolinium-enhanced MRA can

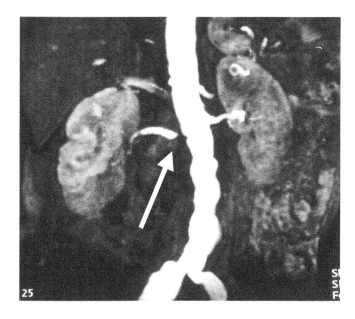

Figure 14.1
*Gadolinium enhanced magnetic resonance imaging of renal arteries showing a right sided ostial stenosis. The left renal artery is normal. Reproduced with permission from McLaughlin et al. BMJ 2000; **320**: 1124–7.*

provide haemodynamic data about relative renal perfusion but is not practical for routine use.[13] The use of isotope scans to assess renal perfusion and function can help define the relative perfusion and function of each kidney.[14,15] The most commonly used isotope is technetium-labelled diethylenetriamine-penta-acetic acid (DTPA) which is a marker of glomerular filtration. The sensitivity and specificity of the isotope scan for detecting renal artery disease can be greatly improved by prior administration of a single oral dose of the ACE-inhibitor captopril which will reduce glomerular filtration on the side of a significant renal artery lesion.[15] This reduction in filtration manifests itself as a delayed and reduced uptake of DTPA. These scans are most useful in the presence of a unilateral lesion in that they help define the contribution of each kidney to overall renal function.

The following findings on isotope scanning post-captopril enhancement are consistent with the presence of a functionally significant RAS:

- Decreased relative uptake by the involved kidney such that it contributes less than 40% of the overall renal function.
- A reduced rate of uptake of the isotope on the affected side. The usual peak uptake occurs at approximately 5 minutes. This will be doubled in the presence of RAS.
- A delay in washout of the isotope on the affected side is also consistent with the diagnosis of a functionally significant RAS.

An alternative functional test is the "captopril provocation test".[16] This test indirectly measures the activity of the renin-angiotensin-aldosterone axis. In the presence of a haemodynamically significant RAS, treatment with a single dose of the short acting ACE-inhibitor captopril (50 mg) will promote an exaggerated rise in plasma renin activity

(PRA) and a fall in systemic blood pressure. The response of PRA to this captopril provocation test has been suggested to have a sensitivity of 100% for haemodynamically significant RAS in people without diabetes and a specificity of 95%. After oral administration of captopril 50 mg, blood pressure is measured at 15-minute intervals for the next hour and the criteria for a positive test are:[8]

- A stimulated PRA of 9.3 pmol/ml/h or more *and*
- An absolute rise in PRA of 7.7 pmol/ml/h *and*
- A 150% increase in PRA if the baseline PRA value is greater than 2.3 pmol/ml/h (a 400% increase if the baseline PRA is less than 2.3 pmol/ml/h).

When this test was recently applied to 85 people with type 2 diabetes and hypertension, no patient had a positive test according to PRA criteria.[7] Interestingly, baseline and stimulated PRA activity were low in patients with hypertension and type 2 diabetes. It is conceivable that this hyporeninaemic state in type 2 diabetes limits the usefulness of this test. Moreover, in 14 of the 85 patients with proven RAS by MRA, the baseline PRA was low and not predictive and the captopril provocation test failed to demonstrate that the lesion was functionally significant. This suggests that even when structurally significant RAS is detected by imaging, it is not always possible to confirm functional significance. What remains unclear is whether functional significance or otherwise, in terms of the captopril test, predicts the response to intervention.

The "gold standard" for diagnosis is percutaneous renal angiography. This is usually reserved to confirm or refute a diagnosis suggested by previous tests (i.e., renal ultrasonography and Doppler studies) in those patients in whom active intervention is being contemplated. It should be emphasized that this procedure is not without hazard. Besides the recognized complications of percutaneous angiography, i.e., local bleeding and the rare late complication of femoral artery aneurysm, there is also the possibility of promoting cholesterol embolization (Fig. 14.1) either to the kidney or lower limbs. There is no definitive data on the risk of this complication but it is my clinical impression that renal artery embolization is understated as a complication of selective renal angiography, particularly when accompanied by angioplasty.

Unless there is strong clinical suspicion based on the criteria highlighted in Table 14.2, it would not be appropriate to consider diabetes *per se* as an indication for active investigation of RAS in a patient with hypertension.

Clinical management of RAS
Medical therapy

These patients are usually severely hypertensive and multiple therapies in combination will be required. The hypertension in these patients is strongly angiotensin II dependent. Consequently, diuretics which activate the renin-angiotensin system can on occasions induce a paradoxical rise in blood pressure. Drugs that block the renin-angiotensin system, i.e., ACE-inhibitors. angiotensin II receptor antagonists and β-blockers, are all particularly effective at reducing blood pressure.[17] However, because glomerular perfusion and filtration is dependent on angiotensin II in the affected kidney, there is a risk of precipitating acute or chronic renal ischaemia and acute renal failure in the kidney affected by the RAS. This is particularly true in patients who are volume contracted. Thus, when drugs that block the renin-angiotensin system are used to treat patients with RAS, they should only be initi-

ated by specialists and usually only to treat refractory hypertension in patients with unilateral RAS. They must be used with caution and renal function must be monitored closely. In my practice, I do not use these agents in the presence of bilateral RAS. In patients with unilateral RAS, I use ACE-inhibition when the function of the affected kidney is less than 25% of the overall function and when the kidney on the affected side is small and unlikely to be salvaged by surgical or angioplasty intervention to improve renal blood flow.

Angioplasty or surgical intervention

Many patients with RAS now undergo intervention, i.e., angioplasty or more rarely surgery to improve renal blood flow. Nevertheless it is important to reflect on a number of key points before contemplating intervention of this kind. Is intervention indicated and what will it achieve? Which kind of intervention is most appropriate? What is the local operator expertise? This latter point is very important in that the intervention procedures, whether surgical or via angioplasty require considerable skill and experience and are best undertaken at specialist centres.

Intervention should certainly be considered in three groups of patients:

1. Refractory heart failure and flash pulmonary oedema associated with bilateral renal artery stenosis. The occurrence of flash pulmonary oedema in a patient with risk factors for RAS should prompt screening for the presence of bilateral RAS. It is a diagnosis that is frequently missed. Such patients will rarely improve without intervention to improve their renal blood flow and as such this presentation is an absolute indication for intervention.
2. Declining renal function where the cause is

likely to be renal ischaemia. This is still an area of uncertainty with regard to management. A previous retrospective study (not in diabetic patients) has shown that in patients with bilateral RAS, the overall mortality rate is high (about 40% at 2 years and 45% at 5 years).[18] The average rate of decline in GFR was 4 ml/min/yr but decline in GFR was not inevitable even in the presence of severe stenosis. This suggests that the extensive collateral renal blood supply that often develops in these patients is sufficient to preserve function in some cases (Fig. 14.2). Angioplasty has been suggested to improve function in 40% of patients and stabilize function in 40%. Some however, experience a decline in function. However the majority of patients in these studies had non-ostial lesions, thus those with the latter (which are much more common) are less likely to do this well.[19-21] Studies are ongoing with renal artery stenting and it seems likely that this will be more effective than angioplasty alone, especially for ostial lesions but this awaits confirmation. A recent prospective randomized clinical trial in 106 patients with atherosclerotic renovascular disease compared medical therapy with angioplasty. This study used an intention to treat analysis and demonstrated that angioplasty offered little advantage over medical therapy with regard to blood pressure control and the preservation of renal function, although the group treated with angioplasty required less antihypertensive therapy.[22]

It is difficult to be prescriptive in recommendations in this area as each case needs to be assessed individually based on the extent of the renal impairment, the size and appearance of the kidneys (i.e., small scarred kidneys are less likely to recover significant function), the general condition of the patient and the complexity of the intervention being contemplated. There remains real uncertainty as to the relative merits of a conservative medical approach versus intervention in such circumstances.

3. Severe and refractory hypertension. This indication is particularly relevant to patients with diabetes in that uncontrolled hypertension has such devastating consequences. As such, any approach that might ease the management of refractory hypertension must be considered carefully. Nevertheless, the results of intervention in terms of improving blood pressure control have been mixed and are largely unpredictable and successful blood pressure control postprocedure is certainly not guaranteed.[23-25] If there is an RAS that is amenable to angioplasty and stenting in diabetic patients with severe, refractory hypertension it is my practice to recommend intervention, largely because in such patients, the consequences of poor blood pressure control are so predictably depressing.

Angioplasty and stenting

No data specific to diabetic patients is available but there are some general principles that are likely to be applicable. The success of angioplasty is dependent on the site and type of lesion. It is more likely to be successful if the vessel is incompletely occluded, where the stenosis is short (<10 mm) and when the lesion does not involve the ostium. In patients with unilateral RAS due to atherosclerotic disease, the immediate technical success rate with angioplasty is about 70% and the cure rate in terms of blood pressure control varies considerably.[26-30] Cure rates are much worse for ostial lesions and even poorer in patients with bilateral disease, particularly if one or both kidneys are atrophic. Even when the procedure is an immediate technical success, recurrence of the lesion is common (30% for

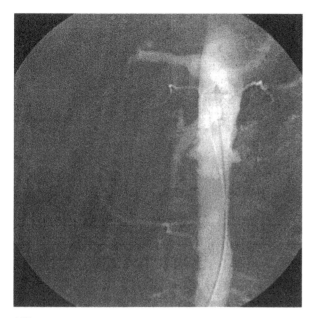

Bilateral renal artery
occlusion due to
atherosclerotic
renovascular disease

Dialysis
dependent

(A)

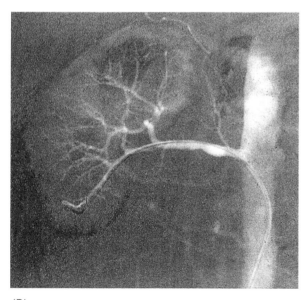

Post percutaneous
stenting of renal
arteries

Dialysis
independent

(B)

Figure 14.2
*(A) Percutaneous renal angiogram showing bilateral renal artery stenosis in a patient who is dialysis-dependent. Note the extensive collateral blood supply to the kidneys which can preserve renal tissue despite a loss of GFR. (B) Percutaneous stenting of the renal artery on the right restores renal blood flow. Subsequently, the patient recovered renal function and became dialysis independent. Reproduced with permission from McLaughlin et al. BMJ 2000; **320:** 1124–7.*

non-ostial lesions and over 50% for ostial lesions). Moreover restenosis often occurs early (up to 30% by two years).

In our practice, we have been so disappointed by the high recurrence rate following angioplasty, that if angioplasty is undertaken, we now routinely place intravascular stents. Early reports (see above) have suggested that stenting is very useful to prevent recurrence, particularly for ostial lesions, although to date, the follow up in the reported studies is too short (less than 2 years) to comment on longer-term success rates.

Renal artery stenosis in patients with diabetes: friend or foe?

Although RAS is undesirable due the resulting hypertension, heart failure and ischaemic nephropathy, there are compelling reasons why RAS may on occasions, protect the affected kidney from haemodynamic damage and diabetic nephropathy. The pathogenesis of diabetic nephropathy is greatly accelerated by haemodynamic stress within the kidney. This is one of the reasons why the treatment of systemic hypertension has proved to be so effective at arresting the rate of decline in renal function in patients with diabetic nephropathy. RAS prevents the transmission of high systemic pressures to the kidney on the affected side. This in effect imposes crude autoregulation of blood flow to the affected kidney. This protects the glomerulus from barotrauma and thus injury, particularly in patients with early diabetic nephropathy. In support of this hypothesis, experimental data from diabetic rats has shown that the induction of unilateral RAS (Goldblatt 2 kidney – 1 clip hypertension) resulted in advanced glomerular disease in the kidney with the unclipped renal artery – the kidney exposed to elevated systemic pressures. In contrast, in the kidney on the same side as the clipped renal artery, there was much less glomerular structural damage.[31] These experimental data are supported by observations in humans. In a case report of a diabetic patient with hypertension due to unilateral atherosclerotic RAS, histological analysis of the two kidneys at autopsy revealed unilateral diabetic nephropathy contralateral to the RAS.[32] Thus, despite the fact that both kidneys were exposed to the diabetic milieu, only the kidney exposed to increased systemic blood pressure developed diabetic nephropathy. It is unknown whether correction of RAS in a patient with diabetic nephropathy would lead to accelerated renal injury due to the increase in glomerular perfusion pressure.

Implications for therapeutic manipulation of the renin–angiotensin system

In a diabetic patient with hypertension, progressive renal impairment and proteinuria, alternative diagnoses to RAS need to be considered. Indeed, the most likely diagnosis remains diabetic nephropathy. Such patients would benefit from blockade of the renin–angiotensin system and must not be denied this treatment based on the unfounded assumption that the patient with diabetes is much more likely to develop clinically significant renovascular disease. Patients with diabetes and hypertension who do not have clinical features to suggest a high probability of RAS (see Table 14.1) can be safely treated with drugs that block the renin-angiotensin system (ACE-inhibitors or angiotensin II receptor antagonists) but should have their serum urea, electrolytes and creatinine levels

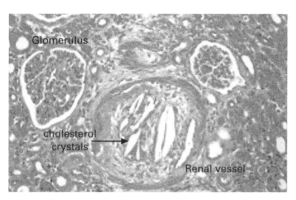

Figure 14.3
*Histological appearance of cholesterol emboli
visible as discrete crystals in this renal biopsy
from a patient with atherosclerotic renovascular
disease. Reproduced with permission from
McLaughlin et al. BMJ 2000; **320:** 1124–7.*

measured before and again within 2 weeks of commencing treatment. It is important to note that blockade of the renin-angiotensin system in patients with diabetes will almost invariably result in some decline in glomerular filtration rate. This is because diabetes is associated with glomerular hyperfiltration and in the absence of overt renal injury, these patients often have an elevated GFR.

Patients with a high clinical suspicion of RAS should be screened by renal ultrasound and colour Doppler studies to assess whether RAS is present. If these studies are negative, the patient should be treated as suggested above. If the screening tests suggest the likely presence of RAS, it is our practice to proceed to renal angiography, particularly if we are contemplating intervention. In general, an appropriate level of clinical vigilance and simple clinical assessment of diabetic patients with hypertension should identify most of those at risk of RAS and thus ensure that the many patients who would benefit from ACE-inhibition or angiotensin II receptor antagonists are not denied access to them based on an unsubstantiated fear of a high prevalence of RAS in diabetic patients with hypertension. As indicated above, patients with atherosclerotic renovascular disease are at very high risk of a premature cardiovascular death and exhibit evidence of extensive target organ damage. As such, they should qualify for additional secondary preventive strategies such as low dose aspirin therapy (once blood pressure control has improved) and statin therapy to maintain a total serum cholesterol level below 5 mmol/l. The latter may be important because cholesterol emboli are frequently observed in small renal vessels and represent an important cause of progressive renal ischaemia (Fig. 14.3). Whether these additional treatments will ultimately reduce the rate of progression of renovascular disease *per se*, and reduce the likelihood of progressive ischaemic nephropathy due to cholesterol embolization from the unstable atherosclerotic plaque is unknown but warrants investigation.

References

1. Sawicki PT, Kaiser S, Heinemann L et al. Prevalence of renal artery stenosis in diabetes mellitus – an autopsy study. *J Intern Med* 1991; **229**: 489–92.
2. Ritchie CM, McGrath E, Hadden DR et al. Renal artery stenosis in hypertensive diabetic patients. *Diabet Med* 1988; **5**: 265–7.
3. Munichoodappa C, D'Elia JA, Libertino JA, Gleason R, Christlieb AR. Renal artery stenosis in hypertensive diabetics. *J Urol* 1979; **121**: 555–8.
4. Courreges JP, Bacha J, Maraoui M et al. Renal artery stenosis prevalence in non-insulin dependent diabetes and hypertension. *Diabetilogia* 1995; **38** (Suppl 1): A269.
5. Isaksson H, Danielsson M, Rosenhamer G et al. Characteristics of patients resistant to antihypertensive drug therapy. *J Intern Med* 1991; **229**: 421–6.
6. Courreges JP, Bacha J, Aboud E. Prevalence and profile of renovascular disease in type II diabetic patients with severe hypertension. *Arch Mal Coeur Vaiss* 1997; **90**: 1059–63.
7. Valabhji J, Robinson S, Poulter C et al. Prevalence of renal artery stenosis in subjects with type 2 diabetes and coexistent hypertension. *Diabetes Care* 2000; **23**: 539–43.
8. Missouris CG, Buckenham T, Cappuccio FP et al. Renal artery stenosis; a common and important problem in patients with peripheral vascular disease. *Am J Med* 1994; **96**: 10–14.
9. Wachtell K, Ibsen H, Olsen MH et al. Prevalence of renal artery stenosis in patients with peripheral vascular disease and hypertension. *J Human Hypertens* 1996; **10**: 83–5.
10. Jean WJ, al Bitar I, Zwicke DL et al. High incidence of renal artery stenosis in patients with coronary artery disease. *Cathet Cardiovasc Diagn* 1994; **32**: 8–10.
11. Gedroyc WMW, Neerhut P, Negus R et al. Magnetic resonance angiography of renal artery stenosis. *Clin Radiol* 1995; **50**: 436–9.
12. Olbricht CJ, Paul K, Prokop M et al. Minimally invasive diagnosis of renal artery stenosis by spiral computed tomography angiography. *Kidney Int* 1995; **48**: 1332–7.
13. Nally JV. Provocative captopril testing in the diagnosis of renovascular hypertension. *Urol Clin North Am* 1994; **21**: 227–34.
14. Mann SJ, Pickering TG. Detection of renovascular hypertension. State of the Art. *Ann Intern Med* 1992; **117**: 845–53.
15. Pederson EB. Angiotensin converting enzyme inhibitor renography. Pathophysiological, diagnostic and therapeutic aspects in renal artery stenosis. *Nephrol Dial Transpl* 1994; **9**: 482–92.
16. Muller FB, Sealey JE, Case DB et al. The captopril test for identifying renovascular disease in hypertensive patients. *Am J Med* 1986; **80**: 633–44.
17. Ram CVS, Clagett GP, Radford LR. Renovascular hypertension. *Semin Nephrol* 1995; **15**: 152–74.
18. Baboolal K, Evans C, Moore RH. Incidence of end-stage renal disease in medically treated patients with severe bilateral atherosclerotic renovascular disease. *Am J Kidney Dis* 1998; **31**: 971–7.
19. Canzanello VJ, Millan VG, Spiegel JE. Percutaneous transluminal angioplasty in management of atherosclerotic renovascular hypertension. Results in 100 patients. *Hypertension* 1989; **13**: 163–72.
20. Greco BA, Breyer JA. Atherosclerotic ischaemic renal disease. *Am J Kidney Dis* 1997; **29**: 167–87.
21. Sos TA. Angioplasty for the treatment of azotaemia and renovascular hypertension in atherosclerotic renovascular disease. *Circulation* 1991; **83** (Suppl 1): 162–6.
22. van Jaarsveld BC, Krijnen P, Pieterman H et al. The effect of balloon angioplasty on hypertension in atherosclerotic renal artery stenosis. Dutch Renal Artery Intervention Cooperative (DRASTIC) Study group. *N Engl J Med* 2000; **342**: 1007–14.
23. Ramsay LE, Waller PC. Blood pressure

response to percutaneous angioplasty: an overview of published series. *BMJ* 1990; **300**: 569–72.

24. Plouin PF, Chatellier BD, Raynaud A, for the ESSAI multicentrique medicaments vs angioplastied (EMMA) study group. Blood pressure outcome after angioplasty in atherosclerotic renal artery stenosis. A randomized trial. *Hypertension* 1998; **31**: 823–9.

25. Webster J, Marshall F, Abalalla M et al. Randomized comparison of percutaneous angioplasty vs. continued medical therapy for hypertensive patients with an atheromatous renal artery stenosis. Scottish and Newcastle renal artery stenosis collaborative group. *J Human Hypertens* 1998; **12**: 329–35.

26. van de Ven PJ, Beutler JJ, Kaatee R. Transluminal vascular stent for ostial atherosclerotic renal artery stenosis. *Lancet* 1995; **346**: 672–4.

27. Blum U, Krumme B, Flugel P. Treatment of ostial renal artery stenosis with vascular endoprostheses after unsuccessful balloon angio-plasty. *N Engl J Med* 1997; **336**: 459–65.

28. Novick AC. Treatment of ostial renal-artery stenoses with vascular endoprostheses after unsuccessful balloon angioplasty [editorial comment]. *J Urol* 1997; **158**: 983.

29. Dorros G, Jaff M, Mathiak L et al. Four year follow up of Palmaz-Schatz stent revascularization as treatment for atherosclerotic renal artery stenosis. *Circulation* 1998; **98**: 642–7.

30. Harden PN, Macleod MJ, Rodger RS et al. Effect of renal artery stenting on progression of renovascular renal failure. *Lancet* 1997; **349**: 1133–6.

31. Mauer SM, Steffes MW, Azar S et al. The effects of Goldblatt hypertension on development of Glomerular lesions of diabetes mellitus in the rat. *Diabetes* 1978; **27**: 738–44.

32. Berkman J, Rifkin H. Unilateral nodular diabetic glomerulosclerosis (Kimmelstein-Wilson): report of a case. *Metabolism* 1973; **22**: 715–22.

III Treatment of Hypertension in Diabetic Subjects

15

The management of hypertension and diabetes: guidelines and blood pressure targets

Munavvar Izhar and George L Bakris

Introduction

It is well established that reduction in arterial pressure and good glycemic control are two prime factors responsible for reducing the incidence of both cardiovascular events and renal disease progression among patients with diabetes.[1-3] Results of clinical trials, such as the Diabetes Control and Complication Trial (DCCT), and the United Kingdom Prospective Diabetes Study (UKPDS) have helped define the level of blood glucose needed to avoid systemic complications of diabetes.[4,5] Likewise, the UKPDS, the Hypertension Optimal Treatment (HOT) and the Appropriate Blood Pressure Control in Diabetes (ABCD) trials, randomised people with hypertension and type II diabetes to different levels of blood pressure control, and thus, helped solidify new guidelines for blood pressure reduction in such individuals.[6-8] The recently published updates on the final outcomes of the Appropriate Control of Blood Pressure in type 2 Diabetes (ABCD) studies[9,10] will further help clarify the optimal blood pressure goal for patients with hypertension and diabetes who are receiving antihypertensive therapy. These trials all demonstrated that those randomised to more intensive lowering of blood pressure (i.e. achieved diastolic pressure <81–82 mmHg), had more marked reductions in cardiovascular events when compared with those randomised to more conventional blood pressure control

(i.e. diastolic pressures between 86 and 92 mmHg).

Current recommendations by both the Joint National Committee (JNC) Report VI and the WHO guidelines suggest that lower blood pressure goals, i.e. <130/85 mmHg, be obtained in order to preserve renal function and reduce cardiovascular risk.[2,11] This is true for people who have either diabetes and/or renal insufficiency. Specifically, the recommendations suggest that while it is desirable to lower blood pressure levels to <140/90 mmHg, ample literature supports the rationale for achieving even lower blood pressure goals, i.e. <130/85 mmHg in these groups. The most recent position statements from the American Diabetes Association have recommended even lower blood pressure goals of <130/80 mmHg for patients with type 2 diabetes treated for hypertension.[12,13] The statements acknowledge that achieving these goals will not be easy, that multiple drugs are likely to be required. Moreover, for patients with isolated systolic hypertension and systolic BP >180 mmHg, the statement recommends that the initial goal of therapy should be to gradually lower the blood pressure 'in stages' and that if initial goals are met and well tolerated, then further blood pressure lowering may be indicated.

Patients with diabetes and blood pressure levels of >140/90 mmHg have relatively higher cardiovascular event rates as compared with the general population. Moreover, data from the Multiple Risk Factor Intervention Trial (MRFIT) suggest that a 15/10 mmHg elevation in arterial pressure above 140/90 mmHg confers a two-fold greater risk for cardiovascular disease.[14,15] Thus, it is not sufficient to have blood pressure close to goal; it must be at goal or below. More recently, retrospective data from thousands of people with hypertension and renal disease in the Veteran's Administration (VA) hospitals have solidified this observation, not only for cardiovascular events, but also progression of renal disease.[1] Moreover, the VA data also demonstrate that systolic blood pressure is a major contributor to renal disease progression.

The purpose of this chapter is to review the data available on level of blood pressure reduction and its impact on diabetic cardiovascular disease and renal disease progression. Additionally, there is a discussion of the pros and cons of various 'antihypertensive cocktails' that may be used to achieve a lower level of blood pressure.

Blood pressure levels and nephropathy progression

Many of the observations that have underscored the importance of blood pressure control in preventing or delaying the progression of target organ damage in diabetes were derived from the study of diabetic nephropathy. Moreover, much of the data that has guided the selection of specific antihypertensive drug therapies has been extrapolated from the study of diabetic nephropathy. It is therefore important to review the evolution of these concepts and how they have shaped the resulting recommendations.

The NHANES III survey[2,16] documented that only 27 per cent of American people with hypertension actually achieve a blood pressure goal of <140/90 mmHg. This low percentage of blood pressure control does not include the elderly or high-risk groups, such as those with diabetes. This is important, since those with diabetes and renal insufficiency are recommended to achieve even lower blood pressure levels (Table 15.1).[2] Moreover, blood pressure control is invariably more difficult in those with diabetes and/or established target organ damage. If these groups were included in the survey, it is estimated that the control rate for blood pressure would be <3 per cent. This failure to achieve adequate blood pressure control may in large part explain why the trend for development of both renal disease and cardiovascular disease is not being substantially reduced.

Early knowledge about blood pressure levels and progression of renal disease is derived either from *post hoc* analyses of prospective trials or case control studies. The first small study that retrospectively evaluated the effect of the level of blood pressure control on progression of nephropathy among patients with type I diabetes was reported from the Steno Diabetes Clinic.[17] These investigators noted a greater slowing in the decline of glomerular filtration rate (GFR) among those with a systolic blood pressure of ≤130 mmHg when compared with the group that averaged a systolic pressure of ≥140 mmHg. In this small retrospective study, all patients were treated with beta-blockers and diuretics. More recent data from Dillon in over 100 patients with diabetic nephropathy followed for almost 2 years confirm this observation.[18] Additionally, data from a retrospective analysis of over 300 type I diabetic patients followed for 3–21 years, further support the concept that mean arterial pressure (MAP) levels of ≤98 mmHg provide optimal protection against renal disease progression (HH Parving, personal communication). Taken together, these data provide

Trial	Primary end-point	BP control levels	Outcome
AASK[32]	Rate of decline in GFR	102–106; <92 mmHg, MAP	To be completed in 2002
HDFP[31]	Cardiovascular events	Usual control; diastolic <90 mmHg	<90, slower decline in serum creatinine
HOT[6]	Cardiovascular events	Diastolic <90, <85, <80 mmHg	<80, slowest decline in GFR and lowest CV events
MDRD[19,20]	Rate of decline in GFR	102–106, <92 mmHg, MAP	<92, slower decline in GFR*
UKPDS[7]	Cardiovascular events	<180/105, <150/85	<150/85 lower CV events and retinopathy
ABCD[8]	Decline in creatinine clearance	Diastolic 80–89 vs 75 mmHg	No difference in creatinine clearance

AASK, African-American Study on the Progression of Kidney Disease; HDFP, Hypertension Detection and Follow-Up Program; HOT, Hypertension Optimal Treatment Trial; MDRD, Modification of Diet in Renal Disease Trial; UKPDS, United Kingdom Prospective Diabetes Study; ABCD, Appropriate Blood pressure Control in Diabetes study; GFR, glomerular filtration rate as measured by iothalamate clearance. *Especially pronounced slowing in African-Americans.

Table 15.1
Randomised clinical trials that evaluate different levels of blood pressure control with a primary end-point of either renal or cardiovascular morbidity or mortality.

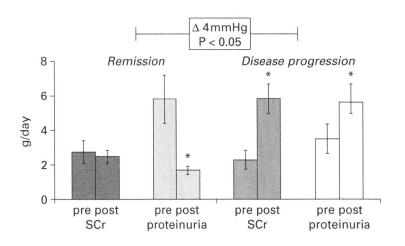

Figure 15.1
*The effects of ACE inhibition and blood pressure level on progression of nephropathy in patients with type I diabetic nephropathy. *P< 0.05 compared with baseline (pre) values. SCr, serum creatinine.*

support for the hypothesis that lower levels of blood pressure are needed to optimally reduce cardiovascular and renal events in diabetic patients.

In the Modification of Dietary protein in Renal Disease (MDRD) trial, hypertensive people with renal insufficiency of various causes were randomised to two levels of blood pressure control.[19] One group had a goal mean arterial pressure (MAP) of <92 mmHg, and the other an MAP of 102–106 mmHg. A *post hoc* analysis of this trial revealed that two subgroups had slower declines in renal function at the lower randomised blood pressure level;[20] these subgroups were African Americans and those with >1 g of proteinuria. Unfortunately, the primary end-point of the study was not focused on blood pressure level and hence, it was not powered to evaluate progression of renal disease as a function of blood pressure level.

It has been suggested from multiple clinical trials, primarily among people with type 1 diabetes, that control of blood pressure with ACE inhibitors slows progression of nephropathy to a greater extent than blood pressure control with other classes of agents. However, differences in the level of blood pressure control also contribute to this outcome. Differences of 4–5 mmHg in diastolic pressure translate into significant differences in renal and cardiovascular outcomes in people with diabetes.[21] This contention is supported by the findings of a *post hoc* analysis of the captopril trial.[22] This analysis evaluated the renal outcomes and change in proteinuria among the group of people with the most advanced nephropathy in this trial, i.e. those with nephrotic syndrome and serum creatinine values of ≥1.5 mg/dl. The group that manifested significant reductions in proteinuria had 'remission' of renal disease. In contrast, the group that had progressive worsening of renal function demonstrated an increase in proteinuria (Fig. 15.1). More importantly, however, independent of the ACE inhibitor component in this trial, there was a difference of 4 mmHg in arterial pressure between these two groups (Fig. 15.1). This was statistically significant and cannot be ignored as a contributing factor to the benefit seen in the patient group with the lower pressure.

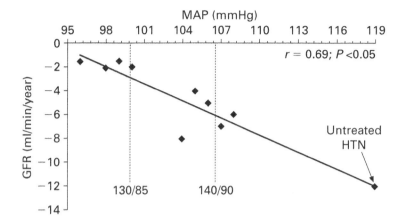

Figure 15.2
Relationship between level of blood pressure reduction and progression of renal disease. Data are derived from randomised clinical studies with a minimum follow-up of 3 years. Adapted from reference 21.

This difference of 4 mmHg in predominantly diastolic blood pressure load has also been noted in other studies and trials, including the UKPDS and the HOT trials, as well as studies in normotensive people with type II diabetes with microalbuminuria.[6,7,23–25] In these trials, there were prolonged periods of time when the group randomised to the ACE inhibitor had an average reduction in diastolic blood pressure of 4–6 mmHg lower than the placebo or control groups. Therefore, it can be argued that the contribution of this small, albeit significantly lower, level of blood pressure may have provided additional protection against renal disease progression.

A recent meta-analysis of 14 major primary prevention trials demonstrated a difference in diastolic blood pressure between the intervention groups and the control groups of only 4–5 mmHg.[26] This difference was associated with a significant reduction in strokes, coronary heart disease events and overall cardiovascular mortality. This was especially evident among elderly patients. *Post hoc* analysis of the Systolic Hypertension in the Elderly (SHEP) Trial supports the contention that if the blood pressure is lowered and sustained within an acceptable range, renal and cardiovascular events are reduced.[27] Thus, blood pressure reduction to appropriate levels by the least intrusive means possible needs to be the physician's goal.

Quality of life studies from the Hypertension Optimal Treatment (HOT) trial and the Syst-Eur trial demonstrate that the best quality of life was achieved in those with the lowest goal blood pressures.[28,29] For the HOT trial it was diastolic blood pressures of <80 mmHg that gave the best quality of life.[28] Therefore, the concept that lower blood pressure values correlate with more side-effects and worse medication tolerability is simply not supported by the data.

Achievement of the recommended blood pressure goals clearly has impact on renal disease progression. This is exemplified by a recent analysis of clinical trials that examines the relationship between the level of blood pressure and progression of renal disease (Fig. 15.2).[3,20] As can be seen, regardless of antihypertensive agents chosen to reduce blood pressure, the decline in renal function is

Group	Blood pressure goal
JNC VI	< 130/85 mmHg (ACEIs should be used as part of antihypertensive medications)
ADA (2002)	< 130/80 mmHg (ACEIs for type 1 or ARBs for type 2 diabetes with nephropathy should be used as part of antihypertensive medications)
NKF	< 130/85 mmHg (ACEIs should be used as part of antihypertensive medications)
ISH	< 130/85 mmHg (ACEIs should be used as part of antihypertensive medications)
WHO	< 130/85 mmHg (ACEIs should be used as part of antihypertensive medications)
Australian/New Zealand	< 130/85 mmHg (ACEIs should be used as part of antihypertensive medications)
BHS	< 140/90 mmHg (All agents suitable. ACEIs used first-line in type I diabetic nephropathy)

JNC, Joint National Committee Report (National Institutes of Health, USA); ADA, American Diabetes Association; NKF, National Kidney Foundation; ISH, International Society of Hypertension; WHO, World Health Organization; BHS, British Hypertension Society.

Table 15.2
Guidelines for control of hypertension in diabetes from various consensus committees around the world.

markedly slower in those who achieve lower blood pressure values.

Evaluation of international guidelines for blood pressure reduction in diabetes

Table 15.2 lists guidelines put forward for blood pressure control by various consensus groups around the world. It is clear from these guidelines that certain groups have tended to be more conservative than others or require more definitive data before accepting that lower levels of blood pressure control are better for reducing cardiovascular or renal events.

Blood pressure thresholds for pharmacological intervention

The international guidelines have reached a unanimous consensus that pharmacological treatment should be offered to patients with type 1 or type 2 diabetes when their blood pressure is consistently ≥140/90 mmHg. It is important to note that this refers to a systolic blood pressure ≥140 mmHg and/or a diastolic blood pressure ≥90 mmHg. Thus, these guidelines have acknowledged the importance of systolic blood pressure in defining the treatment threshold.

Therapeutic goals

While in the past some divergence in recommendations existed between the WHO and the JNC recommendations with regard to the level of blood pressure reduction, for a patient with diabetes or renal insufficiency, the current recommendations seem to be in general agreement with each other. These groups argued that the existing data from studies in people with diabetic nephropathy was strong enough to endorse a lower level of blood pressure control, i.e. <130/85 mmHg. However, other national organisations such as the National Kidney Foundation also argue that use of agents that either reduce or prevent the rise in proteinuria, i.e. ACE inhibitors, should be preferred since they may have greater impact on renal disease progression.[30]

Both the "optimal" blood pressure goals and treatment recommendations have been developed further following the publication of the first clinical trials in patients with type 2 diabetes and nephropathy, using angiotensin II receptor blockers (ARBs). These new developments form the basis of the new position statements from the American Diabetes Association on blood pressure control and choice of therapy, hypertension and nephropathy.[14,15] These most recent recommendations have opted for a lower "ideal" blood pressure target of <130/80 mmHg. They also suggest that the evidence base favours the use of ACE-inhibition for nephroprotection in type 1 diabetes and ARBs in type 2 diabetes, with both classes being interchangeable as an ideal alternative if either is not tolerated.

It is also important to note that there was no J-shaped curve for mortality observed in either the MDRD, HDFP or AASK trials pilot study.[19,31,32] Also, in the recently completed HOT trial there was no evidence of a J-shaped curve, as evidenced by the fact that the group randomised to the lowest level of blood pressure (i.e. diastolic of 80 mmHg) tolerated these pressures well.[6,33] Therefore, these levels of arterial pressure reduction are quite safe, and attainable.

Recommendations to achieve blood pressure goals

It is clear that any patient with either type I or type II diabetes, pre-existing renal disease (serum creatinine ≥1.4 mg/dl), microalbuminuria or

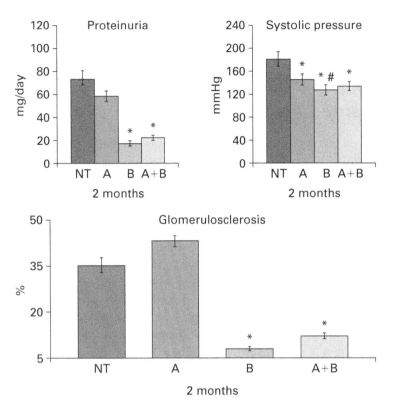

Figure 15.3
*The effects of a dihydropyridine calcium antagonist with and without an ACE inhibitor on blood pressure control, proteinuria and glomerulosclerosis in the rat remnant kidney model. *P< 0.05 compared with NT and/or A; #P< 0.05 compared with A. NT, no blood pressure treatment; A, amlodipine; B, benazepril; A + B, amlodipine with benazepril given in combination, each in lower doses to control pressure.*

proteinuria should have their blood pressure lowered to levels of <130/80 mmHg.[2,14,15,30] The rationale for this comes from the results of multicentered clinical trials that demonstrate an increased risk for development of either cardiovascular or renal disease when blood pressure goes above this level.[4–8,19,22–25,31,32,34] Additionally, it should be borne in mind that failure to achieve these goals results in a less than maximum benefit to the patient. An elevation in blood pressure of 15/10 mmHg above 140/90 actually doubles the risk of a cardiovascular or renal event in any individual with hypertension.[14] Lastly, data from three separate trials demonstrate that achievement of lower blood pressure goal,

i.e. diastolic <85 mmHg, results in substantial cost savings.[35–37]

Moreover, the degree of blood pressure reduction achieved might supersede any unique benefits of a specific class of antihypertensive therapy. This was exemplified in recent animal experiments that compared the effects of two different classes of antihypertensive agents on glomerular scarring. The results clearly demonstrated that in animal models of renal disease at a given level of blood pressure, ACE inhibitors protected against glomerular injury in comparison with dihydropyridine calcium antagonists, but not other antihypertensive agents (Fig. 15.3). Moreover, to garner the benefits of ACE inhibitors at a systolic

An approach to reduce blood pressure to lower than 'usual' levels in a diabetic patient*

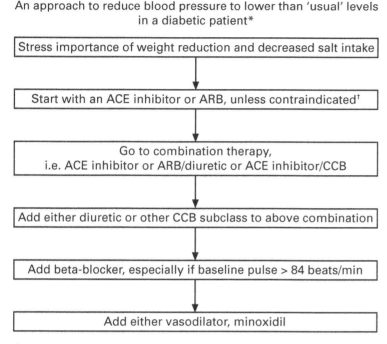

Figure 15.4
Paradigm by which to achieve blood pressure goals in patients with diabetes and/or renal insufficiency.

* Adapted from the JNC VI.
† Contraindications include: development of hyperkalemia after dietary counselling on low potassium intake, development of persistent cough, angioedema. Note: a rise of 30–50 per cent in serum creatinine is NOT a contraindication to ACE inhibitors, if renal function becomes stable within 2–4 weeks after the rise or hyperkalemia develops.

pressure of 140 mmHg, dihydropyridine calcium channel blockers when used alone, would have to achieve a systolic blood pressure of <110 mmHg. The reasons for this apparent lack of nephro-protection by calcium antagonists are beyond the scope of this chapter, but are reviewed elsewhere.[38]

Using the JNC VI and the WHO recommendations as guidelines for a given patient population, a simplified approach for anyone with renal disease or diabetes would be initiation of therapy with an ACE inhibitor, or if poorly tolerated an angiotensin receptor blocker. These agents should be titrated to moderate or high doses as tolerated.

If blood pressure fails to achieve goal after a period of 2–3 months, either a low dose thiazide diuretic or long-acting loop diuretic, such as toresmide (if serum creatinine is ≥1.8 mg/dl) should be added. Diuretics are required to achieve blood pressure goals in most people with diabetes, since they overcome the sodium-retaining effects of insulin.

Alternatively, calcium channel blockers (CCBs) should be considered, especially non-dihydropyridine CCBs, such as verapamil and diltiazem, as they have been shown to reduce cardiovascular mortality as well as slow renal disease progression.[39–41] The non-dihydropyridine CCBs may reduce cardiovascular mortality through a reduction in sympathetic neural tone in contrast to the dihydropyridine agents

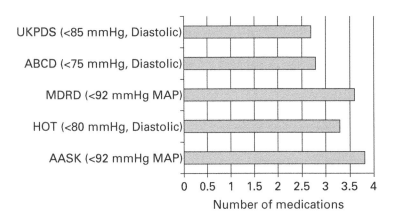

Figure 15.5
Average number of different antihypertensive medications required in studies where intensive blood pressure was a goal.

such as amlodipine that increase sympathetic activity.[42] Additionally, the renal profile of the non-dihydropyridine CCBs is different from the dihydropyridine agents, in that they reduce glomerular permeability, hence the protein-uria.[43–44]

Nevertheless, these potential differences between different classes of CCBs on protein-uria are less relevant when combined with ACE-inhibitors or ARBs as illustrated in some recent studies that have shown greater efficacy of and ACEi-CCB combination than either alone for cardiovascular protection[45] and the common need to add a CCB to an ARB/diuretic combination to improve blood pressure control for nephroprotection.[46]

If the goal blood pressure is not achieved with these medications, then alternative agents should be added (see Fig. 15.4). If three med-ications used in optimal dosages fail to achieve the blood pressure goal, then a fourth medica-tion must be considered. The fourth medica-tions for this group of people should either be a selective beta-receptor blocker, such as metoprolol, or a subclass of CCB not currently being prescribed. For example, if a dihydro-pyridine CCB is already part of the regimen, then a non-dihydropyridine CCB should be added, since these two subclasses of CCB given together have more than additive blood pressure lowering effects.[47,48]

Alternatively, if a dihydropyridine CCB was used initially and the heart rate is in excess of 82 beats per minute, then a selective beta-blocker should be considered to maximally reduce mortality. While beta-blockers have never been shown to be effective in primary prevention trials for reducing cardiovascular risk, data to support their efficacy for cardio-vascular risk reduction in secondary preven-tion trials are overwhelming. Moreover, beta-blockers have been shown to be effective for lowering cardiovascular risk among per-sons with type II diabetes.[7]

Afro-Caribbean patients with hypertension may require more aggressive blood pressure reduction to optimally preserve renal func-tion.[49–51] Thus, the physician should be very aggressive with blood pressure management in Afro-Caribbean patients, as they will reap the benefits of cardiovascular risk reduction and preservation of renal function with blood pres-sure control to <130/80 mmHg.[43,44,47] The results of the African-American Study of Kid-ney (AASK) Disease trial, due by 2002, should establish the level to which blood pressure should be reduced to optimally preserve renal function. Moreover, cost-effectiveness analyses from three separate clinical trials demonstrated that achievement of lower levels of blood pressure, i.e. <85 mmHg, resulted in substantial cost savings.[20,49,50]

In summary, all people with diabetes and especially those with renal insufficiency should have their blood pressures lowered to levels of <130/80 mmHg, which in most cases will require a minimum of three agents (Fig. 15.5). Based on all the trial evidence, ACE inhibitors or ABBs as well as diuretics and CCBs should be included in the 'antihypertensive cocktail' to achieve this goal. Moreover, combinations of certain agents may yield additive benefits on reduction in proteinuria and serve to reduce cardiovascular events.[51–53]

References

1. Perry HM, Miller JP, Fornoff JR. Early predictors of 15-year end-stage renal disease in hypertensive patients. *Hypertension* 1995; **25:** 587–94.
2. Joint National Committee Report on the Diagnosis and Treatment of Hypertension (JNC VI). *Arch Intern Med* 1997; **157:** 2413–46.
3. Bakris GL. Progression of diabetic nephropathy: focus on arterial pressure level and methods of reduction. *Diabetes Res Clin Pract* 1998; **39**(Suppl): 35–43.
4. Diabetes Control and Complications (DCCT) Research Group. Effect of intensive therapy on the development and progression of diabetic nephropathy in the Diabetes Control and Complications Trial. *Kidney Int* 1995; **47:** 1703–20.
5. Effect of intensive blood-glucose control with metformin on complications in overweight patients with Type 2 diabetes (UKPDS 34). UK Prospective Diabetes Study (UKPDS) Group. *Lancet* 1998; **352:** 854–65.
6. Hansson L, Zanchetti A, Carruthers G, et al., for the HOT Study Group. Effects of intensive blood-pressure lowering and low-dose aspirin in patients with hypertension: principal results of the Hypertension Optimal Treatment (HOT) randomized trial. *Lancet* 1998; **351:** 1755–61.
7. UK Prospective Diabetes Group. Tight blood pressure control and risk of macrovascular and microvascular complications in Type 2 diabetes: UKPDS 38. *BMJ* 1998; **317:** 703–13.
8. Estacio RO, Jeffers BW, Hiatt WR, Biggerstaff SL, Gifford N, Schrier RW. The effect of nisoldipine as compared with enalapril on cardiovascular outcomes in patients with non-insulin-dependent diabetes and hypertension. *N Engl J Med* 1998; **338:** 645–52.
9. Estacio RO, Jeffers BW, Gifford N, Schrier RW. Effect of blood pressure control on diabetic microvascular complications in patients with hypertension and type 2 diabetes. *Diabetes Care* 2000; **23** (Suppl 2): B54–B64.
10. Schrier RW, Estacio RO, Esler A, Mehler P. Effects of aggressive blood pressure control in normotensive type diabetic patients on albuminuria, retinopathy and strokes. *Kidney Int* 2002; **61:** 1086–97.
11. 1999 World Health Organization–International Society of Hypertension Guidelines for the Management of Hypertension. Guidelines Subcommittee. *J Hypertens* 1999; **17:** 151–83.
12. American Diabetes Association Position Statement. Treatment of hypertension in adults with diabetes. *Diabetes Care* 2002; **25:** 134–47 and 99–201.
13. American Diabetes Association Position Statement. Diabetic Nephropathy. *Diabetes Care* 2002; **25** (Suppl 1): S85–S89.
14. Klag MJ, Whelton PK, Randall B, et al. Blood pressure and end-stage renal disease in men. *N Engl J Med* 1996; **334:** 13–18.
15. Walker GW, Neaton JD, Cutler JA, Neuwirth R, Cohen JD, for the MRFIT Research Group. Renal function change in hypertensive members of the Multiple Risk Factor Intervention Trial: racial and treatment effects. *JAMA* 1992; **268:** 3085–91.
16. Burt VL, Cutler JA, Higgins M, et al. Trends in the prevalence, awareness, treatment and control of hypertension in the adult US population: data from the health examination surveys, 1960–1991. *Hypertension* 1995; **26:** 60–9.
17. Parving HH, Smidt UM, Hommel E. Effective antihypertensive treatment postpones renal insufficiency in diabetic nephropathy. *Am J Kidney Dis* 1993; **22:** 188–95.
18. Dillon JJ. The quantitative relationship between treated blood pressure and progression of diabetic renal disease. *Am J Kidney Dis* 1993; **22:** 798–802.
19. Klahr S, Levey AS, Beck GJ, for the Modification of Diet in Renal Disease Study Group. The effects of dietary protein restriction and blood pressure control on the progression of chronic renal disease. *N Engl J Med* 1994; **330:** 877–84.

20. Lazarus JM, Bourgoignie JJ, Buckalew VM, et al., for the MDRD Group. Achievement and safety of a low blood pressure goal in chronic renal disease: The modification of diet in renal disease study group. *Hypertension* 1997; **29**: 641–50.

21. Sheinfeld G, Bakris GL. Therapeutic interventions in special hypertensive populations. *Am J Hypertens* 1999; **12** (Suppl): 80–5.

22. Hebert LA, Bain RP, Verne D, for the Collaborative Study Group. Remission of nephrotic range proteinuria in Type I diabetes. *Kidney Int* 1994; **46**: 1688–93.

23. Viberti G, Mogensen CE, Groop LC, Pauls JF. Effect of captopril on progression to clinical proteinuria in patients with insulin-dependent diabetes mellitus and microalbuminuria. European Microalbuminuria Captopril Study Group. *JAMA* 1994; **271**: 275–9.

24. Bakris GL, Copley JB, Vicknair N, Sadler R, Leurgans S. Calcium channel blockers versus other antihypertensive therapies on progression of NIDDM associated nephropathy: results of a six year study. *Kidney Int* 1996; **50**: 1641–50.

25. Ravid M, Lang R, Rachmani R, Lishner M. Long-term renoprotective effect of angiotensin-converting enzyme inhibition in non-insulin-dependent diabetes mellitus. A 7-year follow-up study. *Arch Intern Med* 1996; **156**: 286–9.

26. Chalon S, Brudi P, Lechat P. Arterial hypertension: current large therapeutic trials. *Therapie* 1996; **51**: 631–8.

27. Curb JD, Pressel SL, Cutler JA, et al. Effect of diuretic-based antihypertensive treatment on cardiovascular disease risk in older diabetic patients with isolated systolic hypertension. *JAMA* 1996; **276**: 1886–92.

28. Wiklund I, Halling K, Ryden-Bergsten T, Fletcher A. Does lowering the blood pressure improve the mood? Quality-of-life results from the Hypertension Optimal Treatment (HOT) study. *Blood Press* 1997; **6**: 357–64.

29. Fletcher AE, Bulpitt CJ, Tuomilehto J, et al. Quality of life of elderly patients with isolated systolic hypertension: baseline data from the Syst-Eur trial. *J Hypertens* 1998; **16**: 1117–24.

30. Keane WF, Eknoyan G. Proteinuria, albuminuria, risk, assessment, detection, elimination (PARADE): a position paper of the National Kidney Foundation. *Am J Kidney Dis* 1999; **33**: 1004–10.

31. Hypertension Detection and Follow-Up Cooperative Group. Five-year findings of the Hypertension Detection and Follow-Up Program: II. Mortality by race, sex and age. *JAMA* 1979; **242**: 2572–7.

32. Wright JR, Kusek J, Toto R, et al., for the AASK Pilot Study Investigators. Design and baseline characteristics of participants in the African American Study of Kidney Diseases and hypertension (AASK) Pilot Study. *Controlled Clin Trials* 1996; **17**: 3S-16S.

33. Mallion JM, Pehrsson NG, Raveau-Landon C, Boutelant S, Menard J. Short and long term clinical tolerance of hypertensive treatment during the HOT study. *Arch Mal Coeur* 1996; **89**: 1093–6.

34. Tuomilehto J, Rastenyte D, Birkenhager WH, et al. Effects of calcium-channel blockade in older patients with diabetes and systolic hypertension. Systolic Hypertension in Europe Trial Investigators. *N Engl J Med* 1999; **340**: 677–84.

35. Cost effectiveness of intensive treatment of hypertension. Based on presentations by DS Shepard and D Hodgkin. *Am J Managed Care* 1998; **4**(12 Suppl): S765–9.

36. UK Prospective Diabetes Study Group. Cost effectiveness analysis of improved blood pressure control in hypertensive patients with Type 2 diabetes: UKPDS 40. *BMJ* 1998; **317**: 720–6.

37. Rodby RA, Firth LM, Lewis EJ. An economic analysis of captopril in the treatment of diabetic nephropathy. The Collaborative Study Group. *Diabetes Care* 1996; **19**: 1051–61.

38. Tarif N, Bakris GL. Preservation of renal function: the spectrum of effects by calcium channel blockers. *Nephrol Dial Transplant* 1997; **12**: 2244–50.

39. Makrilakis K, Bakris GL. New therapeutic approaches to achieve the desired blood pressure goal. *Cardiovasc Rev Reports* 1997; **18**: 10–16.

40. Danish Verapamil Infarction Trial II – DAVIT II. Effect of verapamil on mortality and major events after acute myocardial infarction. *Am J Cardiol* 1990; **66**: 779–85.

41. Kloke HJ, Branten AJ, Huysmans FT, Wetzels

JF. Antihypertensive treatment of patients with proteinuric renal diseases: risks or benefits of calcium channel blockers? *Kidney Int* 1998; **53**: 1559–73.

42. Ligtenberg G, Blankestijn PJ, et al. Reduction of sympathetic hyperactivity by enalapril in patients with chronic renal failure. *N Engl J Med* 1999; **340**: 1321–8.

43. Smith AC, Toto R, Bakris GL. Differential effects of calcium channel blockers on size selectivity of proteinuria in diabetic glomerulopathy. *Kidney Int* 1998; **54**: 889–96.

44. Griffin KA, Picken MA, Bakris GL, Bidani AK. Class differences in the effects of calcium channel blockers in the rat remnant kidney model. *Kidney Int* 1999; **55**: 1849–60.

45. Tatti P, Phaor M, Byington RP, et al. Outcome results of the fosinopril versus amlodipine cardiovascular events trial (FACET) in patients with hypertension and NIDDM. *Diabetes Care* 1998; **21**: 579–603.

46. Brenner BM, Cooper ME, De Zeeuw D, et al. Effects of losartan on renal and cardiovascular outcomes in patients with type 2 diabetes and nephropathy. *N Engl J Med* 2001; **345**: 861–9.

47. Saseen JJ, Carter BL, Brown TE, Elliott WJ, Black HR. Comparison of nifedipine alone and with diltiazem or verapamil in hypertension. *Hypertension* 1996; **28**: 109–14.

48. Nalbantgil I, Onder R, Kiliccioglu B, Turkoglu C. Combination therapy with verapamil and nitrendipine in patients with hypertension. *J Hum Hypertens* 1993; **7**: 305–8.

49. Toto R, Mitchell HC, Smith RD, Lee HC, McIntire D, Pettinger WA. 'Strict' blood pressure control and progression of renal disease in hypertensive nephrosclerosis. *Kidney Int* 1995; **48**: 851–8.

50. Bakris GL, Mangrum A, Copley JB, Vicknair N, Sadler R. Calcium channel or beta blockade on progression of diabetic renal disease in African-Americans. *Hypertension* 1997; **29**: 745–50.

51. Bakris GL, Griffin KA, Picken MM, Bidani AK. Combined effects of an angiotensin converting enzyme inhibitor and a calcium antagonist on renal injury. *J Hypertension* 1997; **15**: 1181–5.

52. Bakris GL, Weir MR, DeQuattro V, McMahon FG. Effects of an ACE inhibitor/calcium antagonist combination on proteinuria in diabetic nephropathy. *Kidney Int* 1998; **54**: 1283–9.

53. Epstein M, Bakris GL. Newer approaches to antihypertensive therapy: use fixed dose combination therapy. *Arch Intern Med* 1996; **156**: 1969–78.

16

Non-pharmacological strategies for blood pressure control in diabetic subjects

R Nithiyananthan and Paul M Dodson

Introduction

Hypertension is a common condition in patients with diabetes mellitus; it is twice as common in diabetic individuals as in the normal population.[1–4] In patients who have diabetes and hypertension, 80 per cent of them are also obese.[5] The association between stroke and cardiovascular disease with hypertension is well established. Hypertensive diabetics have an increased risk of stroke which is six times higher than the normal population and it has also been shown that diabetics with hypertension are twice as likely to have stroke compared with diabetics who do not suffer from hypertension.[6] Other studies have demonstrated that hypertension plays a role in the development and progression of diabetic complications such as retinopathy[7,8] and nephropathy,[9] and hence the treatment of these conditions may lead to decrease in morbidity.

It is now established that treating hypertension in diabetic patients should lead to decrease in morbidity and mortality. The benefit of blood pressure lowering has been confirmed in large studies, especially when target organ damage exists, e.g. left ventricular hypertrophy, hypertensive retinopathy or renal damage, and in the presence of other risk factors, e.g. smoking, hyperlipidaemia, family history of premature ischaemic heart disease and diabetes.[10,11] The recent ABCD,[12] HOT,[13] Syst-Eur[14] and UKPDS[15,16] trials demonstrated definite benefit in diabetic subjects treated with modern antihypertensive agents and suggested a target blood pressure (BP) level of <130 mmHg systolic and <85 mmHg diastolic pressure.

The high prevalence of obesity in diabetic subjects, and the potential for some antihypertensive therapy (e.g. thiazides and beta-blockers) to cause deterioration in glycaemic control and adversely affect serum lipid profile,[17–20] support the concept that non-pharmacological intervention should be considered as initial and longer term treatment to achieve normalisation of blood pressure. Non-pharmacological therapies also have the potential to act synergistically with drug therapies, e.g. ACE inhibitors and diuretics.

Syndrome X (Reaven's syndrome)[21] is now a well-established condition in which subjects with type II diabetes have resistance to insulin-stimulated glucose uptake, hyperinsulinaemia, glucose intolerance, hyperuricaemia, hypertension, abnormal lipid metabolism with increase in very low-density lipoprotein (VLDL) triglyceride and decreased HDL-cholesterol. These subjects in particular may benefit from non-pharmacological intervention to lower their blood pressure, as they already have abnormal lipid glucose metabolism, and in addition alterations in carbohydrate intake and weight loss can reduce insulin resistance.

Diet and hypertension

Dietary modification and its influence on blood pressure in diabetics has been studied, but confounding variables are difficult to eliminate. These include the effect of changing diet with resulting weight loss and improved glycaemic control, which are well known to affect blood pressure. There is also difficulty with exact dietary compliance, which is variable depending on the subjects' motivation and according to the palatability of differing dietary regimens. The single dietary modifications that have been studied in diabetics so far have been in sodium, potassium and magnesium intake.

Sodium

The association of hypertension with sodium has long been recognised and has been studied extensively. The findings of the largest study to date (INTERSALT) investigating the relationship of sodium and potassium to blood pressure status in non-diabetic subjects were published in 1988 and 1996.[22,23] Urinary sodium excretion was used as a measure of daily sodium and potassium intake. The study looked at 52 population samples in 32 different countries and recruited 10,079 men and women aged between 20 and 59 years. It demonstrated considerable variation in urinary excretion of sodium from 0.2 to 242 mmol/24 h in the different populations and in individual subjects and showed that increased sodium excretion was significantly related to higher blood pressure levels. It also demonstrated that increased sodium excretion by 100 mmol/24 h was associated with an increase in systolic and diastolic blood pressures on average by 3/0 to 6/3 mmHg respec-

tively, which was still related after correction for body mass in the analysis. The association was greater in the age group 40–59 years. In the cross-population analysis, if 24-hour excretion of sodium was greater by 100 mmol, the systolic/diastolic blood pressure was found to be higher on average by 5–7/2–4 mmHg and estimated mean difference in systolic/diastolic blood pressure at the age of 55 compared with 25 is greater by 10–11/6 mmHg. The INTER-SALT researchers concluded that there was a strong positive association between increasing urinary sodium excretion and increasing systolic blood pressure, and that the high urinary sodium is associated with substantially greater difference in blood pressure in the middle-aged compared with young adulthood. This large study has confirmed the association between salt and blood pressure.

Decreasing the sodium content in the diet has been shown to decrease blood pressure[24,25] and addition of sodium to the diet has been shown to increase blood pressure.[26] Certain lifestyles, such as a vegetarian intake, are associated with absence of hypertension[25–27] and it has therefore been postulated that this might be due to the low sodium and high potassium content of the vegetarian diet. It has also been shown that migration of populations from rural to urban areas has been associated with the development of hypertension.[29]

Seventy-five per cent of consumed salt is obligatory as it is present in processed food. As a result it is difficult for subjects to dramatically lower salt intake without major dietary changes, raising compliance as a potential major problem.

Abnormalities in sodium metabolism may be implicated in diabetic subjects. Diabetic patients have been shown to have increased exchangeable body sodium in both type I and type II diabetic subjects. Insulin increases the absorption of sodium in the renal tubules in normal subjects as well as in diabetic patients. These observations could partly explain the strong association of hypertension to diabetes. Type II diabetic subjects usually have hyperinsulinaemia, and fasting insulin levels are higher in hypertensive diabetics than normotensive diabetics.[30] The findings suggest that alteration in the dietary salt intake could affect blood pressure levels in diabetic subjects, as would be anticipated from studies in non-diabetic normal individuals.

Effects of sodium restriction

Dodson et al. designed a randomised, double-blind, cross-over study of sodium restriction and supplementation in diabetic individuals.[31] They recruited 34 diabetic subjects with systolic blood pressure of >160 mmHg or diastolic blood pressure of >95 mmHg in three consecutive clinic visits, with subsequent randomisation into two groups. Group I had no alteration in their diet and group II had advice on modest reduction of sodium in their diet (avoiding added salt and high salt-containing food) (see Box). Patients who were taking diuretics for hypertension were excluded from the trial in view of the influences of these agents on sodium excretion. Patients were well matched in the two groups for age, duration of diabetes, duration of hypertension, weight and blood pressure at their entry to the study (Table 16.1). After 3 months there was a significant fall in urinary sodium excretion and in the supine and erect blood pressure (Tables 16.2 and 16.3) in the sodium-restricted group of patients (group II). However, there was no significant change in the diastolic blood pressure. Following the 3-month parallel trial period, 13 of the sodium-restricted group of patients received either sodium supplementation (slow sodium tablets, 80 mmol/day) or matched placebo as part of a double-blind,

> Summary of dietary advice given to patients to achieve sodium restriction; adapted from Dodson et al.[31]
>
> Patients were instructed to avoid:
> 1. Adding table salt
> 2. Adding salt in cooking
> 3. Salted meat and smoked fish
> 4. Tinned foods – particularly tinned meats, vegetables, fish and tinned and packed soups
> 5. Salted cheeses
> 6. Oxo, Bovril, Marmite and Bisto
> 7. Bottled sauces and savoury snacks, including crisps and peanuts

cross-over, study for 1 month. These patients were found to have a significant rise in blood pressure with slow sodium supplementation (Table 16.4). The order of sodium supplementation or placebo did not influence the effect, and there were no significant changes in weight, alcohol intake or glycaemic control throughout the whole trial period.

These data suggest that dietary sodium intake has an influence on blood pressure in diabetic subjects, with moderate sodium restriction leading to reduction in blood pressure in type II diabetic subjects. The effect on systolic blood pressure was clinically significant (−19.2 mmHg) and therefore in diabetic patients with mild to moderate hypertension there may not be a requirement for drug therapy as a result. Those subjects with more severe hypertension could have improved control of hypertension as a result of dietary restriction in salt intake. Although it is well known that the majority of salt intake is derived from processed food in the diet, avoidance of high salt-containing foods and added

Characteristics	Moderate sodium restricted group (n = 17)	Control group (n = 17)
Sex	12M:5F	11M:6F
Age (years)	61.9 (7.5)	61.1 (6.3)
% of ideal body weight	126.6 (20.2)	127.5 (24.9)
Duration of diabetes (years)	4.1 (5.2)	5.1 (3.4)
Duration of hypertension (years)	4.1 (3.4)	6.5 (8.0)
Mean erect pre-entry blood pressure (mmHg)	179/98	174/100
Oral treatment (no. of patients) Hypoglycaemic agents Antihypertensive drugs	2 2	4 2

Table 16.1
Clinical details of type II diabetic hypertensive patients; adapted from Dodson et al.[31]

Parameter	Moderate sodium restricted group (n = 17)				Control group (n = 17)			
	Start	Finish	P value	Mean % change	Start	Finish	P value	Mean % change
Blood pressure (mmHg) Supine								
Systolic	179.7 (18.2)	160.5 (22.5)	<0.01	11.0	173.8 (20.3)	167.5 (11.5)	NS	4
Diastolic	91.4 (11.1)	87.6 (10.5)	NS	3.1	92.4 (10.9)	90.4 (5.7)	NS	1
Erect								
Systolic	182.3 (20.1)	160.9 (15.8)	<0.001	12.0	175.9 (17.3)	166.5 (10.8)	NS	4.2
Diastolic	95.2 (9.7)	91.8 (6.9)	<0.05	3.1	100.7 (8)	95 (7.8)	NS	5.1
Weight (kg)	79.9 (13.6)	77.1 (14.3)	NS		79.8 (11.6)	80.6 (11.2)	NS	

NS, not significant.

Table 16.2
Summary of clinical changes recorded in 3-month parallel controlled study; adapted from Dodson et al.[31]

Parameter	Moderate sodium restriction group (n = 17)			Control group (n = 17)		
	Start	Finish	P value	Start	Finish	P value
Urinary electrolyte excretion (mmol/24 h)						
Sodium	198.7 (65.9)	136.8 (37.9)	<0.001	183.2 (62.3)	180.7 (60.4)	NS
Potassium	65.9 (25.4)	63.9 (19.2)	NS	71.8 (27)	67.9 (32)	NS
Sodium:potassium ratio (molar)	3.16 (0.81)	2.31 (0.77)	<0.001	2.8	3	NS
Glycosylated haemoglobin (%)	10.2 (1.95)	10 (2)	NS	10.4 (2.5)	10.9 (2.5)	NS

Table 16.3
Summary of biochemical changes in 3-month parallel control study; adapted from Dodson et al.[31]

salt produced a blood pressure-lowering effect. Whether the diabetic subject is more 'salt sensitive' is conjecture, but is supported by the observation that marked salt restriction is required to lower blood pressure in non-diabetic essential hypertensive subjects.

Meta-analysis of randomised controlled trials and analysis of cross-over trials[32,33] confirms the above findings and supports the use of salt restriction as part of treatment for hypertension. Law et al. analysed 68 cross-over trials and 10 randomised trials of dietary salt reduction.[33] In 45 of these trials where salt reduction lasted ⩽4 weeks reduction in observed blood pressure was less than that predicted, with the difference between observed and predicted reduction being greatest in the trials of shortest duration. In 33 trials that lasted 5 weeks or longer the predicted reduction closely matched the observed reduction in the individual trials. This applied for all age groups. In people aged 50–59 years,

moderate reduction in salt (50 mmol or 3 g of salt) for a few weeks will result in reduction in systolic blood pressure of on average 5 mmHg and 7 mmHg in patients with high blood pressure (170 mmHg); diastolic blood pressure is lowered half as much. It is estimated that such reduction in people in the Western world would result in a reduced incidence of stroke by 26 per cent and ischaemic heart disease by 15 per cent.

A recent study in people with and without hypertension confirmed the power of sodium restriction and dietary modification to lower blood pressure.[25] This study, the Dietary Approaches to Stop Hypertension (DASH), utilised a diet rich in fruits, vegetables and low fat dairy products with reduced fat content. Simultaneously, the study evaluated the effects of different levels of sodium intake, in conjunction with the DASH diet (n = 208) or a normal diet (n=204), on blood pressure in people with and without hypertension. Three

Parameter	Initial value	P value	Sodium supplementation	P value	Placebo
Blood pressure (mmHg)					
Supine					
Systolic	159.9 (19.9)	<0.005	171.4 (17.1)	<0.05	161.7 (17.7)
Diastolic	87.5 (11)	NS	92.4 (10)	NS	87.3 (6.7)
Erect					
Systolic	163.8 (15.9)	NS	165 (18.8)	NS	163.3 (18.3)
Diastolic	95.3 (8.1)	NS	97.3 (8.5)	NS	92.7 (9.7)
Urinary electrolyte excretion (mmol/24 h)					
Sodium	141.5 (47.7)	<0.01	198.8 (37.4)	<0.05	122.6 (50.3)
Potassium	72.3 (20.6)	NS	68.5 (15.3)	NS	52.2 (20.3)
Weight (kg)	77.7 (4.8)	NS	77.7 (4.9)	NS	77 (4.6)

Table 16.4
Summary of mean changes recorded in double blind randomised cross-over study of 1 month of sodium supplementation versus 1 month of placebo in nine subjects; adapted from Dodson et al.[31]

different levels of sodium intake were evaluated in each dietary group; high sodium intake (150 mmol/day), intermediate (100 mmol/day) or low sodium intake (50 mmol/day). Each person in the study was randomly assigned to the three different levels of sodium intake for 30 days in a cross-over design.

Reducing sodium intake markedly reduced both systolic and diastolic blood pressure (see Fig. 16.1). Moreover, there was a stepwise reduction in systolic and diastolic blood pressure as sodium intake was reduced. At very low levels of sodium intake, there was a lower blood pressure in those consuming the DASH diet when compared to those consuming a normal diet (Fig. 16.1). This implies that the combination of a diet rich in fruit and vegetables and low in fat, or a diet low in sodium reduces blood pressure. Moreover the combination of a lower sodium intake with the DASH diet is more effective at reducing blood pressure than either strategy alone. These effects were observed independent of blood pressure status, race or gender. Overall, as compared to the normal diet with a high sodium intake, the DASH diet with a low sodium intake led to a mean systolic pressure that was 7.1 mmHg lower in people without hypertension and 11.5 mmHg lower in those with hypertension.[25] This means that this

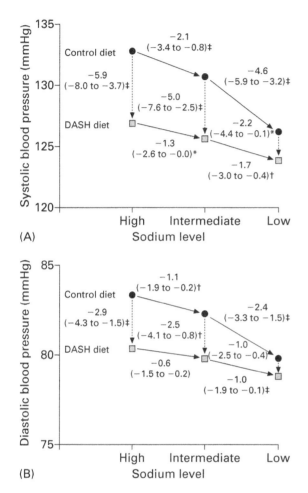

Figure 16.1
The effect on systolic blood pressure (panel A) and diastolic blood pressure (panel B) of reduced sodium intake and the DASH diet. From reference 25. Asterisks (P< 0.05), daggers (P< 0.01). and double daggers (P< 0.001) indicate significant differences in blood pressure between groups or between dietary sodium categories

strategy is about as effective as monotherapy with an antihypertensive drug.

Although the DASH study did not specifically evaluate people with diabetes, the evidence that sodium is likely to play an important role in hypertension in diabetes suggests that the DASH diet combined with a reduced sodium intake is likely to be particularly effective in this patient group.

Potassium supplementation

Potassium is another constituent of diet that has been shown to influence blood pressure. It has been recognised that there is an inverse relationship between urinary potassium excretion and blood pressure.[22,34–36] Vegetarians, who tend to have lower blood pressure than non-vegetarians, have a higher potassium content in their diet and excrete a normal amount of sodium, but a high amount of potassium.[37]

Extensive trials in non-diabetic hypertensive subjects have shown a hypotensive effect of potassium supplementation. For example, MacGregor et al. demonstrated that potassium supplementation with slow release tablets (60 mmol/day) lowered blood pressure by 4 per cent compared with placebo,[38] which is a small but significant fall in blood pressure. In these patients urinary potassium increased to 118 ± 7.4 mmol/24 h compared with patients on placebo who had potassium excretion rates of 62 ± 4.7 mmol/24 h.

There have been no specific trials to investigate whether potassium supplementation alone can influence the blood pressure in hypertensive diabetics. Some studies have assessed potassium supplementation, but in combination with other dietary changes (see section on magnesium below).

In the DASH study,[25] the DASH diet contained approximately 50% more potassium than the control diet. It is thus conceivable that this increased intake of potassium contributed to the overall beneficial effect of the DASH diet on blood pressure.

Magnesium supplementation

Several reports have suggested a blood pressure-lowering effect of magnesium supplementation in the non-diabetic individual. The effect of the magnesium supplement in hypertensive diabetics has been studied by Gilleran et al.[39] They designed a randomised blind trial of replacing added salt (sodium chloride: NaCl) with a salt substitute (50 per cent NaCl, 40 per cent potassium chloride (KCl), 10 per cent magnesium salt (Seltin)), compared to a group with whole added salt. Forty type II hypertensive diabetic patients were recruited and studied over a 9-month period. After 3 months there was a significant reduction of mean systolic blood pressure in the salt-substituted group of patients by 9.6 mmHg ($P < 0.03$) which was maintained at 9 months. There were no significant changes in weight, lipid profile, fasting insulin levels or level of glycaemic control. A greater number of patients withdrew from the study in the whole salt group because of persistent hypertension, with a blood pressure $> 160/95$ (n = 10) compared with the salt substitute group (n = 4), during the trial period. Although there was no significant change in diastolic blood pressure, urinary sodium or magnesium excretion rate, the patients receiving the salt substitute had an increased potassium excretion rate (58.8–77.3; $P < 0.05$). There were no adverse effects reported and the salt substitute was palatable. They concluded that ordinary table salt can be substituted with a mixture of sodium, potassium and magnesium which may lower blood pressure in hypertensive type II diabetic patients. The findings that these patients did not show changed urinary sodium excretion suggests that the observed blood pressure changes were not due to reduction of sodium intake *per se*, but could be due to changes in magnesium and potassium intake. Whilst further study is required to confirm these results, it would appear that magnesium and potassium supplementation is safe and has therapeutic potential.

Calcium

There has been a long recognised negative correlation between hypertensive heart disease and the hardness of the water.[40,41] It has been shown that supplementation of calcium lowers both systolic and diastolic blood pressure in patients with mild hypertension;[42–44] the mechanism for this effect is unclear. However, there is not substantial evidence to either support or dispute the role of calcium in controlling blood pressure. Two studies have demonstrated a fall in blood pressure with calcium supplementation.

In a 4-year clinical trial which recorded calcium loss from bone in hypertensive women, calcium supplementation with 1.5 g/day was given to half the patients in the trial.[45] Blood pressure was measured annually. The calcium-treated group showed reduction in systolic blood pressure of 10 mmHg, while the control group showed no change, with no changes in diastolic blood pressure in either group. Another trial (n = 57) assessed the effects of calcium supplementation in males and females with essential hypertension over 22 weeks.[46] They were given 1 g/day of calcium in the form of calcium carbonate or gluconolactate for 15 weeks. The treatment significantly reduced the systolic and diastolic blood pressure, by 8–6 mmHg and 8 mmHg, respectively.

The concept that calcium supplementation could have an influence on blood pressure in diabetic subjects is of interest, particularly as calcium channels are involved in insulin release, but has not been studied.

Lipids and free fatty acids

Greenland Eskimos whose diet largely comprises seafood do not have a high prevalence of hypertension. It has been demonstrated that there is an association between hypertension and dietary fat intake. A lower fat diet or a diet with a high polyunsaturated to saturated fatty acid ratio (P/S ratio) has been shown to lower both systolic and diastolic blood pressure, with the reduction in blood pressure greater in hypertensive individuals than in normotensive individuals.[47] Dietary supplementation with fish oil has been shown to lower the systolic[48] and diastolic blood pressure.[49] However, there has been no suggested link in diabetic subjects with hypertension who rely on high seafood intake. A higher P/S ratio and low fat dietary intake is recommended as part of the diabetic diet. Although alterations in dietary fat intake or change in P/S ratio have not been studied in diabetic hypertensive subjects as a single dietary change, these changes are an integral part of the diabetic diet, and may be important to studies described later.

Fibre

There is experimental and epidemiological evidence to relate dietary fibre intake and blood pressure. For example, a vegetarian diet comprises a high fibre intake and when meat is incorporated into a vegetarian's diet, higher blood pressure has been observed and conversely when meat intake is withdrawn, blood pressure returns to normal.[50] Although this could relate to alterations in dietary potassium and protein intake, it could also reflect the reduction in fibre intake. Other studies have shown that changing from a low fibre to a high fibre diet resulted in lowering of blood pressure[51] and that changing from a high fibre to a low fibre diet resulted in increasing blood pressure. Anderson and Gustafson studied the effect of a high fibre diet (65 g/day dietary fibre) in type I diabetic patients and found that there was a 10 per cent drop in blood pressure in these subjects, but this was confounded by reduction in insulin dose and weight loss.[52] Whether increasing dietary fibre intake alone is hypotensive in diabetic subjects is unclear,

but such an action may be part of a combined dietary approach. Appel et al. looked at the effect of a diet rich in fruit, vegetables and low-fat dairy food with reduced saturated and total fat content, on blood pressure.[53] They looked at 459 adults with systolic blood pressure of < 160 mmHg and diastolic blood pressure of 80–95 mmHg. For 3 weeks subjects were fed a control diet that was low in fruits, vegetable and dairy products, with fat content typical of the average diet in the USA. They were then randomly assigned to receive a diet rich in fruits and vegetables, or a 'combination' diet rich in fruit, vegetables and low-fat dairy products, with reduced saturated and total fat for 8 weeks. Sodium intake and body weight were maintained at a constant level. They found that a combination diet reduced the systolic and diastolic blood pressure by 5.5 and 3 mmHg respectively versus the control diet ($P<0.001$). The fruits and vegetables diet reduced the systolic blood pressure by 2.8 mmHg ($P<0.001$) and the diastolic blood pressure by 1.1 mmHg compared with the control diet ($P=0.07$). Among the 133 subjects with hypertension, i.e. systolic blood pressure $\geqslant 140$ mmHg and diastolic blood pressure of $\geqslant 90$ mmHg or both, the combination diet reduced the systolic and diastolic blood pressure by 11.4 and 5 mmHg respectively ($P<0.001$), and in the 326 subjects without hypertension the corresponding reductions were 3.5 mmHg ($P<0.001$) and 2.1 mmHg ($P=0.003$). They concluded that a diet rich in fruit, vegetables and low-fat dairy food, with reduced saturated and total fat, can substantially lower the blood pressure, especially in hypertensive subjects. These are important observations, in view of the similarity of the dietary changes to those currently recommended for diabetic subjects.

Parameter	Diet-treated group (n = 25)	Significance between groups	Control group (n = 25)
Blood pressure (mmHg)			
Systolic			
Start	180.5 ± 19.0	NS	170.0 ± 20.0
Finish	165.0 ± 20.7	NS	164.2 ± 17.8
	P<0.001		NS
Diastolic			
Start	96.6 ± 9.3	NS	97.0 ± 7.1
Finish	88.0 ± 10.5	P<0.01	95.4 ± 8.7
	P<0.001		NS
Body weight (kg)			
Start	74.6 ± 13.5	NS	74.2 ± 16.7
Finish	71.7 ± 12.1	NS	73.7 ± 15.9
	P<0.01		NS
Normal blood pressure achieved at 3 months (no. of patients)	10	NS	5

Table 16.5
Summary of clinical changes observed after 3-month controlled trial.[57]

Carbohydrate

Only a few trials have studied the effect of different carbohydrates on blood pressure; studying this aspect of management has been difficult. Complex carbohydrate such as guar gum has been shown to lower the blood pressure in diabetic and non-diabetic individuals,[54] whereas dextrose infusion to normotensive and non-diabetic subjects has been associated with elevation in blood pressure as well as retention of salt and water.

Combination of dietary factors

Although individual dietary manipulations may affect blood pressure (e.g. reduced sodium intake), diabetic patients are recom-mended to make a number of dietary changes which may have multiple effects on lipid metabolism, glucose control and blood pressure.

Trials have been carried out to study the effects of a high fibre, low sodium and low-fat diet, i.e. the diabetic diet, and the effects of this strategy compared to antihypertensive drug therapy, e.g. bendrofluazide and metoprolol.[55,56]

Pacy et al. compared a high fibre, low sodium, low fat diet with metoprolol therapy in 21 hypertensive type II diabetic subjects over a period of 3 months.[55] They found that both groups had significant reduction in both systolic and diastolic blood pressure, and as expected metoprolol also decreased the heart rate significantly. The modified diet had the advantage of reduction in mean glycosylated haemoglobin and weight as well as serum triglyceride levels.

Pacy et al. also compared the effect of a high fibre, low fat, low sodium diet with bendrofluazide (10 mg daily) in 50 diabetic patients with mild hypertension over a 3-month period.[56] There was a similar highly significant decrease in both systolic and diastolic blood pressure in both groups, but weight loss was greater in those receiving dietary therapy, with a reduction in glycosylated haemoglobin levels and at the end of the study patients in this treatment group had a significantly elevated glycosylated haemoglobin level and elevation in HDL level. Bendrofluazide therapy resulted in significant elevation in glycosylated haemoglobin level compared with the diet treatment group. The diet-treated group also demonstrated significant reductions in mean serum cholesterol and triglyceride, while bendrofluazide treatment elevated these mean levels.

These trials suggest that the diabetic diet is hypotensive as well as lowering serum lipid levels and improving glycaemic control without potential side-effects from antihypertensive drugs.

Dodson et al. studied the effect of a high fibre, low fat and low sodium diet for mild hypertension in type II diabetic patients.[57] Fifty hypertensive type II diabetic patients were allocated to a treatment diet of high fibre, low fat and low sodium composition or to a control diet by hospital dietician in a controlled trial.

After treatment for 3 months, the modified diet-treated group showed a highly significant reduction in mean systolic and diastolic blood pressure (Table 16.5). This was accompanied by significant reduction in urinary sodium excretion (183.0 ± 62.1 to 121.7 ± 65.8 mmol/day),

glycosylated haemoglobin (12.4 ± 3.1 to $10.5 \pm 2.9\%$), weight (74.6 ± 13.5 to 71.7 ± 12.1 kg) and serum triglyceride levels ($P < 0.05$).

The mean values of diastolic blood pressure ($P < 0.01$), urinary sodium/potassium ratio ($P < 0.001$) and urinary potassium ($P < 0.01$) were significantly reduced at 3 months. This demonstrated that the modified diet may be an attractive alternative to antihypertensive drug therapy as first-line treatment.

There is compelling evidence for an association between hypertension and obesity. The diabetic diet comprises high fibre, low fat and low sodium content, and therefore encourages weight loss. Other changes, including hypotensive effect and metabolic changes, also favour the diabetic individual with respect to reduction of risk factors associated with excess cardiovascular disease. Therefore this approach can lead to a reduction in drug therapy requirement. This latter aspect has been assessed in non-diabetic subjects. Stamler et al. assessed whether mild hypertensives could discontinue antihypertensive drug therapy, using nutritional means to control blood pressure.[58] This study was carried out in non-diabetic hypertensive patients over a 4-year period; 189 patients were randomised to three groups. Group 1 (n = 97) discontinued drug therapy and reduced weight, excess salt and alcohol; group 2 (n = 44) discontinued drug therapy with no nutritional programme; and group 3 (n = 48) continued drug therapy. In groups 1 and 2 anti-hypertensive drugs were reintroduced if the blood pressure became elevated to a diastolic pressure of $\geqslant 115$ mmHg. Weight loss of at least 4.5 kg was maintained by 30 per cent of group 1 with group mean loss of 1.8 kg; sodium intake fell by 36 per cent and modest alcohol intake reduction was reported. After 4 years 39 per cent of patients in group 1 remained normotensive without drug therapy compared with only 5 per cent in group 2. This demonstrated that a nutritionally based therapy may be substituted for drugs in a significant proportion of mild hypertensives or, if drugs are still needed, there is the potential to avoid unwanted biochemical and side-effects of drug therapy by lowering the dose of medication.

The data from the DASH study,[25] although not in people with diabetes, convincingly shows that a combined dietary intervention comprising an increased intake of fruit, vegetables and fibre and a reduced intake of fat and sodium can markedly reduce blood pressure, equivalent to the effect of monotherapy with antihypertensive medication.

Diet and drugs

Although dietary changes and antihypertensive drugs can significantly lower blood pressure in diabetic individuals, the combined effect of these could have an additive effect on hypertension. As previously quoted in the study by Stamler et al.[58] dietary modification may lead to reduction or even withdrawal of antihypertensive medication. Little et al.[59] looked at the effect of low sodium, low fat, high fibre diet in treated hypertensive patients. They did an observer-blind trial on 196 patients with essential hypertension using a control group, low sodium group, low fat group and a combined diet group (diet low in sodium and fat and high in fibre). They found that the combination diet group showed a larger and highly significant decrease in blood pressure and weight. This group also showed the largest reduction in medication (62.5 per cent, $P < 0.005$) with more patients stopping medication than in the controlled group (57.5 per cent, $P < 0.01$). Reduction in medication also occurred in the control group (32.5 per cent), high fibre group (46.9 per cent), low fat group (38.3 per cent) and low sodium group (44.8 per cent) with even more patients stopping medication in each group (37.5, 32.6 and 36.7 per cent respectively).

A more consistent observation has been apparent with regard to salt restriction when implemented together with pharmacological treatment of hypertension. With the exception of calcium channel antagonists, salt restriction complements the reduction in blood pressure produced by all classes of antihypertensive agents. In many cases satisfactory control of blood pressure can be obtained with lower doses of individual drugs.[60]

Angiotensin converting enzyme inhibition and angiotensin receptor blockers are widely used for the treatment of hypertension in people with diabetes. The antihypertensive efficacy of both drug classes can be enhanced by dietary sodium restriction. It is therefore important to advocate sodium restriction in patients receiving these medications to prevent the response to these medications being blunted by a high sodium intake.

Weight loss

Dietary advice given to diabetic subjects consists of food rich in unrefined carbohydrate, low in salt and high in polyunsaturated fat that is also low in cholesterol. Patients are advised to avoid food rich in refined sugar, high in saturated fat and cholesterol and high in salt (e.g. BDA or EASD regimen). This diet, so-called 'sensible eating' or 'prudent' diet, helps to promote weight loss and lowers blood glucose and insulin requirement, as well as altering lipid metabolism with lowering of cholesterol and triglycerides. These changes should result in altered cardiovascular risk factors in favour of cardioprotection, in addition to a blood pressure-lowering effect.

The potential benefits of major weight loss have been demonstrated by Reisin and his colleagues, who found that a weight loss of 23 lb was associated with mean blood pressure drop of 20 mmHg in diastolic and 25 mmHg in systolic blood pressure, both in patients not on regular antihypertensive medication and in those on regular but inadequate therapy.[61] In the control group blood pressure was unchanged. Experience with the more recent appetite suppressant drugs or weight-promoting pharmacological agents supports these observations.

Alcohol

The association of high alcohol intake with hypertension has been recognised for many years.[62] Saunders et al. found that blood pressure was normalised with abstention from alcohol intake in previous ethanol abuse subjects and hypertension returned in those who recommenced alcohol intake.[63] Potter and Beevers demonstrated the pressor effect of alcohol in patients who were not alcoholic, by demonstrating fall or rise in blood pressure as alcohol was withdrawn or reintroduced under strict conditions in a hospital ward.[64] It is likely that excess alcohol has similar effects in diabetic subjects, with additional consequences of worsening glycaemic control, aggravating hypoglycaemia and adverse effects on lipid metabolism and weight.

Smoking

This is a well-recognised risk factor for cardiovascular disorders including cerebrovascular disorders. The association between smoking and hypertension has not been studied, but cessation of cigarette smoking as part of cardiovascular management is strongly recommended.

Relaxation therapy

Relaxation therapy has been studied as an active part of treatment for hypertension. Some studies found that these therapies were no better than placebo,[65] while others found a modest reduction in blood pressure.[66] One article has reviewed 24 trials of this therapy in 1200 patients.[67] Eleven of the trials looked at the potential of behaviour modification on the blood pressure; none of these trials found a significant change in blood pressure with this approach. In 13 of the trials a significant effect was found, with reduction of mean systolic blood pressure by 26 mmHg and diastolic by 5–15 mmHg. It was also noted that relaxation therapy from a therapist is more effective than programmes without supervision and/or individual psychotherapy,[66] and hence may therefore be considered expensive.

Conclusion

Although drug therapy forms a major component of the treatment of hypertension, it is important to modify lifestyle and dietary habits, in particular low sodium, high fibre, low fat and a dietary regimen in order to achieve control of both hypertension and the metabolic state.[68–70] Non-pharmacology therapy for 3 months is recommended as initial treatment for hypertension associated with diabetes mellitus. Dietary modification offers a cheaper alternative to drug therapy, whereas other forms of therapy such as psychotherapy and behaviour modification tend to be more expensive, and benefits in diabetics are still to be proven. In moderate to severe hypertension, non-pharmacological therapy should be the initial treatment, however, non-pharmacological strategies remain important because they can enhance the efficacy of antihypertensive medication. Potentiation of ACE inhibitors, angiotensin receptor blockers and other drugs by dietary changes, e.g. sodium restriction, may be clinically useful.

Although many trials have shown the hypotensive effect of non-pharmacological therapy, there is no evidence base to show that these measures have an influence on morbidity and mortality in the long term. Although this would be expected to be the case, proven benefit in terms of reducing cardiovascular and total mortality has only been demonstrated with antihypertensive and other drug therapies, e.g. most recently published HOT (hypertensive optimal treatment),[13] ABCD,[12] FACET[71] Syst-Eur[14] diabetes and UKPDS trials.[15,16] It is worth noting that in the HOT study reducing diastolic blood pressure to a mean of 82.6 mmHg had the lowest incidence of major cardiovascular events.[13] With a target of blood pressure reduction to 130/85 mmHg in diabetic subjects, and the requirement of combinations of antihypertensive therapy to achieve this, the role of non-pharmacological therapy may be even more important in respect of synergistic effect and reduction of drug therapy doses. In reality, non-pharmacological and pharmacological approaches to treatment are complementary strategies that are particularly relevant to the diabetic patient with hypertension.

References

1. Pell S, D'Alonzo CA. Some aspects of hypertension on diabetes mellitus. *JAMA* 1967; **202**: 104–10.
2. Kannel WB, McGee DL. Diabetes and cardiovascular risk factors: the Framingham study. *Circulation* 1979; **59**: 8–13.
3. Dupree OA, Meyer MB. Role of risk factors in complications of diabetes mellitus. *Am J Epidemiol* 1980; **112**: 100–12.
4. Turner RC. UK Prospective Diabetes Study. Prevalence of hypertension and hypotension in patients with newly diagnosed diabetes. *Hypertension* 1985; **7** (Suppl II): 8–13.
5. Working Group on Hypertension in Diabetes Mellitus. Statement on hypertension in diabetes mellitus. *Arch Intern Med* 1987; **147**: 830–42.
6. Kuller LH, Dorman JS, Wolf PA. Cardiovascular disease and diabetes. Diabetes in America. US Department of Health and Human Services publication. 1985; **1486**: 1–18.
7. Hostetter TH, Rennke HG, Brenner BM. The case for intracranial hypertension. In the initiation and progression of diabetic and other glomerulopathies. *Am J Med* 1982; **72**: 375–80.
8. Drury PL. Diabetes and arterial hypertension. *Diabetelogia* 1983; **24**: 1–9.
9. Parving HH, Hommel E. Prognosis in diabetic nephropathy. *BMJ* 1989; **299**: 230–3.
10. Management in essential hypertension: Report of the second working party of the British Hypertensive Society. *BMJ* 1993; **306**: 983–7.
11. Guidelines for the treatment of mild hypertension. Memorandum from a WHO/ISH meeting. *Bull World Health Organ* 1986; **64**: 31–5.
12. Estacio RO, Jeffers BW, Hiatt WR, Biggi SL, Gifford N, Schrier RW. The effect of nisoldipine as compared with enalapril on cardiovascular events in patients with non-insulin-dependent diabetes and hypertension. *N Engl J Med* 1998; **338**: 645–52.
13. Hansson L, Zanchetti A, Carruthers G, et al. Effects of intensive blood pressure lowering and aspirin in patients with hypertension: principal results of the Hypertension Optimal Treatment (HOT) randomised trial. *Lancet* 1998; **351**: 1755–62.
14. Tuomilehto J, Rastenye D, Birkenhager WH et al. Effects of calcium channel blockade in older patients with diabetes and systolic hypertension. *N Engl J Med* 1999; **340**: 677–84.
15. UK Prospective Diabetes Study Group. Tight blood pressure control and risk of macrovascular and microvascular complications in type 2 diabetes: UKPDS 38. *BMJ* 1998; **317**: 703–13.
16. UK Prospective Diabetes Study Group. Efficacy of atenolol and captopril in reducing risk of macrovascular and microvascular complications in type 2 diabetics: UKPDS 39. *BMJ* 1998; **317**: 713–20.
17. Murphy MB, Lewis PJ, Kohner E, Schumer B, Dollery CT. Glucose intolerance in hypertensive patients treated with diuretics; a 14 year follow-up. *Lancet* 1982; **2**: 1293–5.
18. Waal-Manning HJ. Metabolic effects of beta-adrenoceptor blockers. *Drugs* 1976; **11** (Suppl II): 121–6.
19. Gundersen T, Kjekshus J. Timolol treatment after myocardial infarction in diabetic patients. *Diabetes Care* 1983; **6**: 285–90.
20. Dodson PM. Lipids and antihypertensive therapy. *Br J Clin Pract* 1982; **20**: 17–20.
21. Reaven GM. Role of insulin resistance in human disease. *Diabetes* 1988; **37**: 1595–607.
22. INTERSALT Co-operative Research Group. INTERSALT: an international study of electrolyte excretion and blood pressure. Results for 24 hour urinary sodium and potassium excretion. *BMJ* 1988; **297**: 319–28.
23. Elliott P, Stamler J, Nicol R, et al. INTERSALT revisited: further analysis of 24 hour sodium excretion and blood pressure within and across population. *BMJ* 1996; **312**: 1249–53.
24. Kempner W. Treatment of hypertensive vascular disease with rice diet. *Am J Med* 1948; **4**: 545–77.

25. Sacks FM, Svetky LP, Vollmer WM, et al. for the DASH-sodium collaborative research group. Effects on blood pressure of reduced dietary sodium and Dietary Approaches to Stop Hypertension (DASH) diet. N Engl J Med 2001; **344**: 3–10.

26. Medical Research Council. The rice diet in the treatment of hypertension. Lancet 1950; **2**: 509–13.

27. Truswell AS, Kennedy BM, Hansen JDL, Lee RB. Blood pressure of Kung bushmen in Northern Botswana. Am Heart J 1972; **84**: 5–12.

28. Vaughan JP. A cardiovascular survey in rural Tansania. East Afr Med J 1978; **55**: 380–8.

29. Poulter NR, Khaw KT, Hopwood BEC, Mugambi M, Peart WS, Sever PS. The Kenyan Luo migration study. Observation on the rise in blood pressure. BMJ 1990; **300**: 967–72.

30. Mbanya JC, Thomas TH, Taylor R, Alberti KGMM, Wilkinson R. Increased proximal tubular sodium reabsorption in hypertensive patients with Type 2 diabetes. Diabetic Med 1989; **6**: 614–20.

31. Dodson PM, Beevers M, Hallworth R, Webberley MJ, Fletcher RF, Taylor KG. Sodium restriction and blood pressure in hypertensive Type 2 diabetics; randomised blind controlled and crossover studies of moderate sodium restriction and sodium supplementation. BMJ 1989; **298**: 227–30.

32. Midgley JP, Matthew AG, Greenwood CM, Logan AG. Effect of reduced dietary sodium on blood pressure – a meta-analysis of randomised controlled trials. JAMA 1996; **275**: 1590–6.

33. Law MR, Frost CD, Wald NJ. Analysis of data from trials of salt reduction. BMJ 1991; **302**: 819–23.

34. Bulpitt CJ. Relationship between potassium and blood pressure in general population samples. In: Whelton PK, Whelton A, Walker WG, eds. Potassium in cardiovascular and renal medicine New York, Marcel Dekker, 355–63.

35. Dai WS, Kuller LH, Miller G. Arterial blood pressure and urinary electrolytes. J Chron Dis 1984; **34**: 75–84.

36. Kesteloot H. Epidemiological studies on the relationship between sodium, potassium, calcium and magnesium and arterial blood pressure. J Cardiovasc Pharmacol 1984; Suppl I: 5192–6.

37. Ophir O, Peer G, Gilad J, Blum M, Aviram A. Low blood pressure in vegetarians; the possible role of potassium. Am J Clin Nutr 1983; **37**: 755–62.

38. MacGregor GA, Smith SJ, Markandu N, Banks RA, Sagnella GA. Moderate potassium supplementation in essential hypertension. Lancet 1982; **2**: 567–70.

39. Gilleran G, O'Leary M, Bartlett WA, Vinall H, Jones AF, Dodson PM. Effects of dietary sodium substitution with potassium and magnesium in hypertensive Type II diabetics: a randomised blind controlled parallel study. J Hum Hypertens 1996; **10**: 517–21.

40. Morris JN, Crawford MD, Heady AJ, Hardness of local water supplies and mortality from cardiovascular disease in the county boroughs of England & Wales. Lancet 1961; **1**: 860–2.

41. Crawford MD, Gardner MJ, Morris JN. Mortality and hardness of local water supplies. Lancet 1968; **1**: 827–31.

42. Akley S, Barrett-Connor E, Suarez L. Dairy products, calcium and blood pressure. Am J Clin Nutr 1983; **38**: 457–61.

43. Strazzulo P, Galletti F, Curillo M, et al. Altered extracellular calcium homeostasis in essential hypertension: a consequence of abnormal cell calcium handling. Clin Sci 1986; **7**: 239–44.

44. Grobee D, Hoffman A. Effect of calcium supplementation on diastolic blood pressure in young people with mild hypertension. Lancet 1986; **II**: 705–6.

45. Johnson NE, Smith EL, Freudenheim JL. Effects on blood pressure of calcium supplementation of women. Am J Clin Nutr 1985; **42**: 12–17.

46. Belizan JM, Villar J, Pinede O, et al. Reduction of blood pressure with calcium supplementation in young adults. JAMA 1983; **249**: 1161–5.

47. Puska P, Iacono JM, Nissinen A, et al. Controlled randomised trial of the effect of dietary fat on blood pressure. Lancet 1983; **I**: 1–10.

48. Norris PG, Jones CJH, Weston MJ. Effect of dietary supplementation with fish oil on systolic blood pressure in mild essential hypertension. BMJ 1986; **293**: 104–5.

49. Bonaa KH, Bjerve KS, Stravrue B, Gram IT,

Thelle D. Effect of eicosapentanoic and docosahexanoic acids on blood pressure in hypertension. *N Engl J Med* 1990; **322:** 781–95.

50. Rouse IL, Beilin LJ. Vegetarian diet and blood pressure. *J Hypertens* 1984; **2:** 231–40.

51. Wright A, Burstyn PG, Gibney MJ. Dietary fibre and blood pressure. *BMJ* 1979; **2:** 1541–43.

52. Anderson JW, Gustafson NJ. Dietary fibre in disease prevention and treatment. *Compr Ther* 1987; **13:** 43–53.

53. Appel LJ, Moore TJ, Obarzarck, et al. A clinical trial of the effects of dietary patterns on blood pressure. DASH collaborative research group. *N Engl J Med* 1997; **336:** 1117–24.

54. Uusitupa M, Tuomilehto J, Karttunen P, Wolf E. Long term guar gum on metabolic control, serum cholesterol and blood pressure in Type 2 diabetic patients with high blood pressure. *Ann Clin Res* 1984; **16:** 126–31.

55. Pacy PJ, Dodson PM, Kubicki AJ, Fletcher RF, Taylor KG. Comparison of hypotensive and metabolic effects of Metoprolol with a high fibre, low fat low sodium diet in hypertensive Type 2 diabetic subjects. *Diabetes Res* 1984; **1:** 201–7.

56. Pacy PJ, Dodson PM, Kubicki AJ, Fletcher RF, Taylor KG. Comparison of hypotensive and metabolic effects of Bendrofluazide therapy and a high fibre, low fat, low sodium diet in diabetic subjects with mild hypertension. *J Hypertens* 1984; **2:** 215–20.

57. Dodson OM, Pacy PJ, Bal P, Kubicki AJ, Fletcher RF, Taylor KG. A controlled trial of a high fibre, low fat, low sodium diet for mild hypertension in type 2 diabetic patients. *Diabetologia* 1984; **27:** 522–6.

58. Stamler R, Stamler J, Grimm R, et al. Nutritional therapy for high blood pressure. Final report of a four year randomised controlled trial – The Hypertension Control Programme. *JAMA* 1987; **257:** 1484–91.

59. Little P, Girling G, Hasler A, Trafford A. A controlled trial of a low sodium, low fat, high fibre diet in treated hypertensive patients: effect on antihypertensive drug requirement in clinical practice. *J Hum Hypertens* 1991; **5:** 175–81.

60. Swales JD, Sever PS, Peart S. *Clinical atlas of hypertension.* London, Gower Medical Publishing, 1991: 10–14.

61. Reisin E, Abel R, Modan M, Silverberg M, Eliahou HE, Modan B. Effect of weight without salt restriction on the reduction of blood pressure in overweight hypertensive patients. *N Engl J Med* 1978; **298:** 1–6.

62. Gillum RF. The association of body fat distribution with hypertension, hypertensive heart disease, coronary heart disease, diabetes and cardiovascular risk factors in men and women aged 18–79 years. *J Chron Dis* 1987; **40:** 421–8.

63. Saunders JB, Beevers GG, Paton A. Alcohol induced hypertension. *Lancet* 1981; **2:** 653–6.

64. Potter IF, Beevers DG. Pressor effect of alcohol in hypertension. *Lancet* 1984; **I:** 119–22.

65. Anon. Relaxation therapy for hypertensive patients. *Drug Ther Bull* 1989; **27:** 77–9.

66. Andrews G, Macmahon S, Austin A, Bryne DG. Comparison of drug and non drug treatments. *BMJ* 1982; **284:** 1523–6.

67. Brauer AP, Horlick L, Nelson E, Farquhar JW, Agras WS. Relaxation therapy for essential hypertension: a Veterans Administration Outpatient Study. *J Behav Med* 1979; **2:** 21–9.

68. Pacy PJ, Dodson PM, Fletcher RF. Effect of a high carbohydrate, low sodium and low fat diet in type 2 diabetics with moderate hypertension. *Int J Obes* 1986; **10:** 43–52.

69. Bain SC, Dodson PM. The pharmacological treatment of obesity and diabetes mellitus. (In: Mogenson CE, Stanol E, eds.) *Pharmacology of diabetes: Diabetes Forum Series*, vol 3. Berlin, De Gruyter, 1991: 163–80.

70. O'Donnell MJ, Dodson PM. The non-drug treatment of hypertension in the diabetic patients. *J Hum Hypertens* 1991; **5:** 287–94.

71. Tatti P, Pahor M, Byington RP, et al. Outcome results of the fosinopril versus amlodipine cardiovascular events randomised trial (FACET) in patients with hypertension and NIDDM. *Diabetes Care* 1998; **21:** 597–603.

17

The pharmacological treatment of hypertension in diabetes
Bryan Williams

Introduction

Despite the compelling rationale for lowering blood pressure in people with diabetes, until recently, the prominence given to antihypertensive therapy within the treatment hierarchy of people with diabetes has been disappointing. There have been many reasons for this, the two most notable being (1) until recently, an absence of prospective randomized clinical trial data confirming the efficacy of antihypertensive therapy in diabetic subjects, and (2) a plague of misconceptions regarding the most appropriate way to treat hypertension in diabetic subjects.

The uncertainties and misconceptions that have surrounded the treatment of hypertension in diabetes have been many. One such concern was that treatment with conventional antihypertensive therapies, i.e. β-blockers and/or thiazide diuretics, might adversely affect the metabolic profile of diabetic subjects and thus negate the presumed benefits of glycaemic control. Furthermore, with β-blockers, there was also concern that they might dangerously mask the symptoms of hypoglycaemia in insulin-treated diabetics. There was anxiety about the use of ACE-inhibitors in type 2 diabetic subjects because of a perceived abundance of occult renovascular disease. More recently, the furore surrounding the ill-founded controversy that calcium channel blockers should not be given to diabetic subjects has led to further apprehension and confusion. Indeed, on reading the literature, it was difficult for practitioners to feel comfortable when prescribing any antihypertensive agent for their patients with diabetes. These concerns were compounded by a lack of clear consensus regarding the appropriate blood pressure threshold at which to initiate antihypertensive therapy and the appropriate target blood pressure to aim for on treatment. This latter point was important because of a widely held view that the over-aggressive lowering of blood pressure might exacerbate 'silent' myocardial ischaemia in diabetic subjects.[1] Added to this were problems of postural hypotension due to autonomic neuropathy and therapy-induced impotence. Thus, in the absence of proven efficacy from clinical trials, misconception and confusion reigned and the treatment of hypertension was not high on the therapeutic agenda in diabetic subjects. The recent emergence of such evidence has been long overdue, eagerly awaited and has been a powerful and crucial impetus for change.

In this chapter, I will first review the key clinical trials that have informed (and on occasion mis-informed!) the decision-making process with regard to the treatment of hypertension in diabetes. This information will then be used to define strategies for the treatment of hypertension in diabetes. Previous chapters have specifically dealt with the treatment of hypertension in patients with diabetic nephropathy, thus in this chapter, the discussion will primarily focus on the treatment of hypertension in people with type 1 or type 2 diabetes without any clinical evidence of nephropathy.

Clinical trials of the treatment of hypertension in people with diabetes

There have actually been very few clinical trials focusing specifically on the treatment of hypertension in diabetes. The vast majority of the studies discussed below represent cohorts of patients with diabetes who have been randomized as part of much larger studies, primarily focused on patients without diabetes. As most blood pressure-lowering trials tend to be conducted on older patient populations, most of the data concerning the treatment of hypertension in people with diabetes have been derived from the study of older patients with type 2 diabetes. In the early studies, the examination of the diabetes cohort tended to be post-hoc. In later studies, such analyses were often pre-specified with targeted recruitment.

The early studies

The hypertension detection and follow-up programme (HDFP) compared stepped care (diuretic-based) with usual community care in 10,940 patients aged 30–69 years, initially over 5 years of follow-up; about 10% of the patients were diabetic, primarily type 2.[2] The systolic hypertension in the elderly programme (SHEP)[3] was a randomized, placebo-controlled, double-blind study that compared chlorthalidone (diuretic)-based care with placebo over an average of 4.5 years in 4736 patients aged >60 years with isolated systolic hypertension, of whom 583 were type 2 diabetics. Post-hoc examination of the diabetic cohorts within these two studies suggested that the benefits of antihypertensive therapy, in terms of reductions in cardiovascular morbidity and mortality, were at least as great in diabetic as in non-diabetic subjects. Indeed, in SHEP, the absolute risk reduction was twice as great in diabetics (101/1000 patient-years) when compared with non-diabetics (51/1000), reflecting the higher risk of the diabetic cohort. These early trials suggested that lowering blood pressure would be beneficial in people with diabetes and they used thiazide-based therapy, which should have dispelled the myth that these agents would be of less benefit or even harmful to people with diabetes. These important early indicators received little prominence and failed to prompt any obvious enthusiasm for antihypertensive therapy in people with diabetes.

More recent studies

The late 1990s heralded a surge in clinical trial evidence in diabetic hypertension. These studies can be considered under two headings: (1) studies confirming that lowering blood pressure was beneficial in people with diabetes; (2) studies examining whether specific classes of antihypertensive therapy were more or less effective than another.

The effectiveness of blood pressure-lowering in diabetes: recent trials

A series of key clinical trials have transformed the treatment of hypertension in people with diabetes. Accepting that lowering blood pressure was likely to be at least as effective in people with diabetes as in the hypertensive non-diabetic population, the first group of trials to be considered examined whether more intensive blood pressure control would be more effective at reducing macrovascular and microvascular complications than less intensive blood pressure control.

The United Kingdom Prospective Diabetes Study (UKPDS)

This large prospective randomized clinical trial reported initially in 1998. The primary objective of the UKPDS was to assess the impact of intensified versus conventional glycaemic control on diabetes-related and other end-points in British subjects with type 2 diabetes.[4] Of the 4297 patients randomized into the main UKPDS, 1544 were receiving antihypertensive therapy or were untreated hypertensives (blood pressure ≥160/95 mmHg), with a mean age of 56 years. Of these, 1148 were recruited into the 'hypertension in diabetes study', embedded within the UKPDS.[5] The 1148 hypertensive patients with type 2 diabetes were randomized to 'less tight' (<180/105 mmHg) ($n = 390$) or 'tight' (<150/85 mmHg) ($n = 758$) blood pressure control. The tight control group was further subdivided into those randomly assigned to an ACE-inhibitor-based regimen (captopril) ($n = 400$) or a β-blocker-based regimen (atenolol) ($n = 358$).[6] The use of ACE-inhibitors or β-blockers was avoided in the group allocated to less tight control of blood pressure. Additional drug therapy included the use of a dihydropyridine calcium antagonist (nifedipine SR), an α-blocker (prazosin) or the centrally acting agent α-methyl dopa. Thiazides were not allowed because of fear that they would compromise glycaemic control and frusemide was used as an alternative. The achieved difference in blood pressure control between the less tight and tight control groups was 10/5 mmHg over a median follow-up of 8.4 years.

In UKPDS the impact of improved blood pressure control on all diabetes-related end-points, macrovascular and microvascular disease was remarkable. The reduction in diabetes-related end-points was 24%. This was twice as effective as that achieved by efforts to improve glycaemic control. Compared with the less tight BP control group, the tight BP control group also showed risk reduction of 32% in death related to diabetes and a 44% reduction in strokes[5] (Table 17.1). These latter two end-points are worthy of comment because tight glycaemic control had no significant impact on the rate of diabetes-related death and no benefit in terms of stroke reduction.[4] Tighter blood pressure control also reduced the risk of heart failure by 56%, a major benefit, mindful of the premature and frequent development of heart failure in diabetic subjects.

The powerful effect of tighter blood pressure control in reducing microvascular disease is worthy of emphasis (Table 17.2), because this was the first large prospective study to assess this important end-point.[5] Microvascular end-points were reduced by 37%, largely due to a reduction in the risk of retinal photocoagulation and progressive retinopathy.

Development of macrovascular disease		
↓ Stroke (CVA)	44%	$p < 0.01$
↓ Fatal stroke	58%	$p < 0.04$
↓ Myocardial infarction	21%	NS
↓ Amputations	49%	NS
↓ Heart failure	56%	$p < 0.004$

NS, not significant; CVA, cerebral vascular accident.

Table 17.1

The impact of more intensive blood pressure control (10/5 mmHg) on macrovascular end-points in patients with type 2 diabetes and hypertension in UKPDS (from reference 5)

Diabetic end-points/macrovascular disease	Reduction	p value
Diabetic-related end-points	24%	<0.005
Diabetic-related death	32%	<0.02
Microvascular disease	37%	<0.01
Retinopathy progression	34%	<0.0004

Table 17.2
The impact of more intensive blood pressure control (10/5 mmHg) on diabetes-related and microvascular end-points in patients with type 2 diabetes and hypertension in UKPDS (from reference 5)

End-point	Intensive glycaemic control (n = 2729)	Intensive blood pressure control (n = 1148)
Any DM end-point	200	61
DM death	–	152
All-cause deaths	–	208
Myocardial infarct	370	204
Stroke	–	196
Microvascular	357	138

(−) = no impact, (-ve) = increase in risk. (Calculated from data in references 4 and 5.)

Table 17.3
The 'numbers needed to treat' to prevent a specified end-point in UKPDS, comparing intensified glycaemic control with intensified blood pressure control

There was an associated 47% reduced risk of deterioration of visual acuity. The impact of tighter blood pressure control on microvascular end-points was more than twice as great as that achieved by tight glycaemic control in the same study (Table 17.3).

UKPDS was a key study in that it confirmed that more intensive blood pressure control (achieved mean blood pressure 144/82 mmHg) was significantly more effective than less intensive blood pressure control (achieved mean blood pressure 154/87 mmHg). Importantly, more than 60% of patients required two or more antihypertensive drugs to achieve tighter blood pressure control. Moreover, at least 30% of patients in the UKPDS blood pressure study received dihydropyridine calcium channel blockers (nifedipine SR, b.i.d).

The Hypertension Optimal Treatment (HOT) study

The primary aim of the HOT study was to define the optimum target blood pressure in treated hypertensive patients.[7] In all, 18,790 patients from 26 European countries were randomly assigned to one of three diastolic blood pressure targets (<90, <85 and <80 mmHg). Blood pressure was titrated to these targets using the dihydropyridine calcium antagonist felodipine as primary therapy, complemented where necessary by other antihypertensive agents (metoprolol, ramipril and/or thiazide diuretic). The patients were followed for a mean of 3.8 years before assessing the impact of different levels of blood pressure control on cardiovascular disease morbidity and mortality. The separation of blood pressure between the three groups was less than anticipated (a spread of only ~4 mmHg) and thus the study was underpowered to address its primary objective. Nevertheless important data emerged.

The results of the HOT study suggested that the treated diastolic blood pressure associated with fewest cardiovascular events across the entire study population was 82.6 mmHg. The 'optimal' treated systolic blood pressure was 139 mmHg, although overall treated hypertensive patients gained little additional advantage from further blood pressure reduction once the treated blood pressure was maintained below 150/90 mmHg.

Within the HOT study there was a large cohort (8%; 1501) of people with diabetes, almost all type 2 diabetes. The outcome in this hypertensive diabetic cohort differed from that of the non-diabetic hypertensive population in one crucially important respect. In the diabetic cohort, there was a significant trend towards greater benefit, the lower the target (and achieved) blood pressure (Fig. 17.1). So much so, that the risk of major cardiovascular events was halved (from 24.4/1000 patient-years to 11.9/1000 patient-years) in the group with a target diastolic blood pressure <80 mmHg (achieved diastolic BP 81.1 mmHg), when compared with the hypertensive diabetic group targeted to <90 mmHg (achieved diastolic BP 85.2 mmHg) (Fig. 17.1). This observa-

tion is complementary to that of UKPDS in that it confirmed that there was definite benefit in targeting lower treated blood pressures in people with diabetes. The HOT study also demonstrated that once again, combinations of drug therapy are required to achieve recommended blood pressure targets in people with diabetes, and even then, achieving these targets is particularly difficult.

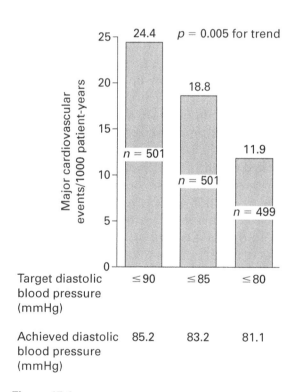

Figure 17.1

The reduction in cardiovascular events in patients with diabetes in the HOT study according to the target blood pressure. The actual number of events is indicated at the top of the columns. The target and achieved diastolic blood pressures are shown below each column. (Drawn from data from reference 7.)

The Systolic Hypertension – Europe Study (Syst-Eur)

At the same time as HOT and UKPDS reported, another study, Syst-Eur, reported key data about the safety and efficacy of treating isolated systolic hypertension in elderly people with type 2 diabetes. This prospective, randomized, placebo-controlled clinical trial was designed to test the efficacy of a dihydropyridine calcium antagonist-based treatment (nitrendipine) versus placebo in elderly patients (mean age 70 years) with isolated systolic hypertension (systolic blood pressure >160 mmHg, diastolic blood pressure <95 mmHg). In all, 4203 patients were randomized to active treatment (nitrendipine ± enalapril ± thiazide) or placebo for a median follow-up of 2 years. The placebo-corrected fall in blood pressure was 10/5 mmHg in the active treatment group. This resulted in a risk reduction of 38% for stroke and 21% for cardiac end-points in the treated patients.[8] This level of risk reduction is consistent with those observed in previous studies of antihypertensive therapy in elderly subjects with isolated systolic hypertension.

Within the Syst-Eur study, there were 492 hypertensive subjects (8.6%) with diabetes, mainly type 2. In this diabetic cohort, the treatment of hypertension was associated with an astounding benefit in terms of cardiovascular risk reduction and reduced mortality, much greater than that observed in the non-diabetic patients.[9] In treated hypertensive diabetic subjects a blood pressure reduction of 10.3/4.5 mmHg was associated with a 55% reduction in total mortality (45.1/1000 patient-years versus 26.4), this compares with a 6% reduction in non-diabetics. There was a 76% reduction in cardiovascular mortality and a reduction in all cardiovascular events combined of 69%. Fatal and non-fatal stroke were reduced by a massive 73% and all cardiac events combined by 63%. When diabetic patients receiving active treatment were compared with the actively treated non-diabetic cohort, there were substantially greater reductions in overall mortality ($p < 0.04$), mortality from cardiovascular disease (CVD) ($p < 0.02$) and all CVD ($p < 0.01$) in diabetic patients. After correction for the impact of other risk factors, the study report concluded that the excess CVD and mortality risk associated with diabetes in this elderly population was completely abolished by the treatment of hypertension. This study unequivocally confirmed that lowering blood pressure in elderly patients with isolated systolic hypertension and diabetes was dramatically effective in reducing cardiovascular events, stroke and mortality. It is also noteworthy that most patients received combinations of therapy, initially with the calcium channel blocker (CCB) nitrendipine, usually combined with a thiazide and/or ACE inhibitor, thereby providing compelling evidence that combination therapy is very effective at reducing cardiovascular events in diabetes.

Appropriate Blood Pressure Control in Diabetes (ABCD)

The ABCD study was conducted in the USA and was a prospective randomized clinical trial designed to test the primary hypothesis that intensive versus moderate blood pressure control would prevent or slow the progression of nephropathy, neuropathy and retinopathy (i.e. microvascular complications) in people with type 2 diabetes, aged 40–74 years. The secondary hypothesis was that a long-acting CCB (nisoldipine Coat Core)-based therapy and an ACE-inhibitor-based therapy (enalapril) would have equivalent effects on the prevention or progression of these diabetic complications. A total of 950 type 2 diabetic

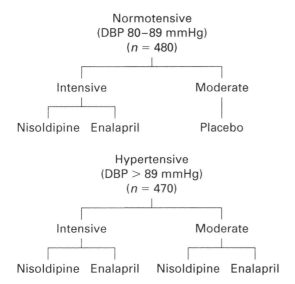

Figure 17.2
Design of the ABCD study. DBP, diastolic blood pressure. (Drawn from reference 10.)

patients was randomized as two distinct cohorts: normotensive ($n = 480$) and hypertensive ($n = 470$).[10] The trial design is shown in Fig. 17.2.

ABCD hypertensive cohort – impact of intensive versus moderate blood pressure control

The hypertensive cohort was randomized to achieve a diastolic blood pressure target of <75 mmHg (intensive group) or 80–90 mmHg (moderate group). The mean blood pressure achieved in the intensive group was 132/78 mmHg and in the moderate group was 138/86 mmHg over a 5-year follow-up. There was no difference between the intensive and moderate groups with regard to changes in creatinine clearance or urinary albumin excretion, irrespective of whether the patients had normoalbuminuria or microalbuminuria at baseline.[11] Moreover, over the 5-year follow-up, there was no difference between the inten-

sive and moderate blood pressure control groups with regard to the progression of retinopathy or neuropathy. However, intensified blood pressure control was associated with a significant reduction in all-cause mortality (intensive 5.5% versus moderate 10.7%, $p < 0.037$). Of interest, however, subgroup analysis did not reveal a statistically significant difference in the myocardial infarction, stroke or congestive cardiac failure to account for this difference in all-cause mortality. Importantly, there was no evidence of a 'J' curve phenomenon with more intensive blood pressure control, confirming the results of the HOT study that intensified blood pressure control is safe in people with type 2 diabetes.[7] Moreover, these results were similar irrespective of whether an ACE-inhibitor or CCB was used as the initial medication.[11]

ABCD normotensive cohort – impact of intensive versus moderate blood pressure control

This cohort within ABCD addressed the very important question as to whether lowering blood pressure in 'normotensive' diabetics (blood pressure <140/90 mmHg) offers any additional benefit with regard to microvascular complications and the incidence of cardiovascular disease. The 480 normotensive type 2 diabetic patients were randomized to 'intensive' (10 mmHg below baseline diastolic blood pressure) versus 'moderate' blood pressure (diastolic blood pressure 80–90 mmHg).[12] Patients randomized to moderate therapy were given placebo therapy, whereas those randomized to intensive therapy were randomized to either enalapril or nisoldipine. If a patient in the 'moderate' group developed a blood pressure ≥160/90 mmHg, they were given either enalapril or nisoldipine according to randomization at entry to maintain the systolic BP <160 mmHg and the diastolic BP between

80 and 90 mmHg. The mean follow-up was 5.3 years and the mean blood pressure in the intensive group was 128/75 mmHg and in the moderate group was 137/81 mmHg. There was no difference in the rate of decline of creatinine clearance but a lower percentage of patients in the intensively treated group progressed from normoalbuminuria to microalbuminuria ($p < 0.012$) and from microalbuminuria to overt proteinuria ($p < 0.028$). The more intensively treated group also had less progression of diabetic retinopathy (34% versus 46%, $p < 0.019$) but there was no difference in the rates of progression of neuropathy. However, there was a 3.3-fold reduction in the incidence of stroke in the intensively treated group (intensive 1.7% versus moderate 5.4%, $p < 0.03$). There were no differences in the rates of non-stroke cardiovascular events between the intensive and moderately treated groups (Table 17.4). Of

interest, these conclusions apply whether the patients were treated with nisoldipine or enalapril, suggesting that once blood pressure is low enough, potential differences between different classes of drug therapy may disappear as a major factor determining outcome.[12]

The Heart Outcomes Prevention Evaluation (HOPE) study

The HOPE study was not designed as a study of antihypertensive therapy in that patients were included in the study if they were 'normotensive' (BP < 140/90 mmHg) at randomization, although almost half of the patients were treated hypertensives. Nevertheless, it is worthy of discussion in this section because the data from HOPE have had a major impact on the use of ACE-inhibition for the treatment of patients at high risk of cardiovascular disease and the study included a large number of patients with type 2 diabetes.

CV outcome	Intensive therapy n = 237 (%)	Moderate therapy n = 243 (%)	OR (95% CI)	p value
Myocardial infarction	19 (8.0)	15 (6.2)	0.75 (0.37, 1.52)	0.43
CVA	4 (1.7)	13 (5.4)	3.29 (1.06, 10.25)	0.03
CHF	12 (5.1)	11 (4.5)	0.89 (0.38, 2.06)	0.78
CV death	13 (5.4)	9 (3.7)	0.66 (0.28, 1.58)	0.35
Death	18 (7.6)	20 (8.2)	1.1 (0.56, 2.12)	0.80
	Nisoldipine n = 234 (%)	Enalapril n = 246 (%)		
Myocardial infarction	18 (7.7)	16 (6.5)	1.20 (0.60, 2.41)	0.61
CVA	11 (4.7)	6 (2.4)	1.97 (0.72, 5.42)	0.18
CHF	11 (4.7)	12 (4.9)	0.96 (0.42, 2.22)	0.93
CV death	8 (3.4)	14 (5.7)	0.59 (0.24, 1.43)	0.23
Death	19 (8.1)	19 (7.7)	1.1 (0.54, 2.05)	0.87

CVA, cerebral vascular accident; CHF, congestive heart failure; CV, cardiovascular.

Table 17.4
Cardiovascular outcomes according to drug therapy and intensive versus moderate blood pressure goals in the ABCD normotensive study (from reference 12)

HOPE was conducted in 19 countries in North and South America and in Europe.[13] A total of 9297 patients, aged 55 years or older, were randomly assigned to treatment with either ramipril (10 mg/day) or matching placebo for 5 years. Patients were randomized into the study if they were at high risk for cardiovascular disease by virtue of a prior history of coronary heart disease, stroke, peripheral vascular disease or diabetes, plus at least one other cardiovascular risk factor (hypertension, elevated total cholesterol level, low HDL-cholesterol level, cigarette smoking or microalbuminuria). Patients with known heart failure or poor systolic function were excluded. Some of the patients also received the antioxidant vitamin E in a 2×2 factorial design. The impact of vitamin E was disappointing and will not be considered further in this discussion. The mean age of the study population was 66 years and a majority were men (~75%). A majority also had a prior history of coronary heart disease (~80%), >40% had evidence of peripheral vascular disease and 11% had a history of stroke or transient cerebral ischaemia.

The primary outcome of the study was a composite of myocardial infarction, stroke or death from cardiovascular causes. Secondary outcomes included death from any cause, the need for revascularization, hospitalization for unstable angina or heart failure and complications related to diabetes.

A total of 651 patients assigned to ramipril reached the primary end-point (14%) compared with 826 (17.8%) assigned to placebo ($p < 0.001$) which represents a significant risk reduction of 22% in favour of ramipril[13] (Fig. 17.3).

Compared with placebo, treatment with ramipril also reduced the rate of death from cardiovascular causes by 26% ($p < 0.001$), reduced myocardial infarction by 20%

($p < 0.001$), stroke by 32% ($p < 0.001$) and death from any cause by 16% ($p < 0.005$). Subgroup analyses suggested that the beneficial effects of ramipril on the primary outcome were consistent in those with or without diabetes, hypertension or microalbuminuria and in younger (<65 years) versus older (>65 years) patients.[13]

Diabetes in HOPE: the MICRO-HOPE study

A detailed analysis was also performed and reported on the large cohort of diabetic patients recruited into the HOPE study.[14] In all, 3654 people with diabetes were randomized into the study (39.3% of the HOPE study population). Of these, 98% were defined as type 2 diabetes. These patients had at least one other cardiovascular risk factor in addition to their diabetes. In addition to the main exclusion criteria specified above, diabetic patients with overt nephropathy (dipstick-positive proteinuria), any other severe renal disease,

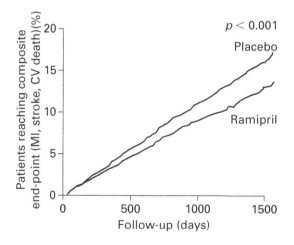

Figure 17.3
The results of the primary end-point of the HOPE trial showing a substantial reduction in risk with ramipril versus placebo in 9297 'normotensive' patients at high risk of cardiovascular disease. (Adapted from reference 13)

hyperkalaemia or uncontrolled hypertension were excluded. There were more women (~1/3) than in the main study and 56% of the diabetic patients were defined as 'hypertensive' at baseline. As part of the diabetic cohort study microalbuminuria was measured as a urinary albumin:creatinine ratio (ACR) at baseline in 98% of the patients and in 86% at the end of the study. Data were also collected on the need for laser therapy for retinopathy. This preplanned substudy was referred to as the MICRO-HOPE study and set out to define whether ramipril delayed the onset of micro-albuminuria, overt nephropathy and microvascular complications in the diabetic cohort.

In the diabetic cohort, ramipril lowered the risk of the composite primary end-point by 25% ($p < 0.0004$) versus placebo. This finding is consistent with the benefits observed in the study overall. Also of interest, the event rates in the diabetic patients receiving placebo were very similar to those observed in the non-diabetic patients receiving placebo (19.8% versus 17.8%). All other risk reductions in diabetic patients for the pre-specified secondary end-points were similar to those observed in the main study (Table 17.5).

Interpreting the data from HOPE
The data from HOPE and the diabetes sub-

study confirm that in high risk patients, ACE-inhibition is better than placebo even in patients with relatively low baseline blood pressure, i.e. mean ~142/80 mmHg (compared with most other trials discussed herein). There has been much debate as to whether the undoubted benefits of ACE-inhibition observed in the HOPE study relate to 'blood pressure-independent' benefits of ACE-inhibition in high risk patients, or whether they may simply be attributable to blood pressure differences between the ACE-inhibitor- and placebo-treated groups.[15] The reported difference in office blood pressure measurements between the two groups was −2.5/1 mmHg in favour of ACE-inhibition in the diabetes cohort. However, it is likely that differences in 24 hour blood pressure load were much greater, mindful of the fact that 24 hour blood pressures are markedly increased in diabetes, despite seemingly normal office blood pressure readings, due to substantial increases in nocturnal blood pressure. In support of this, a small study of the differences in ambulatory blood pressures between ramipril- and placebo-treated patients in the main HOPE study revealed very substantial differences in mean 24 hour blood pressure between the two groups (−17/8 mmHg ramipril versus placebo, $p < 0.001$).[16] Such differences, if relevant to

Parameter	Placebo (n = 1769)	Ramipril (n = 1808)	RR (95% CI)	p value
Primary end-point	19.8	15.3	0.75 (0.64–0.88)	0.0004
Cardiovascular death	9.7	6.2	0.63 (0.49–0.79)	0.0001
Myocardial infarction	12.9	10.2	0.78 (0.64–0.94)	0.01
Stroke	6.7	4.2	0.67 (0.50–0.90)	0.0074
Mortality	14.0	10.8	0.76 (0.63–0.92)	0.004

Table 17.5
Outcomes in the diabetes cohort in the HOPE study (adapted from reference 14)

the whole study and the diabetes cohort, could easily account for the beneficial effect of ramipril observed in the HOPE study. This conclusion is particularly appropriate as a consequence of the aforementioned data from the ABCD study of the treatment of 'normotensive patients' with type 2 diabetes, in whom there are clear benefits with blood pressure reduction in the normotensive range.[12]

Are there drug-specific benefits when treating hypertension in diabetes? Evidence of clinical trials

There has been enormous controversy as to whether a specific drug class (or drug within a class) may be superior to another and may offer specific benefits, over and above the effects of blood pressure control in people with diabetes. This concept was initially generated by the seemingly beneficial effects of ACE-inhibition in patients with diabetic nephropathy and further supported by the Micro-HOPE study.[14] Simultaneously, there was concern expressed by some that CCBs, especially dihydropyridines, might even be harmful to people with diabetes.[17,18] Therefore it is important to consider the studies that have addressed the question of drug superiority/inferiority and have thereby fuelled this debate. The key features of these studies are reviewed briefly below, followed by a discussion of the messages conveyed by the totality of the evidence.

The ABCD study: ACE-inhibition versus calcium channel blockade

As discussed above, the ABCD study examined the effectiveness of CCB-based (nisoldipine) versus ACE-inhibitor-based (enalapril) antihypertensive therapy on the prevention

and progression of complications in people with type 2 diabetes.[10] The data from the normotensive cohort (see above) unequivocally revealed that there was no difference in the primary outcome of the study or multiple secondary outcomes when CCB-based therapy was compared to ACE-inhibitor-based therapy.[12] The authors concluded that 'the specific initial agent used appears to be less important than the achievement of lower blood pressure values in normotensive type 2 diabetic patients'.[12] This conclusion, however, contrasts with the findings in the 'hypertensive' cohort of ABCD.[18]

In the hypertensive cohort ($n = 470$), after 67 months, the data safety monitoring committee observed a significant difference in the cardiovascular event rates between the CCB- and ACE-inhibitor-treated patients and recommended changing hypertensive, nisoldipine-treated patients to open-label enalapril, while continuing blinded therapy in the normotensive groups in ABCD. This decision was based on the fact that the enalapril-treated patients had fewer cardiovascular events than those receiving nisoldipine (Fig. 17.4). This relationship was maintained in the intensively treated group (nisoldipine; 12 fatal/non-fatal myocardial infarctions, versus 3 for enalapril, χ^2, $p < 0.03$) and moderately treated group (nisoldipine, 13 fatal/non-fatal myocardial infarctions versus 1 for enalapril, χ^2, $p < 0.002$). This decision led to a frenzy of controversy fuelled by ill-judged, ill-informed comments by the usual suspects that CCBs were unsafe for people with diabetes. In the absence of a control group (which would have been unethical) what this study certainly could not define is whether CCB treatment was less effective or harmful when compared to no treatment at all. This seemed unlikely because the myocardial infarction (MI) rates in patients assigned to nisoldipine in ABCD were no higher than

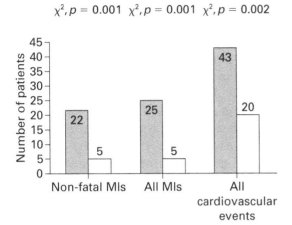

$\chi^2, p = 0.001$ $\chi^2, p = 0.001$ $\chi^2, p = 0.002$

Figure 17.4
Percentage of patients receiving nisoldipine (solid bars) or enalapril (open bars) experiencing a cardiovascular event (cardiovascular death, non-fatal myocardial infarction (MI), non-fatal stroke and congestive heart failure requiring hospitalization) in the hypertensive cohort within the ABCD study. (From reference 18.)

those observed in historical controls with type 2 diabetes at similar or even higher risk of MI. It may thus be more appropriate to conclude that these interim findings of the ABCD study were more likely to reflect a potential 'protective effect' of ACE-inhibition than any detrimental effect of CCBs. Even that conclusion is over-interpretation, mindful of the fact that we are discussing a small number of 'events' in a relatively small study, in which the end-point being examined was not the primary end-point the study was powered to test. Moreover, the findings have not been supported by the results in the normotensive cohort comparing ACE-inhibition with CCB therapy within ABCD, in whom similar rates of MI were observed.[12]

The Fosinopril versus Amlodipine Cardiovascular Events Trial (FACET)

The FACET study compared the effects of fosinopril (ACE-inhibitor) and amlodipine (CCB) on blood pressure control and metabolic parameters, i.e. serum lipids and glycaemic control in 380 patients with type 2 diabetes and hypertension, over 3.5 years.[19] Prospectively defined cardiovascular events were assessed as secondary outcomes. At the end of the study, the two groups were not different with regard to serum lipids and glycaemic control, although amlodipine was more effective at lowering systolic blood pressure. The study report focused on the fact that those receiving fosinopril had significantly lower risk of a combined outcome of acute MI, stroke and hospitalization for angina (fosinopril, 14 out of 189 versus amlodipine, 27 out of 191). However, there was no difference when the individual cardiovascular events were analysed and there was no difference in all-cause mortality. It was only when cardiovascular events were arbitrarily grouped that a result of significance emerged.

Sadly, the FACET study attracted a lot of interest when it was published. It is not clear why. This was an open-label, single-centre study, which is not ideal. The study was small and not powered to test the effects of these two agents on cardiovascular event rates and had the data been appropriately adjusted for multiple comparisons it is most unlikely they would have found a difference. Moreover, review of the original abstract and subsequent study reports suggests that there was considerable cross-over of patients from monotherapy with either drug to a combination of both, suggesting that within 6 months of recruitment ending 35–40% of patients were no longer in their original groups. This meant

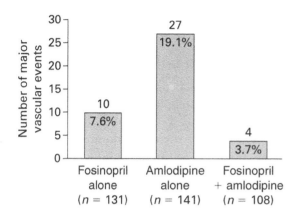

Figure 17.5
Major cardiovascular events according to treatment in the FACET study. (From reference 19.)

that from an early stage in the study almost as many patients were receiving a combination of amlodipine and fosinopril as received either alone (Fig. 17.5). It is of interest then, that the much better outcome of the combination therapy group received little prominence in the discussion of the original article or the accompanying commentary. This finding would not be expected had CCBs been 'harmful' to patients with hypertension and type 2 diabetes. On the contrary, mindful of the fact that most patients with type 2 diabetes require combinations of therapy to achieve blood pressure goal, the FACET data support the use of a CCB as part of an effective combination with ACE-inhibition.

The Swedish Trial in Old Patients with Hypertension-2 Study (STOP-2)

This was a prospective randomized clinical trial of 5 years' duration in 6614 people aged 70–84 years with hypertension who were randomly assigned to conventional therapy (β-blocker or thiazide) or newer therapy

(ACE-inhibitor or CCB).[20] Blood pressure control was equivalent in all groups and the primary outcome of the study (fatal stroke, fatal MI or other fatal cardiovascular disease) was similar for newer therapies when compared to older conventional treatment. The frequency of MI and of congestive cardiac failure was significantly lower in patients treated with ACE-inhibitors when compared with CCB-based therapy in this trial. This lends support to the data from the ABCD study[18] (see above). However, this should be interpreted with caution as 48 statistical comparisons were done, increasing the chance of a significant difference amongst some cohorts. Moreover, there was no evidence that CCBs were less effective in any other way in the prevention of cardiovascular events than conventional drugs or ACE-inhibition.[20]

Importantly, within the study there were 719 patients with diabetes (type 2) at baseline (mean age 76 years) and the treatment effects in these patients with regard to the composite primary end-point did not differ between the three treatment groups.[21] However, there were significantly fewer MIs in those randomized to ACE-inhibitor therapy when compared with those randomized to CCB-based therapy (17 versus 32 events, $RR = 0.51$, CI: 0.28–0.92, $p < 0.025$). This observation followed the trend in the main study and should be interpreted with the same caveats. The main conclusion from the subgroup with diabetes is identical to that for the study as a whole, i.e. there was no obvious advantage of any particular drug class over another.[21]

The Captopril Prevention Project (CAPPP)

This was a prospective, randomized, open, blinded end-point study that evaluated the effects of ACE-inhibitor-based antihypertensive therapy versus conventional therapy (β-blocker/thiazide) on cardiovascular morbidity and mortality in hypertension in patients aged 25–66 years for an average follow-up of 6.1 years.[22] A total of 10,985 hypertensive patients was randomized into the main study, of which 572 (4.9%) had type 2 diabetes at baseline. In this diabetic cohort, the primary end-point of fatal or non-fatal MI or stroke, or other cardiovascular death, was markedly lower in captopril-treated patients when compared with conventionally treated patients (RR = 0.59, $p < 0.018$).[23] Specifically, cardiovascular mortality tended to be lower (RR = 0.48, $p < 0.84$) with no difference between the groups in the rate of stroke. MI was notably less frequent in the captopril group (RR = 0.34, $p < 0.002$) as was total mortality (RR = 0.54, $p = 0.034$). Of interest, these differences were observed despite the fact that on-treatment blood pressures were slightly higher in the captopril (155.5/ 89 mmHg) versus conventional therapy group (153.5/88 mmHg), perhaps because captopril (a relatively short-acting ACE-inhibitor) was given only once or twice per day. The differences were also particularly noticeable in (1) males, (2) those with poorer BP control, and

(3) those with more markedly impaired glycaemic control.[23]

UKPDS – atenolol versus captopril

The UKPDS blood pressure study contained a comparison of atenolol therapy ($n = 358$) with captopril therapy ($n = 400$) in the group of type 2 diabetic patients randomized to tighter blood pressure control.[6] Blood pressure control was similar in both groups. The ACE-inhibitor was significantly better tolerated than the β-blocker and there was more weight gain associated with β-blocker therapy. There was no difference in the primary outcome of any diabetes-related end-point ($p < 0.43$), diabetes-related death ($p < 0.28$) or microvascular disease ($p < 0.30$). As shown in Fig. 17.6, the confidence intervals all overlap 1, because the study was underpowered to test for differences between the two drugs. Nevertheless, it is of interest that the trend for all outcomes is in favour of the β-blocker rather than the ACE inhibitor.[6]

International Nifedipine GITS study (INSIGHT)

This was a prospective, randomized, double-

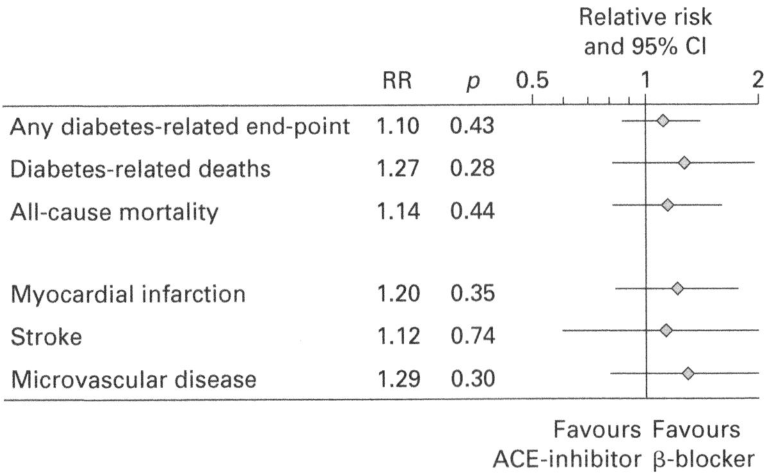

	RR	p	Relative risk and 95% CI
Any diabetes-related end-point	1.10	0.43	
Diabetes-related deaths	1.27	0.28	
All-cause mortality	1.14	0.44	
Myocardial infarction	1.20	0.35	
Stroke	1.12	0.74	
Microvascular disease	1.29	0.30	

Favours ACE-inhibitor   Favours β-blocker

Figure 17.6
The aggregate clinical end-points from the UKPDS 'tighter blood pressure control' arm comparing atenolol with captopril (from reference 6)

blind trial in Europe and Israel in 6321 patients aged 50–80 years with hypertension and at least one additional cardiovascular risk factor.[24] The patients were assigned to either a long-acting formulation of nifedipine or a hydrochlorothiazide/amiloride combination. The primary outcome was the usual composite of cardiovascular death, MI, heart failure or stroke. There was no difference in primary outcome between the two treatment groups (6.3% versus 5.8%, $p < 0.35$). About 20% of patients in the study had diabetes at baseline. The event rates were predictably higher in the patients with diabetes and blood pressures were more difficult to control when compared with the non-diabetic patients. As in the main study, there was no difference in primary event rate between the CCB- (8.3%) and diuretic- (8.4%) treated patients with diabetes. Of interest, new-onset diabetes occurred more commonly in patients receiving the diuretic when compared with the CCB (5.6% versus 4.3%, $p < 0.02$).

Nordic Diltiazem (NORDIL) study

The NORDIL study was a prospective, randomized, open, blinded end-point study that enrolled 10,881 hypertensive patients aged 50–74 in Norway and Sweden.[25] The patients were randomly assigned to either a non-dihydropyridine CCB (diltiazem) or conventional therapy (diuretics and/or β-blockers) for a mean follow-up of 4.5 years. The primary end-point was a composite of fatal/non-fatal stroke, MI and other cardiovascular death. There were 16.6/1000 patient-years in the diltiazem group and 16.2/1000 in the conventional group, indicating no difference in the primary outcome ($p < 0.97$). There were significantly fewer strokes in the diltiazem group (RR = 0.80, CI = 0.65–0.099, $p < 0.04$) and a trend to fewer MIs in the conventional group, ($p < 0.17$). In all, 727 patients had type 2 diabetes at baseline and there was no difference in outcome between the two treatment groups (Table 17.6).

Losartan Intervention For End-Point Reduction in hypertension study (LIFE) – the diabetic cohort

The LIFE study was a prospective, randomized, double-blind, parallel group, end-point-driven trial in 9193 patients with hypertension and ECG evidence of LVH, aged 55–80 years.[26] Patients were assigned to angiotensin

Parameter	Event rate/1000 patient-years		Relative risk (CI)	p value
	Diltiazem	Conventional therapy		
Primary end-point	29.8	27.7	1.01 (0.66–1.53)	0.98
All stroke	13.3	12.3	0.97 (0.52–1.81)	0.92
All MI	11.2	11.1	0.99 (0.51–1.94)	0.99
Cardiovascular death	9.7	7.8	1.16 (0.55–2.44)	0.71
All-cause death	18.1	15.6	1.07 (0.63–1.84)	0.80
Congestive heart failure	8.5	4.2	1.46 (0.57–3.72)	0.43

Table 17.6
The relative risk and occurrence of end-points in 727 patients with type 2 diabetes in NORDIL. The relative risk has been adjusted using the Cox regression model for age, sex, systolic blood pressure and smoking. (Adapted from reference 25)

receptor blocker (ARB)-based therapy (losartan) or β-blocker (atenolol)-based therapy for a mean follow-up of 4.7 years. Most patients received additional therapy, with equivalent additions to both arms of the study, approximately 90% also receiving a thiazide diuretic and 40% a CCB. Thus the only therapeutic difference between the two arms of the trial was the primary drugs being tested, i.e. losartan versus atenolol. The LIFE study contained 1195 patients with type 2 diabetes (mean age 67 years) with a mean baseline blood pressure of 177/96 mmHg.[27] Blood pressure fell on treatment to a mean of 146/79 mmHg with

losartan-based therapy ($n = 586$) and 148/79 mmHg with atenolol-based therapy ($n = 609$). The primary end-point tested was a composite comprising cardiovascular morbidity and mortality (cardiovascular death, stroke or MI).[27]

The primary end-point occurred in 103 patients assigned to losartan and 103 assigned to atenolol (RR = 0.76, CI = 0.58–0.98, $p < 0.03$). There were also dramatic differences in death from cardiovascular disease (losartan 38, versus atenolol 61, RR = 0.63, $p < 0.028$) and all causes (losartan 63, versus atenolol 104, RR = 0.61, $p < 0.002$). There

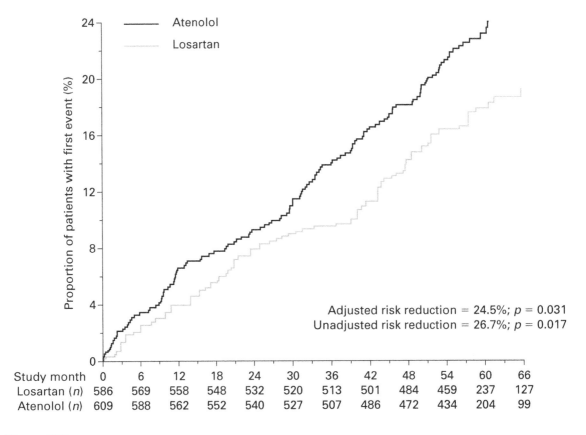

Adjusted risk reduction = 24.5%; $p = 0.031$
Unadjusted risk reduction = 26.7%; $p = 0.017$

Study month	0	6	12	18	24	30	36	42	48	54	60	66
Losartan (n)	586	569	558	548	532	520	513	501	484	459	237	127
Atenolol (n)	609	588	562	552	540	527	507	486	472	434	204	99

Figure 17.7
Primary composite end-point in the diabetic cohort within the LIFE study comparing losartan-based therapy with atenolol-based therapy (n = 1195). (Data from reference 27.)

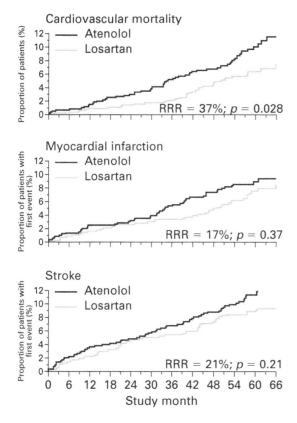

Figure 17.8
Components of the primary composite end-point in the diabetic cohort within the LIFE study. (Data from reference 27.)

was also a trend for a reduction in the rate of MI (RR = 0.81, p < 0.32) and stroke (RR = 0.78, p < 0.19) with losartan-based therapy[27] (Figs 17.7, 17.8 and 17.9).

Most patients randomized into the LIFE study were previously treated with antihypertensive therapy; however, 237 were previously untreated and as shown in Table 17.7, the differences in outcome between the two treatment groups were remarkable, in favour of losartan-based therapy. These differences are particularly striking in view of the fact that

this is not a placebo-controlled trial and both groups of patients received active therapy.[27]

Antihypertensive therapy and new-onset diabetes

Hypertension is associated with an increased risk for developing type 2 diabetes. Data from a large prospective cohort study of 12,550 adults with hypertension who were followed for 6 years confirmed this association.[28] In the 1474 people with untreated hypertension, the risk of developing type 2 diabetes was increased 2.5 times when compared with their normotensive counterparts. Moreover, hypertensive patients who were taking β-blockers had a further 28% increase in risk of developing type 2 diabetes. In contrast, those treated with ACE-inhibitors, CCBs or thiazide diuretics exhibited no increase in risk of developing diabetes, over and above the 2.5-fold increase in risk associated with hypertension per se[28] (Table 17.8).

These findings are consistent with data examining the effects of antihypertensive therapy on insulin sensitivity, which have shown that β-blockers have the most adverse effect of all antihypertensive therapies on insulin sensitivity[29,30] (Fig. 17.10). In this analysis, thiazides appear to have a slight adverse effect, CCBs appear neutral and there is the suggestion that ACE-inhibition and particularly α-blockade may have a slight insulin sensitizing action.

Consistent with these findings, many of the aforementioned head-to-head studies have shown a reduction in new-onset type 2 diabetes in hypertensive diabetic patients treated with ACE-inhibition (HOPE[13]), (CAPPP[22]), angiotensin II antagonists (LIFE[27]), (SCOPE[31]) and CCBs (INSIGHT[24]) when compared with treatment with conventional antihypertensive

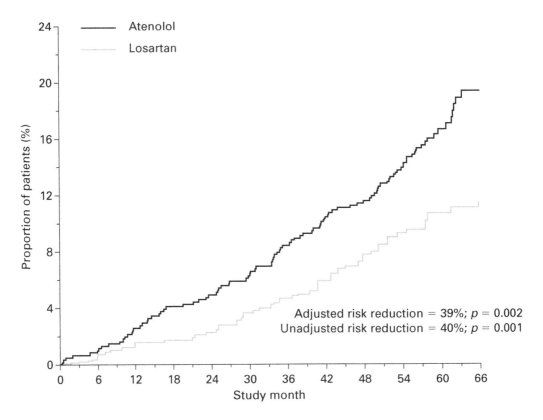

Figure 17.9
Effects of losartan-based therapy versus atenolol-based therapy on total mortality in the diabetic cohort within the LIFE study. (Data from reference 27.)

Parameter	Losartan-based therapy (n = 114)		Atenolol-based therapy (n = 123)	
	Events	Events/1000 patient-years	Events	Events/1000 patient-years
Primary end-point	17	33.3	34	64.7
Cardiovascular death	4	7.2	15	26.6
All-cause death	5	9.1	24	42.6

Table 17.7
Effects of losartan-based versus atenolol-based therapy in 237 hypertensive type 2 diabetics with LVH on ECG but previously untreated for hypertension (adapted from the LIFE study[27])

Antihypertensive medication	Hazard ratio for type 2 diabetes (95% CI)
Thiazides	0.91 (0.73–1.13)
β-Blockers	1.28 (1.04–1.57)*
Calcium channel blockers	1.17 (0.83–1.66)
ACE-inhibitors	0.98 (0.72–1.34)

Data show a multivariate proportional hazards model in 3804 patients treated for hypertension, adjusted for age, sex, race, education, adiposity, exercise and family history of diabetes, showing the independent effect of antihypertensive therapies.* The only therapy associated with significantly increased risk was the β-blocker. (Adapted from reference 28.)

Table 17.8
Risk of developing type 2 diabetes in patients treated with different antihypertensive therapies on a background risk of 2.5-fold excess in people with hypertension when compared with normotensive people

therapy (β-blockers and/or thiazide therapy (Table 17.9).

The studies head-to-head with β-blocker/thiazide therapy are unable to define whether the reduction in new onset diabetes associated with ACE-inhibition, angiotensin II antagonists or CCB-based therapy is a beneficial effect of these drugs in reducing the chances of developing type 2 diabetes or a detrimental effect of conventional therapy, especially β-blockers, on the risk of developing type 2 diabetes. I suspect it may be a combination of both of these factors, especially with regard to RAS blockade. In support of this, the HOPE study demonstrated a marked reduction in new-onset diabetes.[13] Over half of the patients were receiving antihypertensive therapy with combinations of thiazides or β-blockers in the HOPE study. The distribution of therapy appeared to be similar between the

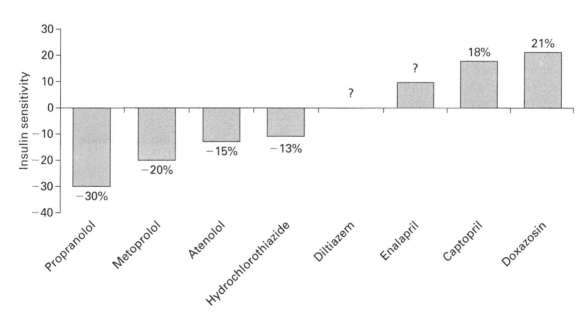

Figure 17.10
The effects of antihypertensive therapy on insulin sensitivity. (Adapted from references 29 and 30.)

Study	Comparators	Reduction in new-onset type 2 diabetes	p value
CAPPP[22]	Captopril vs β-blocker/thiazide	Captopril – 11%	$p < 0.039$
LIFE[26]	Losartan vs atenolol	Losartan – 25%	$p < 0.001$
INSIGHT[24]	Nifedipine GITS vs thiazide	Nifedipine – 20%	$p < 0.02$
HOPE[13]	Ramipril vs conventional therapy	Ramipril – 34%	$p < 0.001$
SCOPE[31]	Candesartan vs placebo ± thiazide	Candesartan – 20%	–

Table 17.9
Reduction in new-onset type 2 diabetes in treatment trials in patients with hypertension but no evidence of type 2 diabetes at baseline

ramipril- and placebo-treated patients, thus suggesting that the presence of ACE-inhibition might have been associated with a direct reduction in risk of type 2 diabetes. It would be of interest to know whether the patients receiving only placebo experienced a similar reduction in risk of developing type 2 diabetes; this has not been reported. Similarly in the recently completed SCOPE study, which compared the angiotensin II receptor blocker candesartan with placebo ± thiazide therapy in elderly hypertensive patients, there was a 20% reduction in rate of new-onset diabetes in those receiving candesartan-based therapy.[31] In that study, 845 patients in the placebo group received no add-on therapy, and 1253 received candesartan alone, thus providing an ideal cohort to test whether RAS blockade reduced the rate of new-onset diabetes in a hypertensive population, without the confounding influence of other antihypertensive therapy.

Despite the seemingly impressive effects of α-blockade on insulin sensitivity, there have been no large-scale studies examining whether this reduces the rate of new-onset diabetes in people with hypertension.

The implications of these findings are important for the long-term treatment of hypertension. It would clearly be undesirable to enhance the otherwise already increased risk of developing type 2 diabetes in a hypertensive population. Such a development would greatly enhance the overall cardiovascular risk burden for the patient despite lowering blood pressure. Consequently, these findings may well be one of the more important observations differentiating newer therapies from conventional antihypertensive therapies.

Summarizing the evidence

Importance of blood pressure control

The SHEP study,[3] the HOT study,[7] UKPDS,[5] Syst-Eur[9] and ABCD[11,12] all confirm that antihypertensive therapy is particularly beneficial in people with diabetes and hypertension across a wide age range (25–80 years) and in people with diastolic and/or systolic hypertension. The main caveat is that the data are almost exclusively for patients with type 2 diabetes. The studies go further and suggest that antihypertensive therapy is more effective at reducing cardiovascular morbidity and mortality and all-cause mortality in people with diabetes and hypertension than in the non-diabetic hypertensive population. This no doubt reflects the higher cardiovascular risk of the diabetic population and their enhanced vulnerability to hypertensive injury.

There are differences in the balance of outcomes in the various studies. For example, HOT showed a reduction in macrovascular events, as did SHEP and Syst-Eur. None of these studies focused on microvascular outcomes. UKPDS demonstrated impressive reductions in macrovascular and microvascular events. The ABCD study of hypertensive patients failed to demonstrate any major effect on microvascular outcomes in the tighter control group but did show a benefit of tighter control on all-cause death. The ABCD normotensive cohort study showed that there was less progression of albuminuria, less retinopathy and less stroke in the tighter BP control group.

It is important not to make too much of these differential outcomes, as they principally reflect differences in trial design, baseline and target pressures, the baseline demographics of the populations studied and above all, the power of the studies to detect differences in specific end-points. Nevertheless the message is clear, with regard to blood pressure control, 'the lower the better' for people with diabetes.

Treatment thresholds and targets

Thresholds
The aforementioned studies lowered blood pressures across a wide range and initiated therapy systolic thresholds ranging from systolic >140 to >160 mmHg and diastolic >90 to >100 mmHg. The ABCD 'normotensive' study was the sole exception in that it initiated therapy in patients with a BP <140/90 mmHg.[12] Importantly, this study confirmed that BP lowering was effective in reducing microvascular disease and stroke when patients with diabetes have their blood

pressure actively lowered within this 'normotensive' range. The HOPE study also supports this conclusion.[13,14] This suggests that treatment with antihypertensive therapy should certainly begin in people with diabetes once their systolic blood pressure is ≥140 mmHg and/or their diastolic blood pressure is ≥90 mmHg. It is likely that patients with diabetes would accrue benefit from antihypertensive therapy even if their blood pressure is normal, i.e. <140/90 mmHg, although further studies are required in patients with blood pressures <140/90 mmHg.

Targets
With regard to blood pressure targets, many studies have struggled to get systolic blood pressure below 140 mmHg, controlling diastolic blood pressure is less of a problem. This is interesting when one considers that most guidelines have recommended a systolic blood pressure target of <130 mmHg. This has only been achieved in one study (ABCD normotensive) and that study enrolled patients who were normotensive at baseline! Nevertheless, a pressure of 128/75 mmHg in that study was associated with less microvascular disease and stroke, suggesting that patients with type 2 diabetes should have their blood pressure lowered to an optimal target of <130/80 mmHg, but the first objective would be to achieve a systolic blood pressure goal of <140 mmHg and a diastolic goal of <80 mmHg.

An important caveat for all of these studies is that aggressive lowering of blood pressure was safe and there was no evidence of a 'J' curve, i.e. no trend to an increased risk with lower blood pressure targets; on the contrary, there was an improved outcome.

The importance of combination therapy

The paradox is that for people with diabetes and hypertension, blood pressure goals are lower than for the non-diabetic population and yet the trials have all shown that blood pressure is actually more difficult to control in people with diabetes.[32] This inevitably means that almost every patient with diabetes and hypertension will require combinations of antihypertensive drug therapy to achieve the more stringent blood pressure goals. With combination therapy of three or more drugs, it will usually be possible to achieve a diastolic target of <90 mmHg, but very much more difficult to lower the systolic pressure below 140 mmHg. Indeed, in the aforementioned trials approximately 90% achieved treated diastolic blood pressures below 90 mmHg but

<50% achieved a blood pressure goal below 140 mmHg[33] (Fig. 17.11). This is particularly true in patients who are older and who have high systolic blood pressures at baseline. Nevertheless, any reduction in blood pressure will be beneficial even if patients do not achieve the exceedingly optimistic goals advocated by most modern guidelines.

Comparison of antihypertensive therapies

The series of studies that compared different therapeutic agents generated some conflicting data but generally allow for some important conclusions. The ABCD study in hypertensive patients suggested that ACE-inhibition-based therapy may be particularly effective at reducing the risk of MI.[18] This is tentatively

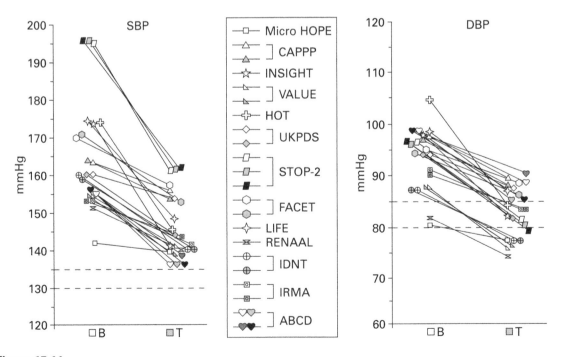

Figure 17.11
Effect of antihypertensive therapies in people with hypertension and diabetes in several clinical trials. Baseline and achieved blood pressures are shown. (From reference 33)

supported by the overall data from STOP-2[20] and more substantially by data from the diabetes cohort within CAPPP.[23] However, in the diabetes cohort within STOP-2, cardiovascular death was similar with CCB therapy, ACE-inhibition or standard therapy.[21] Moreover the superiority of ACE-inhibition in diabetes was not supported by data from the atenolol versus captopril cohort study within UKPDS.[6] However, this was a small study and underpowered to address this question. CAPPP suggested that the differential outcome in favour of ACE-inhibition may be particularly noticeable in those with poorer glycaemic control.[23] This differential effect was not observed in the ABCD normotensive study in which ACE-inhibition appeared to offer no specific advantage once blood pressure was tightly and equivalently controlled.[12] This is unlike the HOPE study, where ACE-inhibition did reduce MI in 'normotensive' people with diabetes and an additional cardiovascular risk factor, but interpretation of this result is confounded by a difference in blood pressure between the ACE-inhibitor and placebo groups.[14]

The LIFE study was one of the best designed comparator studies in patients with hypertension and diabetes.[26,27] In the LIFE study, apart from the primary drugs being tested (losartan versus atenolol), the 'add-on' therapies were similar in both arms of the trial, as was blood pressure control. There were marked reductions in cardiovascular mortality and all-cause mortality in favour of losartan, an angiotensin II receptor antagonist. There were also trends to reduced stroke and MI in favour of losartan in the diabetic cohort. This improvement in survival in favour of renin-angiotensin system blockade is supported by data from the CAPPP study in diabetes, which also showed impressive reductions in total mortality in favour of ACE-inhibition versus conventional therapy.[23] Together

these data suggest that blockade of the renin-angiotensin system offers more than conventional antihypertensive therapy in people with hypertension and diabetes. This may be particularly relevant for people with hypertension and diabetes in whom blood pressure has not been controlled to optimal values (the majority!) and perhaps those with poor glycaemic control. In contrast, the ABCD normotensive study suggests that once blood pressure is optimally controlled, there is no obvious differential effect of RAS blockade on outcomes in people with type 2 diabetes.[12]

The INSIGHT,[24] NORDIL[25] and STOP-2[20,21] studies directly compared CCB-based therapy with conventional therapy (thiazide and/or β-blocker-based therapy) and contained significant numbers of patients with diabetes and hypertension. The primary outcomes of these studies demonstrate that CCB-based therapy is equivalent to conventional antihypertensive therapy in people with diabetes. Moreover, the HOT[7] and Syst-Eur[8,9] studies were based on CCB therapy and, in these studies, there were impressive reductions in cardiovascular events in the cohorts of patients with diabetes. Thus, the notion that CCBs are 'unsafe' and 'may increase risk' in patients with diabetes is not supported by this overwhelming body of data. Moreover, bearing in mind the fact that CCBs are unlikely to be used first-line to treat patients with hypertension in diabetes because of the aforementioned data on the effectiveness of RAS blockade, there is absolutely no evidence that CCB therapy would do anything other than enhance blood pressure lowering and thus efficacy of antihypertensive therapy when used in combination with RAS blockade. In this regard, the limited data from FACET,[19] rather than condemning CCBs, actually support the primacy of combination therapy.

Trial evidence for other antihypertensive therapies

The studies above focus on thiazide diuretics, β-blockade, CCBs, ACE-inhibition and an angiotensin II antagonist. There are no substantial data for other agents for the treatment of hypertension in diabetes. However, this does not mean that such therapies cannot be used as part of a multi-drug treatment cocktail; on the contrary, the over-riding objective is to control blood pressure.

Antihypertensive drugs

The practical issues pertaining to the use of the various antihypertensive drug therapies are discussed below. This discussion is not meant to be exhaustive or comprehensive and physicians should consult specific information provided for each medication before use.

Thiazide diuretics

Thiazides (e.g. hydrochlorothiazide, bendrofluazide) and thiazide-like drugs (e.g. chlorthalidone) act on the luminal aspect of the distal convoluted tubule of the kidney and inhibit the reabsorption of sodium. As this segment of the renal tubule is responsible for only 10% of total renal sodium reabsorption the thiazide diuretics have only a modest natriuretic effect when compared with the loop diuretics. This is appropriate in people with diabetes who often retain sodium. The increased delivery of sodium to the distal tubule promotes sodium:potassium exchange which causes a sustained increase in the renal clearance of potassium, resulting in hypokalaemia. Thiazides also promote the excretion of magnesium and reduce the excretion of calcium and uric acid.

In the acute phase of thiazide therapy, blood pressure is reduced as a result of volume depletion and a reduced cardiac output, which is partially compensated for by an increase in peripheral resistance. With chronic therapy, this acute response is further compensated for by various neurohumoral mechanisms, which leads to a new steady state characterized by a minimal reduction in plasma and extracellular fluid volume, a reduction in total peripheral resistance (which may be due to a vasodilator action) and lower blood pressure.

The hypotensive effect of thiazide diuretics is most pronounced in patients with low plasma renin values, i.e. the elderly and Black hypertensive subjects. It is important to note that the blood pressure response to thiazide diuretic monotherapy is flat and dissociated from the dose effect of thiazides on potassium, glucose and lipid profiles. Hydrochlorothiazide 25 mg once daily or bendrofluazide 2.5 mg once daily appears to be the optimal dose to achieve a maximal antihypertensive effect and minimize the metabolic side-effects of monotherapy. However, in patients with diabetes, thiazides will often be used in combination with RAS blockade when the antihypertensive dose response may not be flat. This is because the increased activity of the RAS which accompanies thiazide therapy and can limit its antihypertensive efficacy is blocked by ACE-inhibition or angiotensin II antagonists. Hence under these circumstances, higher doses of thiazides, i.e. hydrochlorothiazide 50 mg o.d. or bendrofluazide 5 mg o.d., will usually further reduce blood pressure. Higher doses of thiazide diuretics are associated with a reduction in insulin sensitivity but this should not be an obstacle to improving blood pressure control, which has been shown to be very effective in reducing cardiovascular morbidity and mortality and all-cause death. Thiazides are often ineffective in people with impaired renal function and a GFR of <60 ml/min, when loop diuretics are preferred. Thiazides should be avoided in patients with gout and should be prescribed with potassium-sparing diuretics as clinically indicated to reduce the risk of hypokalaemia. This is usually not necessary when thiazides are used in combination with RAS blockade.

The benefits of thiazides for the treatment of hypertension in people with diabetes have been well established in the many studies highlighted above. Thiazide diuretics are cheap, tried and tested, reasonably well tolerated and a key component of any therapeutic cocktail for the treatment of hypertension in people with diabetes. It is often impossible to control systolic blood pressure without them.

Loop diuretics

The antihypertensive mechanism of loop diuretics relates to their action to significantly reduce total body sodium. Loop diuretics can induce significant hypokalaemia, hyponatraemia and volume depletion. Loop diuretics are not recommended for the routine treatment of hypertension in patients with diabetes but they are very useful in patients with clinical evidence of significant sodium and volume retention. They are also preferred to thiazide diuretics in patients with evidence of renal impairment and they are essential in patients with advanced nephropathy, in whom high doses (e.g. frusemide 250–500 mg daily) are often required.

Adrenergic blockers

β-Blockers

β-Blockers are competitive inhibitors of the β-adrenergic receptors. Non-selective β-blockers inhibit β_1 and β_2 receptors whereas 'selective' β-blockers predominantly inhibit the β1 receptor. β-Blockers reduce cardiac output, heart rate and renal blood flow. Although peripheral vascular resistance rises, the net effect of the haemodynamic changes is a fall in systemic blood pressure. β-Blockers also decrease plasma renin activity. β-Blockers have an antiarrhythmic action which may be important in patients with co-existent ischaemic heart disease. They are less effective at lowering blood pressure in 'low renin hypertension', i.e. Black and elderly patients.

β-Blockers are widely used in the treatment of hypertension and are still recommended by all major international guidelines as an appropriate first-line therapy for the treatment of hypertension. Like the thiazides, the β-blockers have been extensively tried and tested in prospective randomized clinical trials, predominantly in non-diabetic hypertensive subjects, and have been shown to reduce cardiovascular mortality, especially post-myocardial infarction. However, they appear to be less effective than thiazide diuretics at reducing stroke in elderly patients. β-Blockers are important for the management of ischaemic heart disease. They are the most effective drug therapy for reducing the symptoms of angina and they reduce mortality post-myocardial infarction. This latter point is important with regard to diabetes because diabetes is associated with increased mortality post-myocardial infarction. β-Blockers have also been shown to be effective in reducing mortality in patients with advanced congestive heart failure.

In the past there has been concern that β-blockers (especially non-selective β-blockers) may blunt the counter-regulatory responses and mask the symptoms of hypoglycaemia in people with diabetes, particularly type 1 diabetes. This appears to be more of a theoretical concern than a major clinical problem in practice. Nevertheless, β-blockers are less well tolerated than other forms of antihypertensive therapy, especially ACE-inhibition or angiotensin II receptor blockade (cf. UKPDS,[5] CAPPP[22] and LIFE[26]) and have been associated with modest weight gain. β-Blockers also impair insulin sensitivity and as discussed above, β-blocker therapy may increase the likelihood of developing type 2 diabetes in people with hypertension when compared with other antihypertensive therapies.[28] Moreover, in the LIFE study, in patients with type 2 diabetes, β-blocker-based therapy was substantially less effective at reducing cardiovascular and all-cause mortality in patients when compared with losartan-based therapy.[27] These observations suggest that unless specifically indicated (i.e. in patients with symptomatic ischaemic heart disease and/or post-myocardial infarction) β-blockers should be avoided in people with hypertension who are at increased risk of developing type 2 diabetes, or as a primary therapy in people with type 2 diabetes.

α₁ Adrenergic blockers

α₁ Adrenergic blockers

Increased central sympathetic nervous system activity is a characteristic feature of insulin resistance. α-Blockers effectively lower blood pressure by decreasing central sympathetic outflow and promoting vasodilatation. The original drug that was widely used in this class was prazosin but this required two to three times daily dosing and was associated with tachyphylaxis. Prazosin has been replaced by longer-acting agents, e.g. doxazosin, which in a sustained release formulation is effective when administered once daily. α-Blockers have a potentially desirable action to improve insulin sensitivity; however, it is unknown whether this is associated with less new-onset diabetes in people with hypertension. Moreover, the effects of long-term α-blocker therapy on the development or progression of microvascular and cardiovascular disease in people with diabetes are unknown. Recently, the doxazosin-treated cohort within a major prospective, randomized clinical study (the

antihypertensive and lipid lowering treatment to prevent heart attack trial: ALLHAT), was discontinued by the data safety monitoring board because of concerns over an enhanced rate of 'hospitalizations due to heart failure' when compared with patients treated with a thiazide diuretic. Separate results for the patients with diabetes have not been reported.[34] The decision to terminate the doxazosin arm of this trial was controversial for a number of reasons[35] and the trial design meant it was unclear whether randomization to doxazosin simply unmasked occult heart failure that was previously treated with alternative drugs, e.g. a diuretic. Regardless, this was a monotherapy, first-line therapy comparison, and this result does not mean that α-blockers should not continue to be used as very useful add-on therapy to optimize blood pressure control in people with diabetes. α-Blockers combine very effectively with ACE-inhibition, angiotensin II antagonists and/or CCBs and are a very useful component of the antihypertensive cocktail in people with diabetes. α-Blockers are also effective at reducing symptoms in males with prostatic outflow obstruction. α-Blockers can cause symptomatic orthostatic hypotension and should be used with caution in diabetic patients with autonomic dysfunction.

Calcium channel blockers

Calcium channel blockers (CCBs) act as vasodilators by inhibiting the influx of calcium into vascular smooth muscle cells via membrane-bound voltage-dependent channels. These channels can be selectively inhibited by the binding of calcium channel blockers to the α1-subunit of these channels. Although often referred to as a single class of agents, the CCBs belong to three distinct chemical groups that have significant differences in their haemodynamic effects. The three chemical groupings are:

1. Dihydropyridines: nifedipine, amlodipine, lacidipine and other '. . . pines'.
2. Benzothiazepines: diltiazem is the only commonly used member of this group.
3. Phenylalkylamines: verapamil is the only commonly used member of this group.

For practical purposes, they are commonly referred to as two groups: the dihydropyridines and the non-dihydropyridines (diltiazem and verapamil). The dihydropyridine group have mainly vasodilator effects with relatively small effects on cardiac contraction and atrio-ventricular (AV) conduction. Only the longer-acting formulations of these drugs should be used to treat hypertension. The main adverse effect of vasodilatation is predictable, i.e. ankle oedema and less commonly, reflex tachycardia.

The non-dihydropyridines have moderate vasodilatory and moderate negative inotropic and chronotropic effects. They have a similar adverse profile to dihydropyridines but are perhaps less likely to cause oedema and tachycardia but have a greater negative inotropic effect and are thus less well tolerated in patients with heart failure. It has been suggested that CCBs may worsen gastroparesis in patients with diabetic autonomic neuropathy. However, the most common gastrointestinal side-effect appears to be constipation, particularly with verapamil. The CCBs are metabolically neutral and in the INSIGHT study,[24] nifedipine GITS was associated with 20% less new-onset diabetes than conventional diuretic-based therapy.

The CCBs are very effective at lowering blood pressure in patients with diabetes. There has been controversy and debate about their safety in patients with diabetes (see above) but this should now be dismissed in the light of data from CCB-based trials such as HOT, Syst-Eur, INSIGHT and NORDIL, all of which reported impressive outcomes in patients with hypertension and diabetes. The CCBs are an effective and important component of the drug combinations required to lower blood pressure and thus microvascular and macrovascular risk in patients with hypertension and diabetes. The CCBs combine very effectively with ACE-inhibition, angiotensin II receptor blockers and α-blockers.

Angiotensin-converting enzyme (ACE)-inhibitors

The renin-angiotensin system has been strongly implicated in the pathogenesis of hypertension and diabetes-related complications in patients with diabetes. ACE-inhibitors have been shown to reduce mortality and the development and progression of complications in patients with diabetes. They also have a favourable effect on the progression of nephropathy (mainly studies in type 1 diabetes), and reduce mortality in patients with heart failure and post-myocardial infarction.

The most common side-effect of ACE-inhibition is cough and more rarely angioedema, the latter being more common in Black patients. ACE-induced cough occurs in about 15% of patients and is more common in the Asia-Pacific region. ACE-inhibitors can also cause hyperkalaemia, notably in patients with advanced renal impairment or when co-administered with potassium-sparing diuretics. ACE-inhibitors are often used as initial therapy for people with hypertension and diabetes but they are not particularly effective at lowering blood pressure in such patients in monotherapy (especially older patients or Black patients). As such, ACE-inhibitors are best used in combination with a diuretic when treating hypertension in people with diabetes.

Angiotensin II receptor blockers (ARBs)

The ARBs provide more selective inhibition of the renin-angiotensin system by selective and specific inhibition of the angiotensin AT_1 receptor. This class of drugs is well tolerated and is as effective as ACE-inhibition at lowering blood pressure. However, unlike ACE-inhibition, ARBs do not cause cough or angioedema any more frequently than conventional antihypertensive therapy. Like ACE-inhibition, ARBs may also cause hyperkalaemia in patients with advanced renal impairment or when used in combination with potassium-sparing diuretics. As discussed in a previous chapter, ARBs have been shown to reduce the progression of nephropathy in type 2 diabetes (IDNT,[36] irbesartan; RENAAL,[37] losartan). With regard to cardiovascular morbidity and mortality outcomes in patients with diabetes, the recent data from the LIFE study[27] have demonstrated that losartan-based therapy was superior to atenolol-based conventional antihypertensive therapy in patients with type 2 diabetes and LVH on ECG. These are the only data thus far with this class of therapy, reporting cardiovascular outcomes in patients with diabetes. ARBs are unlikely to be effective as initial therapy alone to achieve blood pressure goals in people with diabetes and hypertension, and combination with a diuretic is preferred. ARBs also combine effectively with CCBs and/or α-blockers for additional blood pressure lowering.

The question has arisen as to whether the combination of ACE-inhibition and ARBs might be more effective than either alone? There is some evidence that such a combination may be more effective at reducing some surrogate markers such as blood pressure or albuminuria when compared with conventional dosing of the single agents.[38] Whether this would be true if the ACE/ARB combination was compared with much higher doses of the single agents is unknown. Moreover, whether such a combination would offer anything in terms of improved microvascular and cardiovascular outcomes is also unknown.

Other antihypertensive therapies

There are many other classes of drug therapy that effectively lower blood pressure in hypertensive patients. Some of these other drugs are now rarely used in the management of hypertension in diabetes because their side-effect profile renders them less desirable than the aforementioned alternatives. There are also newer classes of drug therapy that may ultimately prove to be useful in hypertensive diabetic subjects but with which clinical experience is currently limited.

Sympatholytic agents

The centrally acting α_2 agonists (clonidine and methyl dopa) inhibit central efferent sympathetic activity. They are very effective at lowering blood pressure in diabetic patients but the high incidence of side-effects, orthostatic hypotension and impotence associated with their use makes them less suitable for the routine management of hypertension in people with diabetes. However, methyl dopa is still used for the management of hypertension in pregnancy because of extensive experience of its safe use in pregnancy. A relatively new addition to the centrally acting agents is moxonidine. This is an imidazoline receptor agonist (specific for the I_1-receptor). These receptors are present in the rostral ventrolateral medulla of the brain and stimulation of the I_1 receptor reduces sympathetic outflow from the brain. Activation of the I_1-receptor as opposed to the α_2-receptor is associated with less of the side-effects of dry mouth, sedation, etc. Inhibition of central sympathetic outflow also improves insulin sensitivity. There are no clinical outcome trials specifically evaluating the effects of moxonidine in hypertensive patients with or without diabetes, but in my own experience, it can be effective as an 'add-on' therapy to achieve blood pressure goals in patients requiring multiple therapies.

Direct vasodilators

These agents (hydralazine and minoxidil) act directly on vascular (predominantly arteriolar) smooth muscle to lower peripheral vascular resistance and thus blood pressure. They induce a profound reflex sympathetic activation (tachycardia and palpitations) and salt and water retention and are therefore usually combined with a β-blocker and a diuretic. Hydralazine has been used extensively to treat moderately severe hypertension, usually as a second- or third-line agent. Its use has declined considerably in recent years due to its propensity to cause a lupus reaction in a significant proportion of patients and the more recent availability of safer and better tolerated agents. The use of minoxidil has always been restricted to those patients with severe hypertension, not readily controlled by combinations of other agents. The current infrequent use of minoxidil is therefore usually best confined to specialist clinicians experienced in the management of severe hypertension.

Aldosterone antagonists – spironolactone

Aldosterone has recently been implicated in the pathogenesis of cardiovascular disease via mechanisms that go beyond its conventional role as a regulator of potassium and volume homeostasis.[39] These actions include enhancement of cardiovascular and renal fibrosis, proteinuria and decreased fibrinolysis, among others. Support for this hypothesis came from the results of the RALES study (Randomized Aldactone Evaluation Study) which examined the effects of spironolactone (25 mg o.d.) on overall morbidity and mortality in patients with severe heart failure when added to an ACE-inhibitor, loop diuretic and digoxin.[40] There was a 30% reduction in all-cause death in the spironolactone-treated patients. Whether spironolactone could enhance survival and reduce complications in hypertensive patients with diabetes is unknown. Nevertheless, in patients with resistant hypertension associated with diabetes, the addition of low dose spironolactone can sometimes help to reduce blood pressure, in some cases substantially, although serum potassium levels need to be monitored, especially in patients who are also receiving ACE-inhibitors or ARBs. Spironolactone is poorly tolerated by some patients due to gynaecomastia in males and menstrual disturbances and/or breast pain in females.

Selective aldosterone receptor antagonists (SARAs) – eplerenone

SARAs effectively inhibit aldosterone (with higher potency than spironolactone) but have much less affinity for androgen and progesterone receptors, thus inducing less side-effects. The first in the class, eplerenone, is currently being evaluated in patients with heart failure, hypertension and renal disease and presently no data are available for patients with diabetes and hypertension.

Vasopeptidase inhibition – omapatrilat

Vasopeptidase inhibitors are single molecular entities that simultaneously inhibit two key enzyme systems involved in the regulation of the cardiovascular system: the renin-angiotensin-aldosterone system (RAS) and the natriuretic peptide system (NPS).[41] RAS inhibition is achieved by inhibition of angiotensin-converting enzyme (ACE) in a manner similar to conventional ACE-inhibition. The activity of the NPS is increased by simultaneous inhibition of neutral endopeptidase (NEP), a key enzyme involved in the degradation of natriuretic peptides. NEP is also involved in the degradation of the natural vasodilator adrenomedullin and bradykinin, the levels of both being increased by NEP inhibition. The net effect is inhibition of the RAS and potentiation of the NPS and bradykinin. As the NPS functions as a natural antagonist of the RAS, its potentiation by vasopeptidase inhibition may potentiate the blood pressure-lowering and cardiovascular structural and functional benefits established for ACE-inhibition alone.

Omapatrilat is a vasopeptidase inhibitor that has undergone the most extensive clinical evaluation thus far. Omapatrilat is a very effective antihypertensive agent; it lowers blood pressure more effectively than monotherapy with other drugs and appears to be particularly effective at lowering systolic blood pressure.[41] However, combining ACE- and NEP-inhibition increases the potential for adverse effects such as angioedema. This is likely to be of particular relevance to Black patients who already experience an enhanced risk of angioedema with ACE-inhibition. If concerns about angioedema are not substantiated and this class of therapy gains a licence for the treatment of hypertension, it would be a useful addition. Soon thereafter, it would be important to confirm its efficacy and safety in diabetic patients with hypertension in a morbidity/mortality outcome trial.

Summarizing treatment recommendations

Various national and international societies have produced recommendations for pharmacological therapy in patients with hypertension and diabetes. It is clear that most of the available evidence applies to patients with type 2 diabetes. Nevertheless, the complications and cause of death are the same for patients with type 1 and 2 diabetes and thus, treatment recommendations are applicable to both patient groups. It is also abundantly clear that the obsession with 'first-line' therapy is futile because all patients, with few exceptions, will require more than one drug to control their blood pressure.

A recent position statement from the American Diabetes Association recommended ACE-inhibition, ARBs, thiazides or β-blockers as appropriate initial therapy for adults with type 2 diabetes and hypertension (without evidence of nephropathy).[42] Their recommendations excluded CCBs as potential *initial* therapy. The European Society of Hypertension in its management update statement adopted a more cautious approach with regard to recommending specific therapeutic classes and acknowledged that ACE-inhibition had been proven to be protective but that there was no consensus as to 'the drug of choice'.[43] This latter statement was written before the more recent LIFE study with the ARB losartan.[27]

As suggested above, the data from the trials demonstrate that blood pressure control is of key importance for microvascular and cardiovascular protection. This cannot be emphasized enough. Most patients will require a cocktail of antihypertensive therapies (often three or more drugs) and even then it will be difficult to achieve recommended blood pressure targets, particularly systolic blood pressure targets. Previous and more recent data in patients with nephropathy have demonstrated the importance of RAS blockade with ACE-inhibition or ARBs as complementary therapy for renoprotection. The evidence from CAPPP, HOPE and LIFE extends this notion to cardiovascular protection and mortality benefits for people with type 2 diabetes and hypertension but without evidence of nephropathy.

Taken together, these new data strongly support the notion that antihypertensive therapy based on ACE-inhibition or an ARB is likely to be more effective at reducing cardiovascular events and mortality than conventional antihypertensive therapy in people with diabetes, especially in those at higher cardiovascular risk by virtue of pre-existing cardiovascular disease and/or LVH. The antihypertensive efficacy of ACE-inhibition or ARBs is greatly accentuated if patients can be encouraged to adhere to a salt-restricted diet.

Accepting that optimal antihypertensive therapy for people with hypertension and diabetes should ideally include an ACE-inhibitor or an ARB as part of the inevitable treatment cocktail, and that these drugs alone are unlikely to control blood pressure, then the next consideration is the appropriate add-on therapy. The logical addition to an ACE-inhibitor or an ARB to improve blood pressure control is a thiazide diuretic. Fixed combinations of ACE-inhibition or an ARB with a thiazide diuretic are available and it seems sensible to use these fixed combinations to reduce the number of tablets and improve concordance with therapy.

Despite the aforementioned evidence that CCBs have been very effective as part of antihypertensive therapy regimes in reducing cardiovascular events and death in people with diabetes, the debate about their safety lingers. CCBs are undoubtedly very effective antihypertensive agents and they are a very useful add-on therapy to help improve blood pressure control as part of a triple therapy cocktail (ACE-inhibition or angiotensin II antagonist + thiazide (or loop) diuretic + CCB). There is then the option of adding either a β-blocker or an α-blocker and thereafter centrally acting agents and/or aldosterone blockade. A suggested treatment algorithm for people with hypertension and

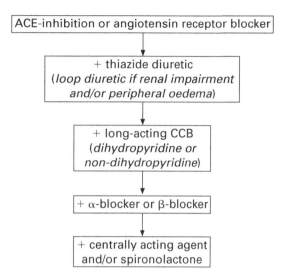

Figure 17.12
Treatment algorithm for patients with hypertension and diabetes. β-Blocker therapy would be promoted in the hierarchy for patients with symptomatic angina, post-myocardial infarction or congestive cardiac failure.

diabetes, based on current evidence, is shown in Fig. 17.12.

In the treatment algorithm above, β-blocker therapy has been relegated because β-blocker-based therapy was clearly inferior to losartan-based therapy in patients with type 2 diabetes and hypertension in LIFE, despite similar blood pressure control. Nevertheless, β-blockers are still very effective drugs for the treatment of diabetic patients with symptomatic angina and post-myocardial infarction. Moreover, the data from LIFE were obtained from an older population and β-blockers are generally more effective antihypertensive agents in younger patients.

Blood pressure goals are more frequently achieved in clinical trials than in clinical practice because they adopt this kind of algorithm approach, often under the direct supervision of a nurse rather than a physician. It is likely that blood pressure control in patients with type 2 diabetes would improve on its current lamentable position if the rigours of the clinical trial setting and treatment algorithm could be replicated in clinical practice. Moreover, antihypertensive therapy in practice frequently fails because physicians fail to use drugs in sufficient doses and/or fail to add-on therapies when blood pressure is not controlled. When specifying which agents within a class to use, it is difficult to be didactic. It is my practice, wherever possible, to follow the trial evidence because such evidence defines the benefits and confirms the safety of the drugs used. This may be particularly relevant to RAS blockade with ACE-inhibition or ARBs because of the implication that in people with diabetes the benefits of these agents may go beyond that

achieved by blood pressure control. In these circumstances, the trials also define the dose of the drug required to replicate the benefits for patients.

The evidence base for treating hypertension in diabetes is now stronger than ever before. It suggests that optimal therapy is a treatment regimen based on RAS blockade as part of a cocktail of antihypertensive drugs designed to lower blood pressure to challenging targets. In the next few years, this evidence base will grow as ongoing clinical trials with large sub-populations with type 2 diabetes conclude and report their findings. These trials include ALL-HAT,[44] ASCOT[45] and VALUE,[46] all of which promise to add to the debate, if not necessarily provide definitive answers.

References

1. Fletcher AE, Bulpit CJ. How far should blood pressure be lowered? *N Engl J Med* 1992; **326:** 251–4.
2. Davis BR, Langford HG, Blaufox MD, et al. The association of postural changes in systolic blood pressure and mortality in persons with hypertension: the Hypertension Detection and Follow-up Program (HDFP) experience. *Circulation* 1987; **75:** 340–6.
3. Curb JD, Pressel SL, Cutler JA, et al. Effect of diuretic based antihypertensive treatment on cardiovascular risk in people with diabetes. Systolic Hypertension in Elderly Program (SHEP) Cooperative research group. *JAMA* 1996; **276:** 1886–92.
4. United Kingdom Prospective Diabetes Study group. Intensive blood glucose control with sulphonylureas or insulin compared with conventional treatment and risk of complications in patients with type 2 diabetes: UKPDS 33. *Lancet* 1998; **352:** 837–53.
5. United Kingdom Prospective Diabetes Study Group. Tight blood pressure control and risk of macrovascular and microvascular complications in type 2 diabetes: UKPDS 38. *BMJ* 1998; **317:** 703–13.
6. United Kingdom Prospective Diabetes Study group. Efficacy of atenolol and captopril in reducing macrovascular and microvascular complications in diabetes: UKPDS 39. *BMJ* 1998; **317:** 713–20.
7. Hansson L, Zanchetti A, Carruthers SG et al. Effects of intensive blood pressure lowering and low dose aspirin in patients with hypertension: principle results of the Hypertension Optimal Treatment (HOT) randomised trial. *Lancet* 1998; **351:** 1755–62.
8. Staessen JA, Fagard R, Thijs L, et al., for the Systolic Hypertension-Europe (Syst-Eur) Trial Investigators. Morbidity and mortality in the placebo-controlled European Trial on Isolated Systolic Hypertension in the Elderly. *Lancet* 1997; **360:** 757–64.
9. Tuomilehto J, Rastenyte D, Birkenhager WH, et al. Effects of calcium channel blockade in older patients with diabetes and systolic hypertension. Systolic Hypertension in Europe Trial Investigators. *N Engl J Med* 1999; **340:** 677–84.
10. Estacio RO, Savage S, Nagel NJ, Schrier RW. Baseline characteristics of participants in the appropriate blood pressure control in diabetes trial. *Controlled Clin Trials* 1996; **17:** 242–57.
11. Estacio RO, Jeffers BW, Gifford N, Schrier RW. Effect of blood pressure control on diabetic microvascular complications in patients with hypertension and type 2 diabetes. *Diabetes Care* 2000; **23** (Suppl 2): B54–64.
12. Schrier RW, Estacio RO, Esler A, Mehler P. Effects of aggressive blood pressure control in normotensive type diabetic patients on albuminuria, retinopathy and strokes. *Kidney Int* 2002; **61:** 1086–97.
13. The Heart Outcomes Prevention Evaluation Study Investigators. Effects of an angiotensin-converting enzyme inhibitor, ramipril, on cardiovascular events in high risk patients. *N Engl J Med* 2000; **342:** 145–53.
14. The Heart Outcomes Prevention Evaluation Study Investigators. Effects of ramipril on cardiovascular and microvascular outcomes in people with diabetes mellitus: results of the HOPE study and MICRO-HOPE substudy. *Lancet* 2000; **355:** 253–9.
15. Williams B. The renin-angiotensin system and cardiovascular disease: Hope or Hype? *J Renin Angiotensin Aldosterone Syst* 2000; **1:** 142–6.
16. Svensson P, de Faire U, Sleight P, et al. Comparative effects of ramipril on ambulatory and office blood pressures: a HOPE substudy. *Hypertension* 2001; **38:** E28–32.
17. Cutler JA. Calcium channel blockers for hypertension – uncertainty continues. *N Engl J Med* 1998; **338:** 679–81.
18. Estacio RO, Jeffers BW, Hiatt WR, et al. The effect of nisoldipine as compared with enalapril on cardiovascular outcomes in patients with non-insulin dependent diabetes

and hypertension. *N Engl J Med* 1998; **338**: 645–52.

19. Tatti P, Phaor M, Byington RP, et al. Outcome results of the fosinopril versus amlodipine cardiovascular events trial (FACET) in patients with hypertension and NIDDM. *Diabetes Care* 1998; **21**: 579–603.

20. Hansson L, Lindholm LH, Ekborn T, et al. Randomised trial of old and new antihypertensive drugs in elderly patients: cardiovascular mortality and morbidity in the Swedish Trial in Old Patients with hypertension-2 study. *Lancet* 1999; **354**: 1751–6.

21. Lindholm L, Hansson L, Ekbom T, et al. Comparison of antihypertensive treatments in preventing cardiovascular events in elderly diabetic patients: results of the Swedish Trial in Old Patients with hypertension-2. *J Hypertens* 2000; **18**: 1671–5.

22. Hansson L, Lindholm L, Niskanen L, et al. Effect of angiotensin converting enzyme inhibition compared with conventional therapy on cardiovascular morbidity and mortality in hypertension: the Captopril Prevention Project (CAPPP) randomised trial. *Lancet* 1999; **353**: 611–16.

23. Niskanen L, Hedner T, Hansson L, et al., for the CAPPP study group. Reduced cardiovascular morbidity and mortality in hypertensive diabetic patients on first line therapy with an ACE inhibitor compared with a diuretic/β-blocker-based treatment regimen. *Diabetes Care* 2001; **24**: 2091–6.

24. Brown MJ, Palmer CR, Castaigne A, et al. Morbidity and mortality in patients randomised to double-blind treatment with long-acting calcium channel blocker or diuretic in the International Nifedipine GITS study: Intervention as a Goal in hypertension treatment (INSIGHT). *Lancet* 2000; **356**: 366–72.

25. Hansson L, Hedner T, Lund-Johansen P, et al. Randomised trial of effects of calcium antagonists compared to diuretics and β-blockers on cardiovascular morbidity and mortality in hypertension: the Nordic Diliazem (NORDIL) study. *Lancet* 2000; **356**: 359–65.

26. Dahlof B, Devereux R, Kjeldsen SE, et al. Cardiovascular morbidity and mortality in the losartan intervention for endpoint reduction in hypertension study (LIFE): a randomised trial against atenolol. *Lancet* 2002; **359**: 995–1003.

27. Lindholm LH, Ibsen H, Dahlof B, et al. Cardiovascular morbidity and mortality in patients with diabetes in the losartan intervention for endpoint reduction in hypertension study (LIFE): a randomised trial against atenolol. *Lancet* 2002; **359**: 1004–10.

28. Gress TW, Nieto FJ, Shahar E, et al. Hypertension and antihypertensive therapy as risk factors for type 2 diabetes mellitus: Atherosclerosis Risk in Communities study. *N Engl J Med* 2000; **342**: 905–12.

29. Hanni A, Andersson PE, Lind L, Lithell H. Electrolyte changes and metabolic effects of lisinopril/bendrofluazide treatment. Results of randomized double blind study with parallel groups. *Am J Hypertens* 1994; **7**: 615–22.

30. Andersson PE, Lithell H. Metabolic effects of doxazosin and enalapril in hypertriglyceridemic, hypertensive men. Relationship to changes in skeletal muscle blood flow. *Am J Hypertens* 1996; **9**: 323–33.

31. Hansson L, on behalf of the Investigators. Study on Cognition and Prognosis in the Elderly (SCOPE). Presentation to European Society of Hypertension. Prague, 2002.

32. Brown MJ, Castaigne A, de Leeuw PW, et al. Influence of diabetes and type of hypertension on response to antihypertensive therapy. *Hypertension* 2000; **35**: 1038–42.

33. Mancia G, Grassi G. Systolic and diastolic blood pressure control in antihypertensive drug trials. *J Hypertens* 2002; **29**: 1461–4.

34. ALLHAT Collaborative Research Group. Major cardiovascular events in hypertensive patients randomized to doxazosin vs chlorthalidone: the antihypertensive and lipid-lowering treatment to prevent heart attack trial (ALLHAT). *JAMA* 2000; **283**: 1967–75.

35. Poulter NR, Williams B. Doxazosin for the management of hypertension: implications of the ALLHAT trial. *Am J Hypertens* 2001; **14**: 1170–2.

36. Lewis EJ, Hunsicker LG, Clarke WR, et al. Renoprotective effect of the angiotensin-receptor antagonist irbesartan in patients with nephropathy due to type 2 diabetes. *N Engl J Med* 2001; **345**: 851–60.

37. Brenner BM, Cooper ME, De Zeeuw D, et al. Effects of losartan on renal and cardiovascular

outcomes in patients with type 2 diabetes and nephropathy. *N Engl J Med* 2001; **345**: 861–9.

38. Mogensen CE, Neldan S, Tikkanen I et al. Randomised controlled trial of dual blockade of renin angiotensin system in patients with hypertension, microalbuminuria and non-insulin dependent diabetes: the candesartan and lisinopril microalbuminuria (CALM) study. *BMJ* 2000; **321**: 1440–4.

39. Young MJ, Funder JW. Mineralocorticoid receptors and pathophysiological roles for aldosterone in the cardiovascular system. *J Hypertens* 2002; **20**: 1465–8.

40. Pitt B, Zannad F, Remme WJ, et al. The effect of spironolactone on morbidity and mortality in patients with severe heart failure. *N Engl J Med* 1999; **341**: 709–17.

41. Weber MA. Vasopeptidase inhibitors. *Lancet* 2001; **358**: 1525–32.

42. American Diabetes Association Position State- ment. Treatment of hypertension in adults with diabetes. *Diabetes Care* 2002; 134–47; 199–201.

43. Kjeldsen SE, Os I, Farsang C, et al. Treatment of hypertension in patients with type-2 diabetes. *J Hypertens* 2000; **18**: 1345–6.

44. Davis BR, Cutler JA, Gorson DJ, et al. Rationale and design for the Antihypertensive and Lipid Lowering treatment to prevent Heart attack Trial (ALLHAT). *Am J Hypertens* 1996; **9**: 342–60.

45. Dahlof B, Sever PS, Poulter NR, et al. The Anglo Scandinavian Cardiac Outcomes Trial (ASCOT). *Am J Hypertens* 1998; **11**: 9A.

46. Mann, Julius S. The Valsartan Antihypertensive Long-Term Use Evaluation trial (VALUE) of cardiovascular events in hypertension. Rationale and design. *Blood Pressure* 1998; **7**: 176–83.

18

Pharmacological treatment of hypertension in pregnant diabetic subjects

Joanna C Girling, Andrew H Shennan and Aidan WF Halligan

Introduction

Diabetes mellitus occurs in four per thousand women aged 20–40 years, and 80–90 per cent are treated with insulin.[1] However, at > 30 years of age and especially in non-Caucasian women the prevalence of type II diabetes rises greatly.[2] Therefore, although the average obstetric unit delivering 3000 babies each year might expect around 10 women with diabetes to deliver, in some areas where there is a high proportion of IndoAsian women, there may be considerably more.

Hypertension occurs in up to one-third of women with type I diabetes, and is frequently associated with nephropathy; it is more common in women who have long-standing diabetes.[3] Hypertension occurs in over one-half of white subjects with type II diabetes, but the prevalence is lower in other ethnic groups despite strong risk factors (for hypertension) such as obesity and severe insulin resistance. Therefore in pregnancy the combination of type II diabetes and hypertension is uncommon, as in general white women develop type II diabetes beyond the usual age for childbearing.[2] Hypertension also occurs in various endocrine conditions which are associated with diabetes, e.g. Cushing's syndrome, Conn's syndrome, phaeochromocytoma. Onset of these conditions is uncommon in pregnancy, but should be considered in the rare case of 'resistant' hypertension where ges-tational diabetes (GDM) has also developed. They will not be discussed further in this chapter. The management of hypertension in women with gestational diabetes will not be discussed separately, as in general it is no different from that of pregnant women without GDM.

Hypertension may accelerate both macrovascular and microvascular complications of diabetes.[4] Therefore the threshold for treating hypertension is lower in diabetes than in the non-diabetic population, and this philosophy should persist in pregnancy. However, there is no need to obtain a further decrement in blood pressure during pregnancy: physiological changes of pregnancy (see below) procure this, and there is some evidence that if blood pressure is too low perfusion of the uteroplacental bed may be impaired.[5]

Maternal physiological adaptations to pregnancy

There are significant physiological adaptations to pregnancy that influence both diabetes and hypertension. It is essential to understand these physiological changes of normal pregnancy in order to understand the problems of diabetic, hypertensive pregnancy.

Physiological changes in the cardiovascular system during normal pregnancy

Substantial cardiovascular changes occur in pregnancy.[6] They commence soon after conception and comprise an increased heart rate, increased cardiac output, increased stroke volume and decreased systemic vascular resistance.[6] There are also important changes in blood pressure (as measured using mercury sphygmomanometry) and Korotkoff phase IV reaches a nadir by 14 weeks' gestation, and which increases gradually towards prepregnancy levels from 24 to 28 weeks onwards.[7] More recently, 24-hour ambulatory blood pressure recording, using the Spacelabs 90207 device, which has been validated for use in pregnancy,[8] has confirmed a similar pattern of blood pressure change in normal primiparous pregnancy. However, it is likely that the nadir is reached as early as 9 weeks' gestation and that significant increases do not begin until 33 weeks gestation. Day-time systolic pressure falls by 3 mmHg and day-time diastolic pressure falls by 6 mmHg in the first and second trimester when compared with measurements taken 6 weeks postnatally.[9] Therefore changes in antihypertensive medication and assessment of 'baseline' blood pressure should be made accordingly.

Recently attention has been drawn to the numerous problems of mercury sphygmomanometry, including sampling error, digit preference, threshold avoidance, inadequate calibration and oxidation of mercury.[10] Doubt has also been expresssed about the use of Korotkoff phase IV (K4, muffling of the sound) (as recommended by the World Health Organization, International Society for the Study of Hypertension in Pregnancy, and British Hypertension Society) rather than Korotkoff phase V (K5, disappearance of the sound) for the measurement of diastolic blood pressure in pregnancy.[11] It is now clear that K5 is more reproducible during mercury sphygmomanometry than K4[11] and it should be adopted as the recommended sound for measuring diastolic blood pressure in pregnancy. However, there may also be inaccuracies if automated monitors that have not been validated in pregnancy are introduced.[12]

Physiological changes in renal function during normal pregnancy

During pregnancy, there is a marked increase in renal blood flow (by 60–100 per cent) and glomerular filtration rate (by 50 per cent) commencing soon after conception.[13] This results in a rise for creatinine clearance and a fall in plasma creatinine: a typical mean second trimester value for creatinine clearance is 154 ml/min, and for plasma creatinine 54 μmol/l.[14] This pregnancy-induced glomerular hyperfusion is probably due to increased glomerular flow without glomerular hypertension.

Tubular function is also altered, accounting in part for the increase in proteinuria found in normal pregnancy: albumin constitutes 10 per cent of total urinary protein excretion in pregnancy. Both these factors increase in the second half of pregnancy, when the upper limits of normal are 29 mg/24 h and 261 mg/24 h respectively (compared with 22 mg/24 h and 220 mg/24 h prior to 20 weeks gestation), but non-pregnant controls were not included.[15] A small increase in albuminuria and proteinuria is therefore likely in diabetic subjects, although this has not been extensively studied; changes during pregnancy in women with microalbuminuria or nephropathy are discussed later.

Physiological changes in glucose metabolism in normal pregnancy

Normal pregnancy is a diabetogenic state. The physiological changes provide a metabolic environment that allows maternal fat deposition early in pregnancy and optimises fetal growth later. Hormonal changes of pregnancy are important for modifying insulin action. Decreased insulin sensitivity occurs in normal pregnancy, resulting in an increased fasting insulin and a three-fold increase in the insulin responses to both oral and intravenous glucose.[16] By late pregnancy, insulin sensitivity is 45–70 per cent less than outside pregnancy, values being similar to those seen in type II diabetes.[17] The effect of this insulin resistance is an increase in synthesis of intact insulin (rather than biologically less active moieties such as proinsulin, or decreased insulin metabolism). In addition, marked islet beta cell hypertrophy and hyperplasia occur.[18]

There is therefore a fall in fasting glucose but a rise in postprandial glucose. This facilitates postprandial transfer of glucose to the fetus and enhances maternal fat deposition. These changes increase with advancing pregnancy and are thought to be under the influence of placental hormones such as human placental lactogen (HPL) and progesterone, and increased levels of the maternal hormones prolactin and cortisol. In addition, HPL has a lipolytic action which increases circulating free fatty acids, which themselves directly decrease insulin sensitivity, although this has only been investigated outside pregnancy.[19]

The cellular mechanisms of this decreased insulin sensitivity of pregnancy are unclear. Outside pregnancy, a major influence on insulin sensitivity is insulin-mediated glucose uptake in muscle.[20] However, in pregnancy, insulin binding to skeletal muscle[21] and to hepatocytes[22] is unaffected, although binding

to adipocytes is decreased;[23] therefore it is likely to be due to a post-receptor binding effect.[21]

However, the fall in fasting glucose that has occurred by 8 weeks' gestation predates these metabolic changes. It is thought to be due to increased renal clearance of glucose[24] and to decreased availability of gluconeogenic precursors such as alanine.[25] Later in pregnancy, haemodilution is an additional factor.

The postprandial increase in maternal glucose concentrations allows transfer to the fetus, a process named 'facilitated anabolism'.[26] The term 'accelerated starvation' has been used to describe the maternal adaptation to fasting hypoglycaemia which allows her to switch from glucose to fat catabolism: this is enhanced by the preferential deposition of nutrients as fat rather than glycogen, which is secondary to the lesser insulin resistance in adipose tissue compared with skeletal muscle (see above).

Effect of physiological changes of pregnancy on established diabetes and on hypertension

Glycaemic control

The dose of insulin required by women with type I diabetes increases 2–3-fold during pregnancy, reflecting the physiological changes of pregnancy. If they are able to achieve tight glucose control (fasting glucose < 5.5, postprandial < 7.5 mmol/l) the metabolic changes are likely to be similar to those in non-diabetic pregnancy.[27]

It is clear that this tight control is beneficial to the fetus in terms of reducing congenital anomaly[28] and spontaneous abortion[29] and minimising the incidence of accelerated fetal growth.[30] It is also important for minimising deterioration in retinopathy, although initial rapid reduction in maternal glucose may cause a reversible worsening.[31] However, there is little evidence that during pregnancy tight glycaemic control in established diabetes results in less hypertension or even, indirectly, in less deterioration in nephropathy (see below).

Hypertension

It is probable that the blood pressure of normotensive women with uncomplicated diabetes shows a similar pattern of change during pregnancy to that of non-diabetic normotensive women. It is also likely that hypertensive diabetic women can attain the same blood pressure changes as a normotensive woman.[32,33] However, a large study by Peterson et al.[27] has suggested conflicting results. They studied 312 women with diabetes and 356 women without diabetes from 5 weeks' gestation until the third trimester. The mean blood pressure readings, taken by mercury sphygmomanometry, were higher in the diabetic women than in the non-diabetic women, although the maximum difference between the means was only 8/5 mmHg, which is of questionable clinical significance. The diabetic women had a small, steady increase in systolic and diastolic blood pressure from 6 weeks' gestation, whereas the non-diabetic women showed the expected pattern of a fall until 20 weeks and then an increase from 28 weeks' gestation. However, the diabetic women included a significant subset whose pressor response to gestation was different from the rest of the group, as indicated by a widening standard deviation, from 8 mmHg at 5 weeks' gestation to 12 mmHg at term (for the mean arterial pressure). (In the control group the standard deviation remained 9 mmHg throughout pregnancy.) The aetiology of this is unclear, but presumably may reflect autonomic neuropathy, underlying microvascular disease or an increased propensity towards pre-eclampsia (see later). The study does not state whether the groups were of comparable parity, or how many were either hypertensive in early pregnancy or developed pre-eclampsia, or what diabetic complications the study group had, all factors that may have an important bearing on the blood pressure changes during pregnancy and therefore the interpretation of results. Neither is it clear that the data were normally distributed, despite the use of parametric statistical analysis.

Renal function

In diabetic pregnancy, similar changes in glomerular filtration rate to those in normal pregnancy are achieved.[34] However, in hypertensive diabetic pregnancy, poorly controlled hypertension may exacerbate the glomerular hyperfiltration of diabetes, particularly if renal autoregulation is impaired. Although it has been hypothesised that optimal blood pressure control may restrict glomerular damage, this is still not proven.

Diabetic women without microalbuminuria prior to pregnancy show the same small increase in proteinuria during pregnancy as non-diabetic women.[35] Diabetic women with pre-existing microalbuminuria show a greater proportional increase in albuminuria during pregnancy than their non-microalbuminuric counterparts, but in both groups it returns to normal postpartum.[36] However, although one-third of hypertensive women with diabetic nephropathy are able to increase their glomerular filtration rate during pregnancy, more than three-quarters of these women have a transient (but often dramatic) increase in proteinuria. There is no evidence that pregnancy hastens the long-term decline in renal function. One-third also developed new onset hypertension or worsening of pre-existing hypertension.[37]

Interaction between hypertension, diabetes and pregnancy

In pregnancy, diabetic women may have 'pregestational' hypertension, 'pregnancy-induced' hypertension or both; the former predisposes to the latter. There are two specific concerns in pregnancy in hypertensive diabetic women. First, the influence of pregnancy on hypertension and diabetes, and second, the effect of hypertension and diabetes on the fetus. These are discussed below.

Complications of pre-eclampsia
Cerebral haemorrhage
Eclampsia
Cortical blindness
HELLP syndrome
Hepatic rupture
Acute renal failure
Disseminated intravascular coagulopathy
Adult respiratory distress syndrome
Pulmonary oedema
Abruptio placentae
Fetal 'distress' or intrauterine death

Importance of hypertension in pregnancy

Pre-eclampsia (PET) is a major cause of maternal mortality in the UK.[38] It has been estimated to account for 50 per cent antenatal care beyond 20 weeks' gestation and up to 24 per cent of all antenatal admissions to hospital.[39] Furthermore, it is the commonest cause of iatrogenic prematurity, resulting in 23 per cent of very low birthweight singletons (as the ultimate 'treatment' of PET is delivery of the baby).[40] It may affect any maternal system, and complications include eclampsia, disseminated intravascular coagulopathy, liver haematoma, pulmonary oedema, etc. (see Box). The problems with placentation that are likely to underlie PET may result in intrauterine growth restriction, oligohydramnios, abnormal uteroplacental blood flow or placental abruption.[32]

The pathophysiology of pre-eclampsia is disputed. The placenta plays a central role in PET, and it is probable that poor placental perfusion is a unifying factor. However, neither the aetiology of this nor the way in which it causes the maternal syndrome are clear. Although poor second-wave trophoblast inva-

sion of the maternal spiral arteries early in the second trimester may be involved resulting in failure of their vasodilation,[41] this is not universally accepted.[42]

Maternal vascular endothelial damage is a possible underlying cause of the widespread maternal problems, resulting in platelet aggregation, activation of clotting cascades and reduced release of endothelial-derived vasodilators such as nitric oxide,[43] causing the widespread vasoconstriction which is typical of PET. The cause of the endothelial damage is disputed, but may involve placental release of a circulating factor[44] or an abnormal serum lipid profile with reduced antioxidant levels and increased free radical generation by the placenta,[45] or deported placental syncytiotrophoblast,[46] thereby linking with the theories which centralise the placenta.

It is not known why women with diabetes are at increased risk of pre-eclampsia. However, arachidonic acid metabolism is altered in diabetes, resulting in decreased prostacyclin synthesis and increased synthesis of thromboxane A2 by platelets.[47] These are also features of pre-eclampsia, and therefore it is possible that diabetes may in some way exacerbate the tendency towards pre-eclampsia.

Definitions of and terminology regarding pre-eclampsia

There is not a universally accepted definition for pre-eclampsia. Current definitions are based either on absolute thresholds, selected arbitrarily, or on an incremental rise of blood pressure from a baseline determined in the first half of pregnancy.[48,49] The physiological changes that occur during normal pregnancy (see above) further confound these definitions.

As blood pressure is a continuum, it is a somewhat arbitrary concept that a single cut-off point can distinguish between normal and abnormal values, particularly as blood pressure varies with gestation. Indeed, data from Oxford show that before the onset of labour, > 20 per cent of a large unselected obstetric population have had a blood pressure recording ≥140/90, which is one of the commonly used defining levels, although the majority are not at any increased risk.[32] However, intervention when a threshold is breached may result in iatrogenic morbidity in association with, for example, induction of labour, Caesarean section or prematurity.

Neither is there agreement about the best terminology relating to hypertensive problems in pregnancy. The term pre-eclampsia usually signifies a multisystem disorder of the second half of pregnancy which is characterised by hypertension and usually either proteinuria, intrauterine growth restriction or suggestion of involvement of any of the other body systems (Box and Table 18.1) which resolves following delivery. Redman and Jefferies use the term 'pre-eclampsia' when both a threshold of blood pressure and an incremental rise from a baseline in the first half of pregnancy have been reached,[48] implying that proteinuria is not essential for the diagnosis. The term 'pregnancy-induced hypertension' is sometimes used to signify hypertension without proteinuria.[50] The International Society for the Study of Hypertension in Pregnancy (ISSHP), which has adopted the recommendations of Davey and MacGillivray,[51] uses the term 'gestational hypertension' to refer to all pregnant hypertensive women whether proteinuric or not who have been previously normotensive and non-proteinuric. If women with gestational hypertension are proteinuric then this is assumed to be pre-eclampsia until proved otherwise. Subdivisions according to whether the hypertension occurs in the antenatal period, in labour or in the puerperium are also specified in the ISSHP classification, as time of presentation may have very different prognostic significance and management implications. Chronic hypertension is defined as raised blood pressure prior to 20 weeks' gestation; if proteinuria develops it is said to be 'superimposed pre-eclampsia'. A further category of 'unclassified hypertension' is used when the clinical scenario does not allow a clear distinction between chronic and gestational hypertension. Patients in this category can be retrospectively allocated to the correct group in the postpartum period.

The National High Blood Pressure Education Program Working Group (NHBPEPWG) Report on High Blood Pressure in Pregnancy defines a woman as having pre-eclampsia when a given blood pressure threshold is met or an incremental rise has occurred[49] (see below). Proteinuria is said to 'bolster' the diagnosis, but is not an absolute requirement for the diagnosis. In order to have pre-eclampsia superimposed on a diagnosis of chronic hypertension (i.e. raised blood pressure before 20 weeks), a rise of blood pressure

	Davey and MacGillivray[51]	Redman and Jefferies[48]	NHBPEPWG*[49]
Endorsed by	ISSHP WHO	–	ACOG
Proteinuria	Yes	No	'Bolsters' the diagnosis
Systolic/diastolic	Diastolic	Diastolic	Either
Threshold	90 mmHg (110 mmHg × 1)	90 mmHg *and* incremental rise	140 mmHg systolic *or* 90 mmHg diastolic *or* incremental rise
Severe hypertension	110 mmHg (×2) 120 mmHg (×1)	–	160 mmHg systolic, 110 mmHg diastolic
Number of measurements	Confirm (≥4 h)	One	Average of two
Korotkoff sound	Phase IV	Phase IV	Phase I & V
Incremental rise	No	25 mmHg	30 mmHg systolic *or* 15 mmHg diastolic
Baseline	N/A	Initial measure	Average before 20 weeks
Superimposed pre-eclampsia	Chronic HT + proteinuria	–	Chronic HT + 30/15 mmHg rise + proteinuria *or* oedema

Table 18.1
Comparison of different systems for defining pre-eclampsia.

of 30 mmHg systolic or 15 mmHg diastolic should occur, together with the appearance of either proteinuria or oedema. 'Transient hypertension' is used to signify isolated hypertension in someone who has not previously been hypertensive (Table 18.1).

Diabetes and pre-eclampsia

Women with chronic hypertension of any aetiology have an increased risk of developing pre-eclampsia, as do those in their first pregnancy, the obese and women with a strong family or personal history of the disease.[32] In women with diabetes, with or without hypertension, the incidence of pre-eclampsia is increased. In a large Canadian study, with clear definitions of pre-eclampsia and stringent attempts to differentiate chronic hypertension and nephropathy from pre-eclampsia, the incidence of pre-eclampsia was 4.3 per cent in non-diabetic controls, 8.9 per cent in diabetic women without chronic hypertension or nephropathy, and 30 per cent in women classified as White class D, F and R.[52] Perinatal mortality was greatly increased in the presence of pre-eclampsia, reaching 60 per 1000 births for women with diabetes and pre-eclampsia, compared with 3.3 per 1000 births for normotensive diabetic pregnancies; all deaths were associated with prematurity, with pre-eclampsia occurring in the late second trimester. Maternal morbidity was not discussed.

Attempts to predict which diabetic women will develop pre-eclampsia have been as fruitless as those in non-diabetic subjects. Prepregnancy albumin excretion, parity and second trimester blood pressure were independently associated with the development of pre-eclampsia in diabetic women, although an unconventional definition of PET was used and parity had an unusual classification.[53] These results are not surprising, as they are well established risk factors for the development of pre-eclampsia. Attempts in this study to provide clinically useful cut-off points for each parameter were unsuccessful.

Differentiation between pre-eclampsia and pre-gestational hypertension

Women with diabetes may have hypertension which predates the pregnancy, and this may occur in conjunction with nephropathy. Alternatively, or in addition, they may have pregnancy-induced hypertension or pre-eclampsia, and indeed are at increased risk of this compared with non-diabetic and normotensive women.

The clinical differentiation of worsening hypertension with or without nephropathy from superimposed pre-eclampsia is difficult, as both are associated with increasing blood pressure and proteinuria, intrauterine growth restriction and deteriorating blood markers of renal impairment. A low platelet count ($< 100 \times 10^9$/l), signs of disseminated intravascular coagulopathy abnormal liver function tests support the diagnosis of pre-eclampsia. Conversely, the absence of uterine artery waveform abnormalities (such as a 'notch' or high resistance) at 20–24 weeks' gestation has a high (97 per cent) negative predictive value for pre-eclampsia, and makes worsening of nephropathy a more likely diagnosis. Unfortunately, however, the positive predictive value for severe pre-eclampsia is only 6 per cent (Fig. 18.1, Table 18.2).[54] Ultimately, however, delivery of the baby may be required in both scenarios because of either fetal compromise or deteriorating maternal condition.

Influence of glycaemic control on hypertension during diabetic pregnancy

Only one randomised study has addressed the issue of the benefits of tight glycaemic control on any aspects of outcome in diabetic

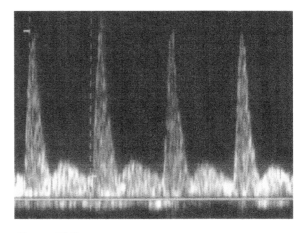

Figure 18.1
Uterine artery Doppler at 20 weeks' gestation showing presence of a 'notch'.

Maternal investigations	Fetal investigations
Full blood count (platelet, film)	Cardiotocograph
Clotting screen	Ultrasound (liquor volume, fetal size)
Creatinine	Umbilical artery Doppler
Urate	
Liver enzymes	
Mid-stream urine	
24-hour urine collection for protein quantification	
Uterine artery Doppler	

Table 18.2
Investigations in suspected pre-eclampsia.

pregnancy;[55] none have specifically addressed the effect of glycaemic control on blood pressure. Sixty women with type I diabetes were randomly allocated in the first trimester to one of three groups: very tight, tight or moderate glucose control (daily mean blood glucose < 5.6 mmol/l, 5.6–6.7 mmol/l, 6.7–8.9 mmol/l respectively). It is not clear whether the groups were comparable in terms of obstetric and diabetic risk factors for adverse outcome nor whether their carers were blinded to their group allocation, although the latter seems unlikely. The 'moderate control' group had bigger babies, a higher Caesarean section rate and more neonatal respiratory distress syndrome, but less maternal hypoglycaemia. Only four women in the study developed hypertension, and this was not influenced by diabetic control. Four other women developed pre-eclampsia, one in the 'very tight' group and three in the 'moderate' group, producing the unsatisfactory 'conclusion' that 'moderate' control results in significantly more pre-eclampsia than 'tight' control, but not 'very tight' control. Neither hypertension nor pre-eclampsia are clearly defined in this study.[55] It

is not justified from these data to establish (or refute) a link between glycaemic control and hypertension.

There are some data from observational studies to suggest that glycaemic control might influence the development of hypertension in diabetic pregnancy. Siddiqi et al. prospectively studied 175 women with type I diabetes: 23 of 175 (13%) women developed pregnancy-induced hypertension and 20 per cent of those with pre-existing hypertension developed superimposed pregnancy-induced hypertension, compared with 5.6 per cent of the general obstetric population.[56] This was associated with nulliparity, more severe White classification, higher mean preprandial glucose values in the first trimester and higher glycohaemoglobin concentrations at 14 and 20 weeks' gestation. The authors hypothesise that hyperglycaemia in the first trimester adversely influences the development of the placenta. However, others have found conflicting evidence: Leveno et al. suggested that hypertension was associated with poor glycaemic control prior to delivery[57] and Martin et al.[58] and Garner et al.[52] found no correlation with diabetic control. The Diabetes Control and Complications Trial Research Group briefly alluded to the development of pre-eclampsia: they found the same incidence in women with conventional or intensive control prior to conception.[59]

Pharmacological management of hypertension in diabetic pregnancy

In practice, all commonly used antihypertensive agents are probably safe during the period of conception, and therefore changes in treatment can be instituted once the woman is pregnant. It is important that she reports early in pregnancy so that this can be carried out. Some women will not need antihypertensive treatment during the first half of pregnancy, because of the physiological decline in blood pressure which occurs then (see above). Blood pressure should be measured fortnightly, and treatment only (re)-instituted when readings are greater than 135/85.

When considering treatment for use in pregnancy, ideally we should know whether a drug can cross the placenta, whether it is teratogenic and whether the immature fetal renal and hepatic systems will be able to metabolise and excrete it effectively. The effect on the uteroplacental circulation is also important, as hypoperfusion may be associated with significant adverse fetal effects. In practice, the answers to many of these questions are not known, and therefore, caution is required when prescribing for a pregnant woman. The first-line choice of treatment for chronic hypertension is usually methyldopa, with second-line agents being nifedipine, labetolol or hydralazine. Rapid control of severe hypertension may be required if fulminating pre-eclampsia becomes superimposed on chronic

hypertension: this is usually achieved with either oral nifedipine, intravenous hydralazine or intravenous labetolol (see below): each obstetric unit should have an agreed policy for the management of this situation.

If the pregnancy has been complicated by pre-eclampsia, blood pressure should be monitored closely in the first few days after delivery, as it sometimes rises during this time before it begins to return to the prepregnant level. It may take up to 3 months until blood pressure has completely reached normal readings; during this time, women who are usually normotensive may require treatment, and those who have established hypertension may require additional treatment. Pre-eclampsia does not cause, or worsen, chronic hypertension: blood pressure which requires long-term treatment after pregnancy represents either coincidental new onset hypertension or the medical recognition of a long-standing problem.

Methyldopa

Methyldopa is the first choice oral antihypertensive agent for chronic control of hypertension in pregnancy. It is a centrally acting antihypertensive and has received the most detailed investigation in pregnancy of all antihypertensive drugs. It crosses the placenta and concentrations in umbilical cord blood are similar to those in the maternal circulation,[60] but this has not been shown to have any adverse clinical effects. Treatment between 16 and 20 weeks' gestation causes an insignificant reduction in neonatal head circumference. Neonates have also been found to have a small insignificant reduction in systolic blood pressure.[61] Extensive follow-up of these children has failed to reveal any significant action, and this includes development assessment of the offspring to the age of 7 years.[62,63] No other adverse effects have been found.

The maximum dose is 3 g taken in three or

four divided doses. Most women feel tired when they commence it, and some may feel depressed, reflecting its action as a central nervous system depressant; it has no major maternal side-effects. However, because of these effects, it should be stopped after delivery and substituted with the antihypertensive agent used prior to pregnancy.

Angiotensin-converting enzyme (ACE) inhibitors

Prepregnancy advice is essential for all women with diabetes, in order to optimise their glycaemic control and therefore minimise the risk of congenital abnormality or miscarriage.[64] In addition, for women with pre-existing hypertension it is an important time to discuss management of blood pressure control. The majority of women will be taking ACE inhibitors. Although there have been case reports of teratogenicity in association with these compounds,[65] it is generally believed that they are not harmful in early pregnancy.[66] However, they are associated with oligohydramnios and fetal renal impairment if taken later in pregnancy.[67] Therefore, diabetic women should discontinue treatment with these agents as soon as they know they are pregnant. Although ACE inhibitors also have an important role in slowing the deterioration of diabetic nephropathy, their cessation for 9 months of pregnancy is unlikely to have an important effect in this respect. They may be taken during lactation.

Nifedipine

Nifedipine is a dihydropyridine calcium blocker. Its major effect is to cause a reduction in systemic and pulmonary vascular resistance; it does not affect venous beds, including the uteroplacental circulation; it does not affect umbilical circulation.[68] It also reduces the amplitude and frequency of myometrial con-

tractions and reduces the basal tone, making it an effective tocolytic agent.[69] Nifedipine does cross the placenta and into breast milk, but in greatly lower concentrations than in the mother.[70] It is not teratogenic, and may be taken when breastfeeding.[71]

The sustained release (rather than the immediate release) preparation should be used for chronic administration in hypertensive pregnancy: although its peak concentration is lower and clearance faster than in non-pregnant or normotensive women, it is the most likely of the two formulations to provide antihypertensive treatment throughout the 24-hour period.[70] It is frequently used as a second-line agent in the control of hypertension in pregnancy. The immediate release form is useful for urgent control of severe hypertension, and should usually be taken orally rather than sublingually: the latter may be associated with such a profound drop in blood pressure that significant maternal and fetal side effects occur.[72]

Hydralazine

Hydralazine works directly on the intact endothelium of the blood vessel, to cause vasodilatation. In pregnancy it is sometimes used as a second- or third-line agent for chronic control of hypertension. However, it is most frequently used intravenously for urgent control of severe hypertension (e.g. mean arterial pressure > 140 mmHg for 15 min, or MAP > 125 mmHg for 45 min), and is the recommended treatment in this scenario.[73] It may be associated with maternal tachycardia, flushing, tremors or nausea. It may also cause reduced placental perfusion[74] and fetal distress,[75] probably because of increased resistance in the uterine vessels.

A typical and widely used regime is shown (Fig. 18.2) [adapted from ref 76]. It is important that, if undelivered, the maternal circula-

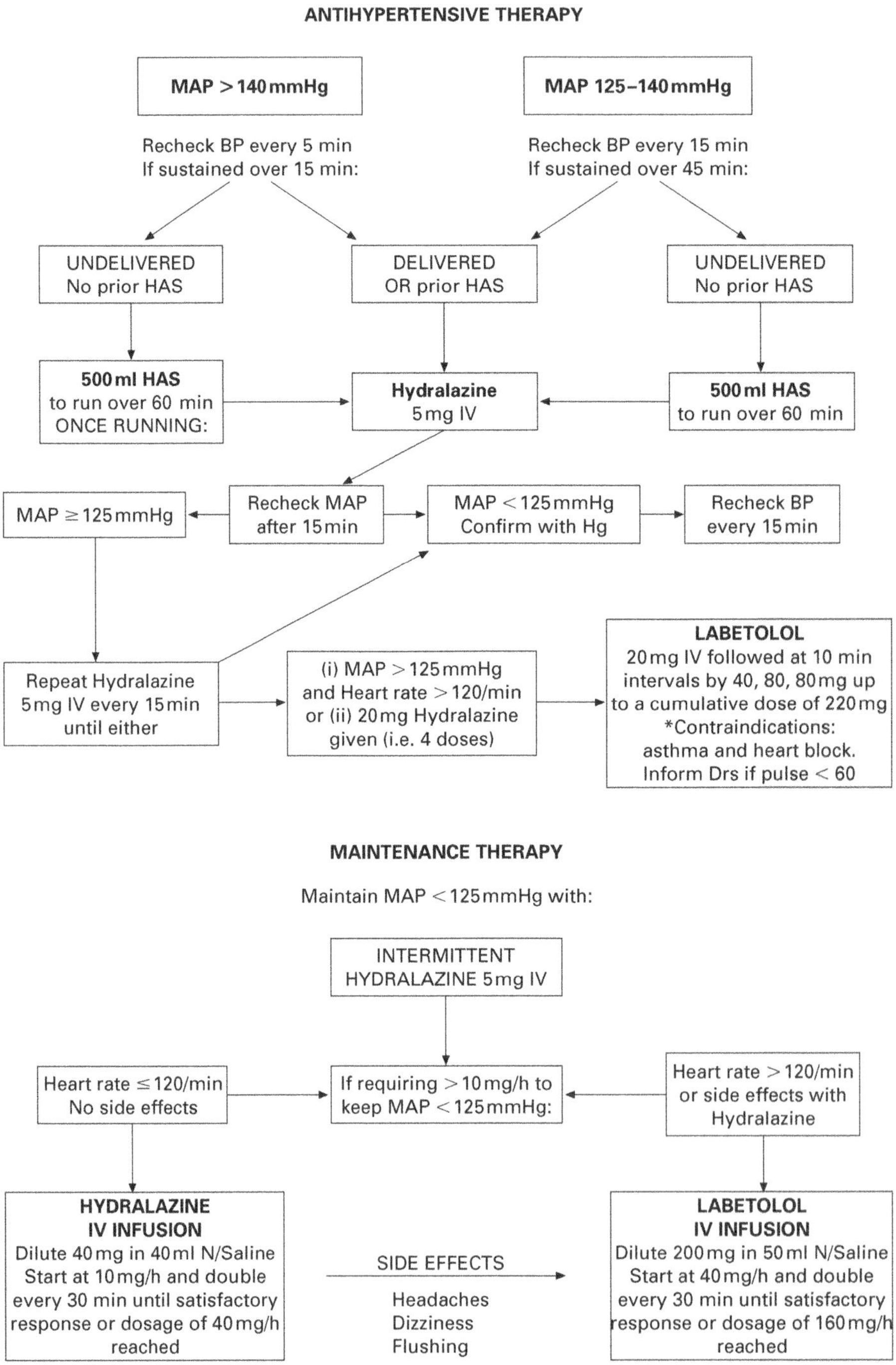

ANTIHYPERTENSIVE THERAPY

MAP > 140 mmHg	MAP 125–140 mmHg

Recheck BP every 5 min
If sustained over 15 min:

Recheck BP every 15 min
If sustained over 45 min:

UNDELIVERED No prior HAS	DELIVERED OR prior HAS	UNDELIVERED No prior HAS

500 ml HAS to run over 60 min ONCE RUNNING:

Hydralazine 5 mg IV

500 ml HAS to run over 60 min

MAP ≥ 125 mmHg

Recheck MAP after 15 min

MAP < 125 mmHg Confirm with Hg

Recheck BP every 15 min

Repeat Hydralazine 5 mg IV every 15 min until either

(i) MAP > 125 mmHg and Heart rate > 120/min or (ii) 20 mg Hydralazine given (i.e. 4 doses)

LABETOLOL
20 mg IV followed at 10 min intervals by 40, 80, 80 mg up to a cumulative dose of 220 mg
*Contraindications: asthma and heart block. Inform Drs if pulse < 60

MAINTENANCE THERAPY

Maintain MAP < 125 mmHg with:

INTERMITTENT HYDRALAZINE 5 mg IV

Heart rate ≤ 120/min No side effects

If requiring > 10 mg/h to keep MAP < 125 mmHg:

Heart rate > 120/min or side effects with Hydralazine

HYDRALAZINE IV INFUSION
Dilute 40 mg in 40 ml N/Saline Start at 10 mg/h and double every 30 min until satisfactory response or dosage of 40 mg/h reached

SIDE EFFECTS

Headaches
Dizziness
Flushing

LABETOLOL IV INFUSION
Dilute 200 mg in 50 ml N/Saline Start at 40 mg/h and double every 30 min until satisfactory response or dosage of 160 mg/h reached

Figure 18.2
Pharmacological management of severe hypertension in pregnancy.

tion is increased with colloid prior to giving hydralazine, to minimise the effects of hypoperfusion on the fetus. Intermittent boluses of 5 mg hydralazine are given, to a maximum dose of 20 mg until blood pressure control is achieved. This is followed by further boluses as required, or if >10 mg/h is used, by a continuous infusion of hydralazine. If hydralazine is not successful in controlling blood pressure, boluses or an infusion of labetolol are added.

Labetolol

Labetolol is both an alpha-1-adrenoreceptor blocker and a weak, non-selective beta-adrenoreceptor blocker (the latter being four times less potent than propranolol). Its main action is by peripheral vasodilatation. It does not compromise the maternal circulation and is able to maintain renal and uterine perfusion.[77] It is usually used as second-line therapy. For long-term control, it is given orally, to a maximum dose of 2.4 g. For rapid control of severe hypertension it is given as either intravenous boluses of 20 mg to a maximum dose of 220 mg, or as an intravenous infusion with a maximum dose of 160 mg/h.

Other antihypertensive agents

The choice of additional medication is largely dictated by consideration of fetal well-being. Although third- or even fourth-line agents may occasionally be used, if hypertension is proving so difficult to control, serious consideration is usually given to the other risk factors relating to the pregnancy, with a view to recommending delivery (or occasionally termination of the pregnancy if it is still at an early gestation).

Many commonly used antihypertensive agents are avoided in pregnancy, although they are only relative contraindicated. There is evidence that beta-blocking agents may cause a significant reduction in weight centile at birth if taken in the first half of pregnancy.[78] The cause of this is unclear, but may be due to prolonged exposure to atenolol during the time of placental development which may affect placental physiology. This is not convincingly borne out by changes in Doppler waveform indices.[79,80] Atenolol in the third trimester is more effective than placebo at controlling blood pressure and was associated with a lower incidence of severe respiratory distress syndrome. It was not associated with an earlier gestation at delivery or a reduction in birthweight.[78] Therefore beta-blockers may be considered for use in the third trimester.

Although diuretics may be used to control hypertension in pregnancy, they are generally avoided in case pre-eclampsia supervenes: PET is a situation of intravascular depletion, which diuretics may exacerbate. However, neither diuretics nor beta-blocking agents are likely to be first choice for management of hypertension in a woman with diabetes.

Second-line agents if methyldopa is insufficient are usually nifedipine followed by either hydralazine or labetolol.[32]

Prevention of pre-eclampsia

In view of the diagnostic difficulties relating to pre-eclampsia, the limited treatment options and the potentially devastating effects it may have for the mother or baby, many attempts have been made to prevent it. Prevention would be especially valuable in hypertensive diabetic women for whom pregnancy may be particularly complicated. A wide range of prophylactic measures have been suggested, including fish liver oils, calcium supplementation and low dose aspirin (approximately 75 mg daily). Only the latter has been subjected to large, well-organised and double-blind randomised studies, meta-analysis of which suggests that aspirin may reduce the incidence of PET by 22 per cent.[81] It therefore has a role in the prevention of PET in women who are at increased risk, including diabetic hypertensive women. It is also clearly safe to take throughout pregnancy: it does not have adverse fetal or maternal effects. These women should commence it as soon as they know they are pregnant.

Monitoring the hypertensive diabetic woman throughout pregnancy

In addition to good glycaemic control, these women should have their blood pressure monitored carefully (either weekly or every 2 weeks), especially in the second half of the pregnancy. A rise in blood pressure may be physiological or due to superimposed pre-eclampsia.

These patients should have a uterine artery Doppler assessment at 20 weeks' gestation and fetal growth scans from 26 weeks' gestation. In the absence of diabetic nephropathy, they should test their urine at home on a daily basis, as detection of proteinuria may signify the development of pre-eclampsia. 'Baseline' bloods for pre-eclampsia should be performed (Table 18.2).

Preterm delivery of hypertensive diabetic women

These women are at increased risk of preterm delivery, on both fetal and material grounds. If delivery is necessary prior to 34 weeks' gestation, advanced neonatal care facilities may be needed and provision should be made for transfer to an appropriate centre if this is not available locally. One of the major concerns relating to such early delivery is the develop-

ment of neonatal respiratory distress syndrome (RDS), in association with insufficient fetal surfactant production. This may be more prominent in diabetic pregnancies than non-diabetic pregnancies, particularly if glycaemic control is poor.[82] The pathogenesis has been postulated to be due to fetal hyperinsulinaemia inhibiting the synthesis of the phospholipid component of surfactant,[83] although this theory is not universally accepted.[84]

It is clearly established that maternal treatment with steroids which are able to cross the placenta improves fetal lung maturity and reduces the incidence of RDS by half: typically two doses of dexamethasone 12 mg intramuscularly 12 h or 24 h apart are given.[85] For women with diabetes, this is associated with a considerable, but temporary, increase in insulin requirements, which may require additional boluses of short-acting insulin.

It is not uncommon for steroids to be given in combination with tocolysis. If beta-sympathomimetics such as ritodrine or salbutamol are used there is a significant increase in insulin requirements, due to their synergistic effect on hepatic glycogenolysis and insulin resistance. Diabetic ketoacidosis may be precipitated if appropriate changes to the insulin regimen are not instituted.[86] Pregnancy-induced lipolysis already makes the diabetic woman more susceptible to diabetic ketoacidosis, which can develop quickly and at relatively low levels of hyperglycaemia;[87] if untreated it is associated with high fetal loss[88] and maternal morbidity. Rarely, pulmonary oedema may be precipitated or even myocardial ischaemia in the presence of coronary artery disease (which although unusual in a hypertensive diabetic woman of childbearing age should be considered). When possible therefore, this combination of steroids and beta-sympathomimetics should be avoided in diabetic women. However, a number of obstetric scenarios will warrant it, in order to optimise neonatal outcome. Women should be changed to a sliding scale of intravenous short-acting insulin, titrated against hourly capillary measurements of glucose.

Hypertension and retinopathy in diabetic pregnancy

In a prospective study of diabetic women, raised diastolic blood pressure had a greater effect on progression of retinopathy in the pregnant group than the non-pregnant group.[89] In another prospective study, both pregnancy-induced hypertension and chronic hypertension were each independently associated with progression of retinopathy during pregnancy.[90] However, as yet there is no evidence to suggest whether tighter control of blood pressure is able to ameliorate pregnancy-induced changes in retinopathy.

Conversely, the possibility that proliferative retinopathy prior to pregnancy is associated with the onset of pre-eclampsia has been made. Price et al.[91] reviewed 31 pregnancies in 23 women: no cases of pre-eclampsia occurred in 14 pregnancies without retinopathy; but pre-eclampsia occurred in one of 10 pregnancies with background retinopathy and five of seven pregnancies with proliferative retinopathy. Unfortunately this retrospective survey did not define pre-eclampsia, or describe other diabetic (such as pre-existing hypertension or nephropathy) or obstetric risk factors for pre-eclampsia (parity, previous history of pre-eclampsia, etc.). It is most likely that advanced retinopathy is associated with other risk factors for pre-eclampsia rather than being itself a predisposing factor.

Hypertensive diabetic women with nephropathy

The prognoses for the mother and baby are poorer in the presence of chronic renal disease than when diabetes and hypertension occur alone.

Data from studies of chronic renal disease in general rather than diabetic renal disease specifically, suggest that plasma creatinine is a helpful marker for determining pregnancy outcome. Thus if plasma creatinine in the first trimester is $< 125 \, \mu mol/l$, one-quarter of women will experience some problems in pregnancy, but > 90 per cent will have successful pregnancy outcomes and very few will have long-term deterioration in their renal function. However, if the creatinine is $> 250 \, \mu mol/l$, then < 50 per cent have a successful outcome, and > 50 per cent will have long term deterioration in their renal function; most will experience problems during pregnancy.[14] When chronic renal disease is combined with hypertension, the outcome is even worse. In another study of chronic renal disease, the risk of intrauterine growth restriction was increased five-fold, of pre-term delivery was doubled and of renal deterioration increased five-fold in hypertensive rather than normotensive women.[92]

Meta-analysis of the specific effects of diabetic nephropathy on pregnancy suggest that, even in the presence of preserved renal function, both fetal and maternal outcome are worse when compared with non-diabetic glomerular disease.[93] By late pregnancy, > 75 per cent of women had diastolic hypertension (diastolic $> 90 \, mmHg$). Worryingly, > 50 per cent of women experienced accelerating hypertension and in > 35 per cent there was a temporary decline in renal function. Intrauterine growth restriction (IUGR) occurs in almost 50 per cent of pregnancies where both accelerated hypertension and impaired renal function occur, in 15 per cent where either occur and in only 5 per cent where neither are present. It is hoped, but not proven, that control of hypertension may reduce the occurrence of IUGR. Preterm delivery occurs in almost one-third of diabetic women with nephropathy, and in 50 per cent of cases this is due to hypertension, either accelerated or due to pre-eclampsia. Accelerated hypertension remains difficult to distinguish from pre-eclampsia (see above).

Ultimately, the decision to deliver the baby must be individualised, depending upon the perceived balance of fetal well-being *in utero* against prematurity *ex utero*, and the likely effect of delivery on modifying the maternal disease: experienced obstetricians with an interest in maternal medicine should be closely involved in this decision-making process.

Although it is difficult to be proscriptive regarding the safety of embarking on a pregnancy, diabetic women with significant hypertension and renal dysfunction should think very carefully before doing so; for some, pregnancy would be an inadvisable course of action.

Conclusion

Hypertension in diabetic pregnancy has a number of important implications for the mother and baby. There is an increased risk of pre-eclampsia, intrauterine growth restriction, perinatal mortality, temporary deterioration in nephropathy and possibly a reversible progression in retinopathy. Although the goals of blood pressure control in pregnancy are similar in the non-pregnant situation, the anti-hypertensive agents used are different.

The management of hypertensive diabetic pregnant women is complex, because of the additional physiological burden of pregnancy and because of the conflict which sometimes arises with the needs of the second patient, the fetus. It requires the combined expertise of a physician and an obstetrician with an interest in the field.

References

1. Neill HAW, Gatling W, Mather HM, et al. The Oxford Community Diabetes Study: evidence for an increase in the prevalence of known diabetes in Great Britain. *Diabetes Med* 1987; **4**: 539–43.

2. Mather HM, Keen H. The Southall diabetes survey: prevalence of known diabetes in Asians and Europeans. *BMJ* 1985; **291**: 1081–4.

3. Microalbuminuria Collaborative Study Group. Risk factors for the development of microalbuminuria in insulin dependent diabetic patients: a cohort study. *BMJ* 1993; **306**: 1235–9.

4. Stamler JS, Vaccaro O, Neaton JD, et al. Diabetes, other risk factors and 12 year cardiovascular mortality for men screened in the Multiple Risk Factor Intervention Trial. *Diabetes Care* 1993; **16**: 434–44.

5. Greiss FC. Pressure-flow relationship in the gravid uterine vascular bed. *Am J Obstet Gynecol* 1966; **96**: 41–7.

6. Robson SC, Hunter S, Bvoys RJ, Dunlop W. Serial study in the factors influencing changes in cardiac output during human pregnancy. *Am J Physiol* 1989; **256**: H1060–5.

7. MacGillivray I, Rose GA, Rowe B. Blood pressure survey in pregnancy. *Clin Sci* 1969; **37**: 395–407.

8. Shennan AH, Kissane J, de Swiet M. Validation of the SpaceLabs 90207 ambulatory blood pressure monitor for use in pregnancy. *Br J Obstet Gynaecol* 1993; **100**: 904–8.

9. Halligan A, O'Brien E, O'Malley K, et al. Twenty-four-hour ambulatory blood pressure measurement in a primigravid population. *J Hypertens* 1993; **11**: 869–73.

10. Shennan AH, Halligan AWF. Blood pressure in pregnancy: room for improvement. *Mat Child Health* 1996; **21**: 55–9.

11. Shennan AH, Gupta M, Halligan A, Taylor DJ, de Swiet M. Lack of reproducibility in pregnancy of Korotkoff phase IV as measured by mercury sphygmomanometry. *Lancet* 1996; **347**: 139–42.

12. Gupta M, Shennan AH, Halligan A, Taylor DJ, de Swiet M. Accuracy of oscillometric blood pressure monitoring in pregnancy and pre-eclampsia. *Br J Obstet Gynaecol* 1997; **104**: 350–5.

13. Dunlop W. Serial changes in renal haemodynamics during normal human pregnancy. *Br J Obstet Gynaecol* 1981; **88**: 1–9.

14. Davison J, Baylis C. Renal disease. In: de Swiet M, ed. *Medical disorders in obstetric practice*, 2nd edn. Oxford, Blackwell Science, 1995.

15. Higby K, Suiter CR, Phelps JY, Siler-Khodr T, Langer O. Normal values of urinary albumin and total protein excretion during pregnancy. *Am J Obstet Gynecol* 1994; **171**: 984–9.

16. Buchanan TA, Metzger BE, Freinkel N, Berman RN. Insulin sensitivity and beta-cell responsiveness to glucose during late pregnancy in lean and moderately obese women with normal glucose tolerance or mild gestational diabetes. *Am J Obstet Gynecol* 1990; **162**: 1008–14.

17. Kuhl C. Insulin secretion and insulin resistance in pregnancy and gestational diabetes. Implications for diagnosis and management. *Diabetes* 1991; **40** (Suppl 2): 18–24.

18. Van Assche FA, Aerts L, de Prins F. A morphological study of the endocrine pancreas in human pregnancy. *Br J Obstet Gynaecol* 1978; **85**: 818–20.

19. Bonadonna RC, Groop LC, Simonson DC, DeFronzo RA. Free fatty acid and glucose metabolism in human aging: evidence for operation of the Randle cycle. *Am J Physiol* 1994; **266**: 501–9.

20. DeFronzo RA. Lilly Lecture 1987. The triumvirate: beta cell, muscle, liver: a collusion responsible for non insulin dependent diabetes. *Diabetes* 1988; **37**: 667–87.

21. Damm P, Handberg A, Kuhl C, et al. Insulin receptor binding and tyrosine kinase activity in skeletal muscle from normal pregnant women and women with gestational diabetes. *Obstet Gynecol* 1993; **82**: 251–9.

22. Davidson M. Insulin resistance of late pregnancy does not include the liver. *Metabolism*

1984; **33**: 532–7.

23. Ciraldi TP, Kettel M, El-Roiey A, et al. Mechanisms of cellular insulin resistance in human pregnancy. *Am J Obstet Gynecol* 1994; **170**: 635–41.

24. Lind T. Metabolic changes in pregnancy relevant to diabetes mellitus. *Postgrad Med J* 1979; **55**: 353–7.

25. Metzger BE, Agnoli FS, Hare JW, Freinkel N. Carbohydrate metabolism and pregnancy. X Metabolic disposition of alanine by the perfused liver of the fasting pregnant rat. *Diabetes* 1973; **22**: 601–12.

26. Freinkel N. Banting Lecture 1980: of pregnancy and progeny. *Diabetes* 1980; **29**: 1023–35.

27. Peterson CM, Jovanovic-Peterson L, Mills JL, et al. The diabetes in early pregnancy study: changes in cholesterol, triglycerides, body weight and blood pressure. *Am J Obstet Gynecol* 1992; **166**: 513–78.

28. Rosenn M, Miodovnik M, Combs CA, Khoury J, Siddiqi T. Glycemic thresholds for spontaneous abortion and congenital malformations in insulin-dependent diabetes mellitus. *Obstet Gynecol* 1994; **1994**: 515–20.

29. Dicker D, Feldberg D, Samuel N, et al. Spontaneous abortion in patients with insulin-dependent diabetes mellitus: the effect of preconceptional diabetic control. *Am J Obstet Gynecol* 1988; **158**: 1161–4.

30. Schwartz R, Gruppuso PA, Petzold K, et al. Hyperinsulinemia and macrosomia in the fetus of the diabetic mother. *Diabetes Care* 1994; **17**: 640–8.

31. Chew EY, Mills JL, Metzger BE, et al. Metabolic control and progression of retinopathy. *Diabetes Care* 1995; **18**: 631–7.

32. Redman CWG. Hypertension in pregnancy. In: de Swiet M, ed. *Medical disorders in obstetric practice*, 2nd edn. Oxford, Blackwell Science, 1995.

33. Wallenburg HCS. Hemodynamics in hypertensive pregnancy. In: Ruben PC, ed. *Hypertension in pregnancy*. Amsterdam, Elsevier, 1988: 66–101.

34. Krutzen E, Olofsson P, Back SE, Nilsson-Ehle P. Glomerular filtration rate in pregnancy: a study in normal subjects and in patients with hypertension, pre eclampsia and diabetes.

Scand J Clin Invest 1992; **52**: 387–92.

35. McCance DR, Traub AI, Harley JMG. Urinary albumin excretion in diabetic pregnancy. *Diabetologia* 1989; **32**: 236–9.

36. Biesenbach G, Zazgornik J, Stoger H, et al. Abnormal increases in urinary albumin excretion during pregnancy in IDDM women with pre existing microalbuminuria. *Diabetologia* 1994; **37**: 905–10.

37. Reece EA, Winn HN, Hayslett JP, Coulehan J, Wan M, Hobbins JC. Does pregnancy alter the rate of progression of diabetic nephropathy? *Am J Perinatol* 1990; **7**: 193–7.

38. HMSO Report on Confidential Enquiries into Maternal Deaths in the United Kingdom 1991–1993. London, HMSO, 1996.

39. Rosenberg K, Twaddle S. Screening and surveillance of pregnancy hypertension – an economic approach to the use of day care. *Baillieres Clin Obstet Gynaecol* 1990; **4**: 89–107.

40. Ales KL, Frayer W, Hawk G, Auld PMcF, Druzin ML. Development and validation of a multivariance predictor of mortality in very low birthweight. *J Clin Epidemiol* 1988; **41**: 1095–103.

41. Khong TY, De Wolf F, Robertson WB, Brosens I. Inadequate maternal vascular response to placentation in pregnancies complicated by pre-eclampsia and by small-for-gestational age infants. *Br J Obstet Gynaecol* 1986; **93**: 1049–59.

42. Pijnenborg R, Anthony J, Davey DA, et al. Placental bed spiral arteries in the hypertensive disorders of pregnancy. *Br J Obstet Gynaecol* 1991; **98**: 648–55.

43. Roberts JM, Redman CW. Pre-eclampsia: more than pregnancy-induced hypertension. *Lancet* 1993; **341**: 1447–51.

44. Smarason AK, Sargent IL, Starkey PM, Redman CW. The effect of placental syncytiotrophoblast microvillus membranes from normal and pre eclamptic women on growth of endothelial cells in vitro. *Br J Obstet Gynaecol* 1994; **101**: 559.

45. Hubel CA, Roberts JM, Taylor RN, Musci TJ, Rogers GM, McLaughlin MK. Lipid peroxidation in pregnancy: new perspectives on pre-eclampsia. *Am J Obstet Gynecol* 1989; **161**: 1025–34.

46. Girling JC, de Swiet M. 'Pre eclampsia'. *Update* 1996; **53**: 338–42.

47. Tomas V, Strano A, Orlandi M, et al. Are the vascular complications of diabetes mellitus preceded by an altered thromboxane/prostacyclin ratio? *Med Hypotheses* 1986; **19**: 224.

48. Redman CW, Jefferies M. Revised definition of pre-eclampsia. *Lancet* 1998; **1**: 809–12.

49. National High Blood Pressure Education Program Working Group Report on High Blood Pressure in Pregnancy. *Am J Obstet Gynecol* 1990; **163**: 1691–712.

50. Greer IA. Hypertension. In: *High-risk pregnancy*. Oxford, Butterworth Heinemann, 1992: 31–93.

51. Davey DA, MacGillivray I. The classification and definition of the hypertensive disorders of pregnancy. *Am J Obstet Gynecol* 1988; **158**: 892–8.

52. Garner PR, d'Alton ME, Dudley DK, Huard P, Hardie M. Pre eclampsia in diabetic pregnancies. *Am J Obstet Gynecol* 1990; **163**: 505–8.

53. Winocour P, Taylor RJ. Early alterations of renal function in insulin dependent diabetic pregnancies and their importance in predicting pre eclamptic toxaemia. *Diabetes Res* 1989; **10**: 159–64.

54. Bower S, Schuchter K, Campbell S. Doppler ultrasound screening as part of routine antenatal scanning: prediction of pre-eclampsia and intrauterine growth retardation. *Br J Obstet Gynaecol* 1993; **100**: 989–94.

55. Farrag OAM. Prospective study of 3 metabolic regimens in pregnant diabetes. *Aust NZ J Obstet Gynaecol* 1987; **27**: 6–9.

56. Siddiqi T, Rosenn B, Mimouni F, Khoury J, Miodovnik M. Hypertension during pregnancy in insulin-dependent diabetic women. *Obstet Gynecol* 1991; **77**: 514–19.

57. Leveno KJ, Hauth JC, Gilstrap LC, Whalley PJ. Appraisal of 'rigid' blood glucose control during pregnancy in the overtly diabetic woman. *Am J Obstet Gynecol* 1979; **135**: 853–62.

58. Martin FIR, Heath P, Mountain KR. Pregnancy in women with diabetes mellitus. Fifteen years' experience: 1970–1985. *Med J Aust* 1987; **146**: 187–90.

59. The Diabetes Control and Complications Trial Research Group. Pregnancy outcome in the diabetes control and complications trial. *Am J Obstet Gynecol* 1996; **174**: 1343–53.

60. Jones HMR, Cummings AJ, Setchell KDR, Lawson AM. A study of the disposition of alpha methyl dopa in newborn infants following its administration to the mothers for the treatment of hypertension during pregnancy. *Br J Clin Pharmacol* 1979; **7**: 433–40.

61. Whitelaw A. Maternal methyl dopa treatment and neonatal blood pressure. *BMJ* 1981; **282**: 471.

62. Cockburn J, Moar VA, Ounsted M, Redman CWG. Final report of study on hypertension during pregnancy: the effects of specific treatment on the growth and development of the children. *Lancet* 1982; **I**: 647–9.

63. Ounsted MK, Moar VA, Good FJ, Redman CWG. Hypertension during pregnancy with and without specific treatment; the children at the age of 4 years. *Br J Obstet Gynaecol* 1980; **87**: 19–24.

64. Steel JM. Personal experience of prepregnancy care in women with insulin dependent diabetes. *Aust NZ J Obstet Gynaecol* 1994; **34**: 135–9.

65. Thorpe-Beeston JG. Pregnancy and ACE inhibitors. *Br J Obstet Gynaecol* 1992; **100**: 692–3.

66. Lip GYH, Churchill D, Beevers M, Auckett A, Beevers DG. Angiotensin converting enzyme inhibitors in early pregnancy. *Lancet* 1997; **350**: 1446–7.

67. Rosa FW, Bosco LA, Graham LFCF, Milstein JB, Dreis M, Creamer J. Neonatal anuria with maternal angiotensin-converting enzyme inhibition. *Obstet Gynecol* 1989; **74**: 371–4.

68. Danti L, Valcamonica A, Soregaroli M. Fetal and maternal doppler modifications during therapy with antihypertensive agents. *J Mat-Fet Invest* 1994; **4**: 19–23.

69. Childress CH, Katz VL. Nifedipine and its indications in obstetrics and gynaecology. *Obstet Gynecol* 1993; **83**: 616–24.

70. Manninen AK, Juhakosi A. Nifedipine concentrations in maternal and umbilical serum, amniotic fluid, breast milk and urine of mothers and offspring. *Int J Clin Pharm Res* 1991; **XI**: 231–6.

71. Briggs GG, Freeman RK, Yaffe SJ. *Drugs in pregnancy and lactation*, 3rd edn. Baltimore,

Williams and Wilkins, 1990: 450–3.

72. Walters BNJ, Redman CWG. Treatment of severe pregnancy-associated hypertension with the calcium antagonist nifedipine. *Br J Obstet Gynaecol* 1984; **91**: 330–6.

73. Naden RP, Redman CWG. Antihypertensive drugs in pregnancy. *Clin Perinatol* 1985; **12**: 521–38.

74. Lipshitz J, Ahokas RA, Reynolds SL. The effect of hydralazine on placental perfusion in the spontaneously hypertensive rat. *Am J Obstet Gynecol* 1987; **156**: 356–9.

75. Vink GJ, Moodley J, Philpott RW. The effect of dihydralazine on the fetus in the treatment of maternal hypertension. *Obstet Gynecol* 1980; **55**: 519–22.

76. Robson SC, Redfern N, Walkinshaw SA. Protocol for the intrapartum management of severe pre eclampsia. *Int J Obst Anaesth* 1992; **1**: 222–9.

77. Lund Johansen P. Pharmacology of combined alpha-beta blockade. *Drugs* 1984; **28**: 35–50.

78. Butters L, Kennedy S, Rubin PC. Atenolol in essential hypertension during pregnancy. *BMJ* 1990; **301**: 587–9.

79. Montan S, Liedholm H, Lingman G, Marsal K, Sjoberg NO, Solum T. Fetal and uteroplacental haemodynamics during short term atenolol treatment of hypertension in pregnancy. *Br J Obstet Gynaecol* 1987; **94**: 312–17.

80. Hanretty K, Whittle M, Rubin PC. Influence of atenolol on Doppler waveform velocities in hypertensive human pregnancy. *J Hypertens* 1987; **5**: 767–8.

81. ECPPA: randomised trial of low dose aspirin for the prevention of maternal and fetal complications in high risk pregnant women. ECPPA (Estudo Colaborativo para Prevencao da Pre-eclampsia com Aspirina) Collaborative Group. *Br J Obstet Gynaecol* 1996; **103**: 39–47.

82. Dudley DK, Black DM. Reliability of lecithin/sphingomyelin ratio in diabetic pregnancy. *Obstet Gynecol* 1985; **66**: 521–4.

83. Bourbon JR, Farrell PM. Fetal lung development in the diabetic pregnancy. *Pediat Res* 1985; **19**: 253–67.

84. Fadel HE, Saad SA, Davis H, Nelson GH. Fetal lung maturity in diabetic pregnancies: relation among amniotic fluid insulin, prolactin, and lecithin. *Am J Obstet Gynecol* 1988; **159**: 457–63.

85. Crowley P. Corticosteroids prior to preterm delivery. In: *Pregnancy and childbirth module of the Cochrane database of systematic reviews*, 1997.

86. Tibaldi JM, Lorber DL, Nerenberg A. Diabetic ketoacidosis and insulin resistance with subcutaneous terbutalin infusion: a case report. *Am J Obstet Gynecol* 1990; **163**: 509–10.

87. Felig P, Lynch V. Starvation in human pregnancy, hypoglycaemia, hypoinsulinaemia and hyperketonaemia. *Science* 1970; **170**: 990–2.

88. Kilvert JA, Nicholson HO, Wright AD. Ketoacidosis in diabetic pregnancy. *Diabetes Med* 1993; **10**: 278–81.

89. Klein BEK, Moss SE, Klein R. Effect of pregnancy on progression of diabetic retinopathy. *Diabetes Care* 1990; **13**: 34–40.

90. Rosenn B, Miodovnik M, Kranias G, et al. Progression of diabetic retinopathy in pregnancy: association with hypertension in pregnancy. *Am J Obstet Gynecol* 1992; **166**: 1214–18.

91. Price JH, Hadden DR, Archer DB, Harley JMcDG. Diabetic retinopathy in pregnancy. *Br J Obstet Gynaecol* 1984; **91**: 11–17.

92. Surian M, Imbascati E, Cosci P, et al. Glomerular disease and pregnancy: a study of 123 pregnancies in patients with primary and secondary glomerular disease. *Nephrology* 1984; **36**: 101–5.

93. Kitzmiller JL, Combs CA. Management and outcome in diabetic pregnancy. In: Dormhorst A, Hadden DR, eds. *Diabetes and pregnancy, an international approach to diagnosis and management.* Chichester, J Wiley and Sons, 1996.

Index

Note: page numbers in *italics* refer to figures and tables

Printed and bound by CPI Group (UK) Ltd, Croydon, CR0 4YY

23/10/2024

01777679-0012